THE ATHLETE'S WAY

THE ATHLETE'S WAY

TRAINING YOUR MIND AND BODY
TO EXPERIENCE THE JOY OF EXERCISE

CHRISTOPHER BERGLAND

ST. MARTIN'S GRIFFIN ⚲ NEW YORK

www.stmartins.com

Illustrations by Daniel Pelavin
Book design by Gretchen Achilles

Library of Congress Cataloging-in-Publication Data

Bergland, Christopher.
    The athlete's way : training your mind and body to experience the joy of exercise / Christopher Bergland.
        p. cm.
    ISBN-13: 978-0-312-35587-6
    ISBN-10: 0-312-35587-4
    1. Exercise—Psychological aspects.   2. Physical fitness—Psychological aspects.   3. Mind and body.   I. Title.

GV481.2.B47   2007
613.7'1—dc22

                                                                              2007009826

First St. Martin's Griffin Edition: June 2008

10 9 8 7 6 5 4 3 2 1

A NOTE TO THE READER

Please consult your doctor before beginning this or any exercise program. Not all exercise programs are suitable for everyone, and this or any other program may result in injury. Any user of this exercise program assumes the risk of possible injury resulting from performance of the exercises or following the advice given herein. The instructions and advice presented through this program are in no way intended as a substitute for medical counseling.

The creator of this program is not a doctor or a medical professional, and he, on his own behalf as well as on behalf of his employees, agents, publisher, and/or his or their affiliates, disclaims any liability or loss sustained in connection with the exercises, or the instructions and advice included herein.

DEDICATED TO DIANE REVERAND

A MILLION THANKS

IN MEMORIAM

RICHARD MONROE BERGLAND, M.D.

(AUGUST 23, 1932–NOVEMBER 9, 2007)

CONTENTS

A NOTE FROM THE AUTHOR

Exercise ferments the humors, casts them into their proper channels, throws off redundancies, and helps nature in those secret distributions, without which the body cannot subsist in its vigor, nor the soul act with cheerfulness.

JOSEPH ADDISON *(THE SPECTATOR, JULY 12, 1711)*

I love to sweat. All told, I have run distances equal to four trips around the world on a treadmill and on the streets of Manhattan where I live. I have biked to the moon and back, dueling it out with a red, blinking pacer light on a LifeCycle control panel or logging countless laps in Central Park. I've even crossed the Atlantic a few times—in the pool—and I've swum in almost every ocean around the world competing in Ironman triathlons. When I am running, biking, or swimming, happiness pours out of me. I am not alone. Everyone who exercises regularly experiences this bliss. And it is available to you, too, anytime you break a sweat. *The Athlete's Way* is an individual process but ultimately a universal experience.

Everything that human beings do for our survival—eating, sleeping, reproducing, and working physically—breaking a sweat—is designed to make us feel good biologically. We are rewarded for doing the things necessary to stay alive. This is a generous biological design, and at the same time, the key to our survival. All animals seek pleasure and avoid pain. Maintaining life in the human body was designed to be an ecstatic experience, as was bonding with other humans. Throughout our evolution, physical exertion and sticking together have produced neurochemicals that scientists are just beginning to identify as being associated with happiness. One reason the psycho-pharmacological business is booming is that our bodies are not designed to be sedentary or isolated behind computer screens. Doctors prescribe pills to make people feel better—I prescribe sweat, community, energy balance, and a sense of purpose. Humans need to move. Organic, self-produced bliss, kinship, and stress reduction are available to all of us, if we are willing to break a sweat, bond with other humans, and chase our happiness down.

While racing, I have sweated my way through many spectacular landscapes. Athletics have taken me to Brazil, Australia, South Africa, New Zealand, Denmark, Austria, Germany, and Hawaii, as well as the White Mountains of New Hampshire, the swamplands of Florida, and the vast emptiness of Death Valley—and many other amazing places. But most of the time, I train inside a New York City gym or in Central Park—which are just as exotic as any landscape for me. The sea of people in front of me is ever changing. People watching and connecting to others gets my juices going. The real joy of sport for me is in the process, the connections to other people, and the places I go inside my head—not the places I go with my physical body.

I have stayed in New York City for my entire athletic career and plugged myself into the energy of humanity here. Central Park is my microscope; international races are my telescope for exploring the athletic process. Luckily the "lab rat" aspect of indoor training triggers the same neurological responses that have evolved for hundreds of millions of years. We feel good when we sweat. I have learned how to find Nirvana on the treadmill, and I am going to teach you my secrets.

TO KNOW IS NOT ENOUGH

I use my single windup, my double windup, my triple windup, my hesitation windup, my no windup. I also use my step-n-pitch-it, my submariner, my sidearmer, and my bat dodger. Man's got to do what he's got to do.

SATCHEL PAIGE

I was born in Manhattan and have lived in the same East Village apartment since 1988. If I train outdoors, I'm usually in Central Park or along the waterways surrounding Manhattan. I love indoor training, too. Treadmills allow me to lose myself in the purest form of running. On a treadmill it is just the simple, repetitive organic motion of running. There is nothing to navigate, nowhere to get to—just running—and running fills me with the purest bliss of any sport.

My approach to exercise has been influenced by my surroundings, education, and upbringing. Urban, down-to-earth, creative, no-nonsense, cosmopolitan, and left-of-center are words I'd use to describe my philosophy.

This book is quirky in many ways—it breaks the mold. I graduated from Hampshire College in Amherst, Massachusetts, a small nonconformist liberal arts school with no tests or grades, where students design their own curriculum. I wrote my college thesis on "Cultural Imperialism in Developing Countries," basically studying the impact of Big Macs and Mickey Mouse in India. As a college student I traveled to India a few times and spent many hours meditating in ashrams. The Eastern philosophies melded with my athletic and scientific brain at an impressionable period. I am a free thinker and encourage you to "think about your thinking" and take accountability for it. I will teach you everything I know, but you have to participate in the process.

The Hampshire motto is *Non Satis Scire*, which means "to know is not enough." As a writer and coach, I bring this philosophy to my teaching. *The Athlete's Way* program is about taking knowledge and continually adapting it to fit your life in a way that keeps you evolving. I want you to discover ways to apply and expand on the building blocks I will provide through your own trial and error. You will need to discover solutions for yourself, not just plug in a set of rules. I will give you guidance and hold your hand through the process, but ultimately you need to tailor this advice to your personality if you expect it to stick.

MAKE IT YOUR OWN, AND OWN IT

You have your way. I have my way. As for the right way, the correct way, and the only way, it does not exist.

FRIEDRICH NIETZSCHE

This program is practical. It is designed to be used. This book comes from my life experience—it is not a theoretical or academic dissertation. Even the science in these pages has been filtered through my athletic process. I want to bring you inside my athletic mind so that you can understand your own athletic mind. I share everything I have learned in this book, knowledge I wish I had had when I started my athletic career more than twenty years ago. *The Athlete's Way* is a memoir and a manual designed to educate, motivate, and inspire you.

I want you to connect to this book. My goal is to transfer the enthusiasm and passion I have for sport to you so that you will seek exercise—not avoid it. I hope this book becomes one that you keep by your bed stand, drip sweat all over, lug around in your gym bag, and share with friends and family. I want the zest of your athletic experiences to leave a mark on these pages. I want this book to improve your life. I want you to succeed.

I have poured the same amount of hard work, intuition, and attention to detail into crafting this program as I have into every athletic challenge. I have tried to find ways to inspire you to exercise. I want you to seek breaking a sweat with the same motivation as I do. I'll be rooting for you. I am eager to learn from you, too. I encourage you to use the website www .theathletesway.com as an interactive tool. On the Web site you will find updated resources, interactive training tools, and forums to share experiences with other people living their lives the athlete's way. I hope that this book will be a catalyst for getting a conversation started and lead to an exchange of ideas.

Many of the scientific ideas I present here are things I discovered first through life experience, then went back to my father, or medical journals, to get further explanations for. Hopefully, the ideas will get the dialogue going with medical professionals, too, and lead to further scientific research. Many of the ideas I propose in this book push the envelope and are at this point, like so many things in science, still just an educated guess.

The Athlete's Way is a movement and a work in progress—you can influence the future of this program, and other people's lives, by sharing your insights via forums on my Web site. And your insights will help others. This is a program based on a philosophy of individual achievement and community, individualism, and collectivism. We're all in this together.

YOU ARE A LINK IN THIS CHAIN

The fullness of your bliss, I feel—I feel it all.
WILLIAM WORDSWORTH

Joseph Campbell's book *The Power of Myth* has influenced me as an athlete. It was published in 1988, the year I started racing. Myths fueled the idea that it was possible to tap into the fullness of my strength by pushing beyond my own limits and then letting go. As an athlete I could break free of the daily grind if I worked hard physically and used my imagination. Sweat, music, and mythology combined into a mystical brew, a life-giving elixir. Myths grabbed me somewhere deep down inside. They got into my spine. It was a metaphysical experience for me as a teenager, because I realized that I and "the other" were one. This experience of complete connectedness is what I have coined *superfluidity*—the episodic feeling of existing without any friction or viscosity—a state of pure bliss I will explore in this book.

My copy of *The Power of Myth* has taken a licking. This summer I used it as a seat cushion after long, sweaty runs. When I ran in the door and wanted to jot down my insights I would grab that book from the coffee table and sit on it so that I wouldn't wreck the suede upholstery on the sofa. The book is now molded to my butt and I like that. Looking at its warped cover now, I realize that my summer runs merged back into the same pages that had fueled me to get moving in the first place. My sweat marks and the gravity of my body imprinted on the book took the energy full circle. There is a personal history recorded there in the salt stains and warped cover now. You can do this with your copy of *The Athlete's Way* if you want. I hope you leave your personal mark on these pages. Please also share your experiences on www.theathletesway.com and use the World Wide Web to connect with the Athlete's Way community. You can give something back by sharing the lessons you've learned inside the athletic process, and bond with other people. Your insights could inspire someone else to exercise. The more people we have breaking a sweat every day, the better place the world will be.

> Both tears and sweat are salty, but they render a different result. Tears will get you sympathy; sweat will get you change.
>
> JESSE JACKSON

I am confident that *The Athlete's Way* will improve your life by extracting gallons of sweat from your skin in years to come. If you do drip your own sweat into this book—literally or figuratively—you will make a dream for me come true. I want to make you want to sweat. My life success has been about dreaming big, staying honest, working hard, making the most of what I've got to work with, and sweating it out every day. In these pages I will tell you everything I have learned with the hope that it will help you take your life to a higher ground.

CHRISTOPHER BERGLAND

NEW YORK CITY, SEPTEMBER 2006

INTRODUCTION:
THE ATHLETE'S WAY TO
HEALTH AND FITNESS

A RÉSUMÉ
FARTHER, FASTER, HIGHER

Watch your thoughts, they become words; watch your words, they become actions; watch your actions, they become habits; watch your habits, they become character; watch your character, for it becomes your destiny.

FRANK OUTLAW

I am a world-class endurance athlete with multiple triathlon championship titles and a Guinness World Record. I work as a consultant and writer now, but I've also done a lot of coaching. While running a triathlon program at Manhattan's Chelsea Piers, I developed the concept of *The Athlete's Way*. A native New Yorker, I've done almost all of my training for endurance sports either in Central Park or inside a Manhattan gym. I understand what the daily exercise routine entails for most people through observation and personal experience. I train side by side with all kinds of people. I am an expert when it comes to sports and human motivation, and I have incorporated everything I know into a program for people from all walks of life and levels of fitness.

My preference for training indoors, rare for a long-distance runner, enables me to connect to the exercise experience of most people. Today, many of us do our cardiovascular exercise and strength conditioning indoors. I am an expert in the field of indoor training. Treadmills are currently the number one method people use to get exercise, and I know treadmills well.

I hold the Guinness World Record for running farther and faster on a treadmill than any other human being ever has, logging 153.76 miles in twenty-four hours. I have run at least thirty to fifty miles on a treadmill every week since 1984, which adds up to about 50,000 miles. I have won the Triple Iron Man, the longest nonstop triathlon in the world, three times. It includes a 7.2-mile swim, a 336-mile bike ride, and a 78.6-mile run. I have competed in dozens of regular Ironman races—2.4-mile swim, 112-mile bike and 26.2-mile run—all over the world, including five appearances at the Hawaii World Championships. I have finished the Kiehl's Badwater Ultramarathon, a 135-mile run through Death Valley in July, twice. I have spent a lot of my time analyzing and experimenting with the athletic process like a lab rat on an exercise wheel, and I will share everything I've learned with you in this book, so that you can apply it to your daily workouts.

Many people think that ultra-endurance sports are crazy. Even though I loved doing them, I have to agree. This book is not written to teach you how to be an ultra-runner. Unless it is in your blood as something you have to do, I would not encourage you to be an ultra-athlete. It is not good for you. The physical strain on the body is, in fact, probably bad for you. My joints are fine, but my kidneys have been pushed to the verge of shutdown a few times. Twenty to sixty minutes a day is good for you, but running nonstop for twenty-four hours is not. I did it because it was my calling—my life's passion.

Nobody realizes that some people expend tremendous energy merely to be normal.

ALBERT CAMUS

I am not coming back from the depths of Death Valley or the lava fields of Hawaii or the shark-infested waters of South Africa to hand a map and instructions to another crazy conquistador and send him or her off to those places. Instead, I am coming back to what I see as my village to tell you about what I have learned from my explorations and how you can apply it to your day-to-day life. This program is about applying the tools that I've used to do superhuman feats to performing everyday feats, like climbing the Stairmaster for thirty minutes or jogging around the block.

I have always been fascinated by the science and creative process of sport. I want to break new ground, but I believe that the same hard work and discipline that the classical Greeks brought to athletics are essential for us today. This book focuses on the classic core tenets of the athletic process and explains them in terms of my own experiences as an athlete and also in terms of current neuroscientific and psychological research.

THE CORE PHILOSOPHY:
AIM HIGH, WORK HARD, HAVE FUN, AND TRUST YOURSELF

I know very well that many others might, in this matter, as in others, do better than I can; and though I believe that I have not so much of the confidence of the people as I had some times since, I do not know that, all things considered, any other person has more; and, however this may be, there is no way in which I can have any other man put where I am. I am here. I must do the best I can and bear the responsibility of taking the course which I feel I ought to take.

ABRAHAM LINCOLN

All the theory in the world is useless if you can't put it into action. The information here has been road tested by me. Now you have to take it out for a test drive, personalize it, and incorporate it into your life. Exercise is a source of joy, and I hope to persuade you to make it a bigger part of your life. My mission is to get this message to you so that you can use neurobiology and behavioral models to help improve your life through exercise. I am a zealot about the power of sweat to transform people's lives by transforming their minds. My conviction is strong and authentic because I have lived it.

I sweat real sweat and I shake real shakes.

ELIZABETH TAYLOR

Shifting the focus from thinner thighs to stronger minds makes this exercise book unique. *The Athlete's Way* is about the process of creating a healthier mind and happier brain through physical activity and positive psychology. This exercise book does not focus just on sculpting six-pack abs or molding buns of steel. We are more interested in bulking up your neurons and reshaping your synapses to create an optimistic, resilient, and determined mind-set.

The goal is transformation from the inside out. As William James said, "We don't laugh because we're happy, we're happy because we laugh." I would go further: we don't exercise because we are happy; we are happy because we exercise. By taking you inside the athletic mind, *The Athlete's Way* illustrates the characteristics of the "athletic mind-set" and shows you how to incorporate these traits into your daily routine. The program lays the groundwork for attitudinal and behavioral changes through neuroplasticity. Unlike most exercise books, the weight loss and improved physical appearance that will result from this plan are actually by-products of the program, not goals. The goal is to tap your bliss and have an athletic conversion.

NEUROPLASTICITY AND NEUROGENESIS
COMBINING NEUROSCIENCE AND SPORT

What we feel and think and are is to a great extent determined by the state of our ductless glands and viscera.

ALDOUS HUXLEY

All too often, scientific knowledge and brain chemical engineering with drugs is used only to bring people with depression, anxiety, or ADD back to "normal." My goal is to use this information to help people move beyond normal. We can feel better and live better without drugs. Neurochemical improvement is possible through this program. My mission is to help people tap their own biology and apply neuroscience to their own lives so that they can become better athletes and better human beings.

For many people, exercise is a dreaded task rather than a source of bliss. I believe that the joy I find in movement is something I can share. It is universal. No matter how much you dread exercise now, you can transform your attitudes. I aim to convince you that you can rewire your mind to enjoy exercise because of the *neuroplasticity* of the brain.

Yes, you can teach an old dog new tricks. The human brain is not a static organ but rather a malleable web of neurons designed to change shape in response to internal and external stimuli. Neuroplasticity refers to the brain's ability to change its structure and function, by expanding or strengthening the neural circuits that are used, while shrinking or weakening those that are rarely engaged. This process is also called *synaptic plasticity* or *Neural Darwinism*. Neuroplasticity offers a scientific model that shows that we all have the ability to reinvent ourselves. *The Athlete's Way* is going to reshape your brain to think, train, and behave like an athlete—making you a more optimistic, resilient, and intense human being.

The Athlete's Way not only reshapes the mind through the physical experience itself, but also the thoughts and mental signals used in this program to achieve your daily fitness goals weave the neural nets of the athletic mind-set into your daily perspective. According to the laws of Neural Darwinism, when exercise is perceived as a pleasurable experience, these pathways are strengthened, and the neural pathways associating exercise with discomfort and drudgery atrophy.

> *The surface of the earth is soft and impressible by the feet of men; and so with the paths which the mind travels. How worn and dusty, then, must be the highways of the world, how deep the ruts of tradition and conformity!*
>
> HENRY DAVID THOREAU (*WALDEN*)

Recent brain imaging proves that you have the power to reshape your mind by rewiring your brain based on your patterns of thought and your patterns of behavior. With consistent use, networks of neurons get stronger; with lack of use, they get weaker. The stronger networks are where your thoughts and actions will gravitate. The human brain is designed to reshape its circuitry in response to life experience and psychological mind-set. Neuroplasticity is the foundation of all learning and memory. The brain wants to be streamlined and cuts the fat of what is not used. If you never think positive thoughts, those neurons will be cut, and you become a cynic. The good news is you can always wake them up and build new ones. The brain is never fixed, nor are your patterns of behavior.

Be patient. Studies on addictive behavior have shown that if people who are hooked on drugs can stay clean for eight weeks the odds of them staying sober are exponentially greater than people who fall off the wagon after four weeks of sobriety. **Stick with this program consistently for at least fifty-six days (eight weeks) and your brain will be restructured.** You will break old patterns of behavior once and for all because your brain will change. Exercise triggers new cell growth in the hippocampus (memory hub), in the cerebellum (motor function), and in the frontal lobes (executive function), which makes you happier, more agile, sharper, and less stressed out. This growth of new neurons is called *neurogenesis.*

Contrary to the original idea that antidepressants (especially serotonin reuptake inhibitors) work solely by keeping serotonin in circulation longer, the latest research shows that the key to their effectiveness may in fact lie in neurogenesis. Like exercise, antidepressants work by stimulating cell structures associated with antidepression to grow and strengthen.

Whether neurogenesis is caused by antidepressants or by exercise, changes in cell growth take time, which explains why it takes two to four weeks for exercise or antidepressants to kick in. *The Athlete's Way* exercise program triggers changes in brain structure and perception by improving the delivery of neurochemicals that make you feel good, which will make exercise something that you seek regularly, rather than avoid. I will talk about the key neurochemicals behind athletic bliss and athletic calm, namely dopamine, serotonin, adrenaline, endorphin, and the star of the show, **endocannabinoids,** your brain's own cannabis, which is primarily responsible for creating "runner's high."

SO HUMAN AN ATHLETE

I did not want to be a tree, a flower or a wave . . . not the phenomenon of nature, not exotic creatures from another planet, but something of the miracle that is a human being.

MARTHA GRAHAM

In the 1960s, before I was born, my mother worked for René Dubos, a microbiologist, environmentalist, author, U.N. ambassador, and humanist from Rockefeller University. Dubos wrote *So Human an Animal,* which won the Pulitzer Prize in 1969, and my mother typed the manuscript. The humanist ideals of René Dubos seeped deeply into my cells and shaped my earliest view of the world. His idea of our intellectual human selves and our physical, animal selves coexisting in harmony to create complete and wonderful human beings is the core of *The Athlete's Way* philosophy. This program is about maximizing the human and the animal in each of us as athletes and returns to the classical value of a healthy mind in a healthy body: *mens sana in corpore sano.*

The Athlete's Way is a new approach to exercise and the mind-body connection. More than 2,000 years ago Plato wrote that "it is as important to exercise the body as it is to exercise the mind, in order to preserve an equal and healthy balance between them." *The Athlete's Way* updates this timeless message for the twenty-first century. By incorporating modern brain science, positive psychology, behaviorism, and a lifetime of athletic training, racing, and coaching experience, I have created a program that will teach you how to rewire your mind and reshape your brain to enjoy exercise and maximize your human potential in the process. The goal of this book is to improve your mental and physical well-being and get your body and brain into terrific shape so that you can pump up the volume in your life. *The Athlete's Way* is also a method for anything in life. You can transfer the skill set you learn here to your professional and personal life. It's not just about sports.

I owe my successful career as an endurance athlete to my understanding of psychology and neurophysiology, but I am not a scientist. I am an athlete. Even though I haven't had formal training in the sciences, I grew up with neuroscience since my father was both a neurosurgeon and a neuroscientific researcher.

When I was growing up, neuroscience was a constant topic of conversation, and discussions with my father continued over the years. *The Athlete's Way* is based on the hypothesis that humans have two brains: an animal feeling-and-doing athletic brain called the *cerebellum* (Latin: little brain), and a human thinking-and-reasoning brain called the *cerebrum* (Latin: brain).

My dad and I referred to this brain model as **"down brain-up brain."** The up brain is the cerebrum, based on its position north of the mid-brain, which is midway between the two brains. The cerebellum is the down brain, the southern hemisphere in the cranial globe as it were, based on its position south of the mid-brain. The simple names down brain-up brain may sound grammatically incorrect but are a direct and cogent response to the 1970s split-brain model of **"left brain-right brain."** I coined the new names in early conversations with my father about the differences between the cerebrum and the cerebellum, and I like the new terminology for its simplicity.

As I will show you throughout this book, the salient divide in the brain is not from east to west or from right to left. Instead, it is from north to south. New brain imaging unavailable in the 1970s has confirmed the power of the cerebellum (the down brain) to do more than just keep our balance, posture coordination, and proprioception, a sense of body position. The down brain is our emotional and intuitive center and may even hold our personal and collective unconscious mind. It stores all long-term memories, an ancient primal defense mechanism. In trying to decode the cerebellum, I have uncovered new ideas about the mysterious and exotic little brain. The down brain has been hidden under the surface for far too long. This book puts the cerebellum in the spotlight.

THE LAYOUT OF THE BOOK

End in what all begins and ends in—yes.
EDWARD FITZ GERALD

In *The Athlete's Way* I explain the anatomy of athletic process from the psychological, behavioral, and neuroscientific perspectives as these elements intertwine and overlap with mind, body, and brain during exercise. We will look at the "mind mechanics" of the brain under the categories of architecture (structure), electricity (firing rate/brain waves), and chemicals (neurotransmitters). Specific topics we'll cover will be neuroplasticity, neurogenesis, and endocannabinoids as well as mirror cells, olfaction, and the source of human free will, which I call *volition*.

The extensive research I've done on neuroscience is from the perspective of an athlete. I believe this makes me a better communicator to other like-minded athletes. All of the scientific information has been checked with my father, who has been an extraordinary resource and inspiration. I have filtered all the research I've done to keep it accessible and applicable. I comprehend brain science in a practical way. My goal as an author is to make complex ideas of neuroscience simpler, without dumbing them down.

Everything should be made as simple as possible, but not simpler.
ALBERT EINSTEIN

First I will deal with the philosophy and principles of *The Athlete's Way.* I reflect back on my experiences as a coach and my father's role in shaping my perspective on the connection between brain science and sport that I bring to you here. I will show you how to get started by teaching you about fundamentals from buying equipment and joining a gym to creating runner's high. I'll show you how to set up a training log, kick-start your program, and keep tabs on your progress.

The first section will also cover positive psychology. As humans, we have evolved to need individual achievement, and a sense of purpose and community. Optimism, resilience, and determination are innate. We will explore the work of René Dubos, Martin Seligman, and Abraham Maslow, as well as my own trials, tribulations, and triumphs.

Next I will show you how to put theory into action by reshaping your mind-set and behavior. The key to reshaping your mind is to employ cognitive therapy and behaviorism. To reprogram the mind, I take a two-pronged approach. I deal with psychology for reshaping mind-set in the cerebrum, and I use behaviorism for the "animal brain," the cerebellum. Neuroscientific terms will all be explained throughout this book. In order to rewire your mind, I will identify the ideal athletic mind-set by examining the athletic mind and will turn to other professions and even creatures for inspiration you can use to build an alter ego and new athletic mind-set.

All animals seek pleasure and avoid pain. If you make exercise pleasurable, it will become something that you seek. This is called "Pleasure Principle" or "The Law of Effect" as described by the behaviorist Edward L. Thorndike. *The Athlete's Way* includes such behavioral principles as classical conditioning, reward conditioning, contiguity, and token economy as part of making exercise a habit. I will elaborate on these behavioral principles in chapter 10, when we talk more about reprogramming your mind and building an athletic alter ego to help you stick with this program.

Finally, I provide practical athletic advice on cardio, strength, stretching, balance, and nutrition that can apply to any level of fitness. We will look at the importance of sleep and dreaming for improving athletic performance as well as the spiritual aspects of the athletic process. Research has proven that we learn in our sleep by transferring short-term memory to long-term memory. We will examine the importance of REM (rapid eye movement) sleep and circadian rhythms.

In closing I will show you how you can take yourself to the next level—how to create a state of superfluid performance and enlightenment. In this chapter I compare the work of scientists and scholars. I examine the ideas of William James, Joseph Campbell, and the research of Marghanita Laski—who all explored the realm of religious experience, rapture, and ecstasy from different angles. I compare their insights with my own observations inside the athletic process by defining a new term I coined called *superfluidity*. In closing I talk about trance and transcendence as goals you can reach anywhere, anytime either through sport or doing anything so absorbing that you lose yourself.

USING QUOTATIONS AS SIGNPOSTS OFFERS A DIFFERENT POINT OF VIEW

Strong reasons make strong actions.
WILLIAM SHAKESPEARE

I have been collecting quotations that help me inside the athletic process since I started racing more than twenty years ago. I have amassed thousands. Each day the nuggets of thought held in these quotes have inspired me in my workouts and races. They have been a key ingredient in my recipe for success, which is why I share them with you here. Some of the quotes come from athletes, but in general they come from all sorts of people from all generations, and serve to illustrate that the ideals of *The Athlete's Way* are timeless, universal, and transferable.

I have inserted these quotes as signposts throughout the book to complement the text. They are also a subtext that can stand completely on its own. In most cases the quotes relate directly to the text, but I had fun with them, and many are used to create a playful dynamic with the text. I encourage you to read the quotes anytime you need a quick refresher course on *The Athlete's Way*—and to extract them for motivation in your daily life. If a particular quote resonates with you, write it on a notecard and put it somewhere that you will see it often. I include them here so that you can draw inspiration and humor from them, too.

We learn when we sleep. Keep this book on your nightstand and skim the quotes for a few minutes before bed; the nugget of wisdom held in each will meld with your dreams to help shape your athletic mind-set. Their simplicity allows them to slip past the cerebrum's intellectual guard into the subconscious cerebellum. Reviewing important things before bed helps to weave them into your dreams and from there into long-term memory. I find that when I'm exercising that one of these quotes will often pop into my mind—always at the moment that I need it most. They keep me entertained and help me to stay on course and achieve my goals. I hope these quotes reveal themselves to you as well inside your athletic process, bring a smile to your face, and make you charge on. They offer a range of insights and viewpoint that my single perspective alone could not.

PHYSICALITY IS SPIRITUALITY
SWEAT TAKES YOU THERE

A box without hinges, key, or lid, yet golden treasure inside is hid . . . Still round the corner there may wait, a new road or a secret gate.

J. R. R. TOLKIEN

I hate to admit it, but yes, I am a spiritual person, although I am not into the New Age jargon surrounding spirituality. I find it difficult not to feel a religious or mystical aspect to the athletic process. Through sport, I find connections to an outside force inside my own biology—and I connect to that source in other living creatures and nature. This has been my fuel since the beginning. I believe that feeling connected to "God" through sport is directly linked to the electrochemical environment of my brain, but that doesn't make it any less of a mystical experience.

Seating yourself deep inside the underbelly of the brain, down in the cerebellum, is the way to enlightenment and an end to suffering as I see it. We have to use our cerebellum to pierce through to another place; it is the pinhole from the three dimensions of day-to-day reality. If we get deep enough into our brains, we escape from reality. Getting one's consciousness into the cerebellum creates a springboard for piercing through the frontal lobes to another place. It is a state of transcendence. I will explore this topic in the final chapter as the ultimate carrot to inspire you to the next level of deeper understanding and higher sense of connectedness. I will share ways to pierce through the pinhole to this place.

NO GURU, NO METHOD, NO TEACHER
ALL PATHS LEAD TO THE SAME PLACE

God makes the animals, man makes himself.
G. C. LICHTENBERG (GERMAN PHILOSOPHER)

If watching a daily soap opera while you ride the elliptical trainer gets you through every workout every time, use that tool—own it. If you are consciously using TV, music, or reading as a tool to achieve your goal; if you're enjoying the process, engaged and pushing against your own limits, you are doing it *The Athlete's Way*. There is no right or wrong way to be motivated to achieve your goals; use anything at your disposal to get inspired. There is nothing sacred about this program. Not all parts of this book will resonate with everyone. Pick and choose the parts of the program that work for you.

The only thing I ask is that before you dismiss a piece of advice, try it first. When you read this book, odds are that you will be sitting still and the advice may seem dubious from that vantage point. This book was written inside the athletic process, and that is where the insights spring to life. Learn through trial and error. Take the ideas out for a test drive before dismissing them. If something works, use it, stick with it, but always stay flexible. If it stops working, readapt. Stay introspective, be creative—and make it your own. That is *The Athlete's Way*.

I have poured every ounce of my energy, experience, and knowledge into creating a simple book that has potential to improve your life profoundly. Exercise changed my life, and I have invested the same intense passion, drive, and dedication into delivering this program to you as I have invested into my own athletic pursuits for the past twenty years. I hope it is a valuable resource for you.

The process of learning to think and behave like an athlete is universal, but it is also a unique personal experience. No two people are inspired or motivated by the same things. We all have different dreams, passions, and desires. *The Athlete's Way* celebrates this diversity and encourages you to make it your own and find your way to approach the athletic process. Breaking a sweat is the passport to join *The Athlete's Way* community—dedication, commitment, and daily practice are the only dues you pay as a member of this collective. This book is a formal invitation to join the sporting life. The time is now. Start today.

THE ATHLETE'S WAY

CHAPTER ONE

MY STORY

I would not talk so much about myself if there were anybody else whom I knew so well.

HENRY DAVID THOREAU

I have spent the past two decades exploring my own motivation and what motivates other people, and I am excited to share everything I have learned here. This book offers hundreds of reasons that will inspire you to exercise. Sport turned my life around and continues to inform my life—I know the power exercise has to improve daily life and to change your life. That is why I am a zealot about this program.

By pushing against my limits every day for more than twenty years, I have been able to isolate the components that go into maximizing the potential of brain, mind, body, and spirit. I have probably logged more miles on a treadmill than just about any other person on the planet. I run about thirty to fifty miles a week, indoors and outside, and have done so for more than two decades. I also bike, swim, lift weights, and stretch religiously. I know the inside of the athletic process very well.

Now, here, you see, it takes all the running you can do, to keep in the same place. If you want to get somewhere else, you must run at least twice as fast as that!

LEWIS CARROLL

There is one important caveat. When it comes to exercise, more is not necessarily better. I do adventure and ultra-racing because I love it, not because it's good for me. I know I'm a freak. I would never encourage anyone to become an ultra-athlete unless it was his life's passion. There are tonic levels of fitness that can fit into your schedule easily and give all the benefits of exercise.

THE ATHLETE'S WAY *PRESCRIPTIVE FOR A TONIC LEVEL OF FITNESS*

- *Twenty to forty-five minutes of cardio most days*
- *Full-body strength training two to three times a week (twenty to forty minutes)*
- *Stretch-balance three to five times a week (ten to fifteen minutes)*
- *Sleep for seven to eight hours a night*

This adds up to a minimum weekly time commitment of three hours of exercise. There are 168 hours in a week. Just three hours of exercise per week will radically change the other 165 hours of your life. Think about it. That's about 2 percent of your week to feel better the other 98 percent of the time. It's an unbeatable ratio. With just three cumulative hours of exercise a week you feel better, look better, and sleep better. The return on investment is astronomical. Our biological design was generous; relatively little exercise reaps an exponentially huge payback.

SWEAT AND THE BIOLOGY OF BLISS
LIKE A SUNNY DAY IN JUNE

No one has ever drowned in sweat.
LOU HOLTZ

I came up with the title *The Athlete's Way: Sweat and the Biology of Bliss* on a summer afternoon as I was biking in Central Park. If you spend a lot of time in Central Park, you get to recognize the regulars. You see the same faces every day. This June day felt like the first day of summer—everyone was exuding so much energy and a love of life . . . walking, biking, running, in-line skating, skateboarding, horseback riding. I felt that I was with old friends, even though we were technically strangers. The enthusiasm was contagious, and we were all feeding off one another's happiness.

In looking for the X-factor that connected us, I realized that how fast or slow people were going, or if they were particularly svelte or graceful, didn't matter. What mattered was that we were all in the park for the same reason . . . it made us feel good. We were all there because we loved to move, and sport was a chance to feel the excitement of forward movement. None of us were standing still in life. I decided that X-factor was summed up in the words *The Athlete's Way*—we were all doing it our own way, but collectively it could be called the athlete's way. The key to being an athlete was that athletes seek exercise.

I was a link in this chain. I felt connected because I was sweating, too. I know it sounds simple, but it was an epiphany for me at the time. I still look for the athlete's way in people I observe every day on stationary equipment or whizzing by outside. Often, it is the ethereal bursting out of human spirit in a movement that captures the athlete's way. The move of a wrist or hip, the angle of the eyes, the rhythm and grace. I suggest you look for this effervescent X-factor of *the athlete's way* in people you see exercising, or doing anything well. Tag it, and extract the traits that go into the fluidity of their performance so you can imitate it. Feed off others and embrace the solidarity you feel in doing so. Know that others will borrow the same from you when you are exuding this fluidity, too. You become a link in this chain.

The light was perfect that day in Central Park. I looked around and all that caught my eye was this very specific quality of Manhattan summer light reflecting off different shades of skin. To be with these fellow New Yorkers, pushing against our own limits, together against the deep green trees, clear blue skies, and huge skyscrapers to the south was Utopia. The Manhattan skyline and the energy of human possibility collided, as they often do on the roadways and bridle paths of the park.

I came up with the subtitle after doing a few more laps in the park. I was coming down the West Side from the reservoir toward Tavern on the Green, which is mostly downhill, and I was flying. I looked down and saw the sun beaming back at me from the beads of sweat on my own shoulder. I lifted my wrist to my nose and smelled the Coppertone mixed with the chlorine of my swim earlier that day, the delicious smell harbored in my watch wristband of the musk of a year's worth of sweaty workouts, and thought, *that is the essence of sport to me*. Sweat is the common denominator in every workout and every athlete. It is egalitarian. Sweat creates an unspoken bond among all athletes. We get on to the same wavelength.

I always felt free when I ran. I suppose that's what was good about it.
BETTY CUTHBERT (OLYMPIC GOLD MEDALIST)

In soaking in the rapture of sport, I am always reminded of Joseph Campbell, who said, "Follow your bliss," and who often refers to the Sanskrit word *ananda*, which means bliss or rapture. *Ananda* is the root used to name *anandamide*, the endocannabinoid released during exercise, linked now to runner's high more than endorphin. Anandamide is called "The Bliss Molecule" by neuroscientists and is the key to feeling good when we sweat.

I was biking along, and suddenly the idea of sweat and anandamide came together into the words *sweat and the biology of bliss*. It is very basic, but summed up the impetus for my motivation to get a glow on every day and has been a mantra for me ever since. These words reflect my message, too. Sweat on the outside represented anandamide and other brain chemicals pumping on the inside. It was a eureka moment. Sweat=Bliss. The universality of that equation became the foundation of this program. I have never looked at a sweaty person the same way after that day. All I picture now when I see people sweat is the joie de vivre radiating from them in the form of neurochemicals pumping inside their brains symbolized by sweat streaming from their skin.

Sweat and the biology of bliss are human experiences accessible to everyone. The same anandamide, serotonin, and dopamine that flow through you flow through me, too. Anybody can experience this bliss through sweat. My advice is to chase your bliss by breaking a sweat every day. Don't just follow your bliss; reach out and grab it. Chase it down. It's at your fingertips . . . just a few heartbeats, deep breaths, and paces away. Anytime you want bliss, you can come and get it by breaking a sweat.

ONE ATHLETE'S WAY
MY LIFE TAKING SHAPE

Some people create with words or with music or with a brush and paints. I like to make something beautiful when I run. I like to make people stop and say, "I've never seen anyone run like that before." It's more than just a race, it's a style. It's doing something better than anyone else. It's being creative.

STEVE PREFONTAINE (AMERICAN LONG-DISTANCE RUNNING LEGEND)

I started running when I was seventeen and never stopped. It was the summer of 1983. At first I was running away from many things—dysphoria, substance abuse, my parents' divorce, and typical teenage angst. If I was running toward anything, it was the hope of changing my looks. I was initially driven by a teenage mix of despair and vanity, but running became my sanctuary and my salvation. I would go to another place when I ran—as if a trap door unlocked and opened to a magical wonderland in my brain. As I got more and more into running, I would lace up my sneakers every day and run toward this magical place. It became a destination. Over the years running became less about escape and more about adventure and exploring my human potential and bonding with other people. It was, and still is, my daily refuge.

Boarding School Daze
This Is Not Camelot

In the depth of winter, I finally learned that there was in me an invincible summer.

ALBERT CAMUS

My parents had a really bad divorce. Boarding school was the best option for all parties involved, offering a sort of diplomatic immunity for us—an adolescent "Switzerland"—while judges made decisions. My two siblings and I were sent off to different boarding schools—it sucked.

I went to a boarding school in Connecticut called Choate. The place was a magnet for Holden Caulfield types and party animals from wealthy homes. JFK was an alumnus of Choate, and seeing his portrait peering down every day was a constant reminder that my own life could not be further from Camelot. "Peacefulness, Tranquility, Enlightenment" were not a way of life for boarding students in Wallingford, Connecticut. I found a bunch of like-minded kamikazes at Choate, eager to party hard, rebel against authority, and derail our own trains.

Some people are born on third base and go through life thinking they hit a triple.

BARRY SWITZER

Stuck in a stodgy, preppy, Brooks Brothers and country club society, I was coming to grips with being a gay teenager. In the early eighties being gay or "heteroflexible" was in no way considered to be cool. Rather than deal with it, I shut down and used drugs and music to anesthetize myself. I hung out either on the fringe or by myself. Headphones in ears at all times at full blast, Ray-Ban aviators glued on to block out the world. I was either drunk or stoned. I felt dead inside. I was never blatantly ridiculed, but I made myself an outcast. The good news is feeling like a black sheep, like an underdog, has served me well as an athlete, making me more of a trailblazer. I will always fight harder and dig deeper to prove that I'm not a sissy.

> *Be bold. If you're going to make an error, make a doozy, and don't be afraid to hit the ball.*
>
> **BILLIE JEAN KING**

Obviously, all the components of my life make up who I am. I will always overcompensate and push harder than most to prove to myself and others that I am tougher than the rest, which is my trump card for winning races. I will always have something to prove. I can tap a deep source of raw power and block out pain simultaneously. I can be intrepid and introspective simultaneously in daily life and have mastered walking this tightrope as an endurance athlete. And that is my winning formula.

> *The quality of strength lined with tenderness is an unbeatable combination.*
>
> **MAYA ANGELOU**

There's a place inside me that's always safe. It's surrounded by Kevlar-coated one-way glass—I can see out, and I can feel the emotions inside—but nothing can touch me or hurt me when I'm inside that place, unless I decide to let it in. Otherwise, it is deflected, and no one or nothing can penetrate that fortress.

Bright Lights, Big City . . . Igby Goes Down
Acquainted with the Night

> *And when night, darkens the streets, then wander forth the sons of Belial, flown with insolence and wine.*
>
> **JOHN MILTON**

When I finally hit rock bottom as teenager, I landed on a rock in Central Park. The same place that would months later and for the past twenty years become my Bliss Station, Sanctuary, Oasis, Pinhole . . . you name it. That night in 1983, Central Park inspired me to change my life.

Central Park is the lungs of the city, our metropolitan Fresh Air Fund, but this night it was a suffocating place, a netherworld. I was staying at a suite in the Pierre Hotel just off the park with some classmates during an illegal off-campus weekend. I had been out all night at Mudd Club, Paradise Garage, and Save the Robots. We were drinking, smoking, doing cocaine and psychedelic mushrooms. I think it was the psilocybin that pushed the wheels off my bus.

I ended up curled up in a ball, hands to chest, rocking back and forth—alone—having a classic bad trip on a rock by the Rambles just off the boathouse, listening to my Walkman. I don't know if you've ever had a bad trip, but it feels like all the tumblers in your brain are turning and reconfiguring, unlocking doors that should stay shut, closing windows that should stay open, all the while re-etching the blueprints of your psyche and the foundation of your soul, fusing your synapses into new configurations, permanently rearranging the architecture of your mind.

I sat on the rock and watched the water. The sky began to take on light. I was definitely spooked and strung out. I wanted to crawl under a rock and die. Suicide seemed like a viable escape plan.

Most of the people in the park were up early for morning jogs. They seemed so together, but they were like gnats to me, buzzing around in their Nikes and Lycra. I wanted to swat them away or squish them. I resented them for not having been up all night, but of course, I envied them, too, and wanted to trade places. I found my way back to the Pierre and staggered in like a stray dog. This scene had played itself out many times before in one way or another, but this was the last time for me.

Empty and Aching
Razor-Blade Feeling

If you think dope is for kicks and for thrills, you're out of your mind. There are more kicks to be had in a good case of paralytic polio or by living in an iron lung. If you think you need stuff to play music or sing, you're crazy. It can fix you so you can't play nothing or sing nothing.

BILLIE HOLIDAY

I was only seventeen but felt as if I'd been dragged around the block a few times. I had.

And I knew I never wanted that razor-blade feeling in my mouth again. I never wanted to be comfortably numb. That was the turning point for me. I haven't done drugs since. In many ways I was probably self-medicating for a tendency toward depression, and some chemical imbalances in my brain. I medicate with exercise now. I am vigilant about my mental health and don't take it for granted. The endocannabinoids, dopamine, epinephrine, and opioids that I pump through my system now make my life force stronger and more resilient. I try the best I can not to be self-destructive and not to fear success. I refuse to sabotage my life in any way.

> *Drug misuse is not a disease, it is a decision, like the decision to step out in front of a moving car. You would call that not a disease but an error of judgment.*
>
> PHILIP K. DICK

Hitting rock bottom was probably mostly about feeling stuck or trapped in a life that I didn't like and not knowing how to break the patterns. I could have been stuck in some cubicle in an office park somewhere and probably felt just as desperate over time.

Hitting rock bottom often tends to be more of a fizzle. I don't think people realize sometimes that they've bottomed out if there hasn't been a trail blaze to document the downward spiral. We all hit lifetime lows, and when it happens, exercise is a way to pull ourselves up by our sneaker laces and take charge, to break the cycle and get back in the game.

> *Yippee! That may have been a small one for Neil, but it was a big one for me.*
>
> PETE CONRAD (ON THE MOON)

Growin' Up . . . What a Feeling
A Chemical Reaction

> *A rooster crows only when it sees the light. Put him in the dark and he'll never crow. I have seen the light and I'm crowing.*
>
> MUHAMMAD ALI

On a sunny June day in 1983 I bought a pair of clunky gray size-twelve New Balance 990's that weighed about twenty pounds and felt like gun boats, which meant I had to wear two pairs of tube socks to keep them on my feet. My coming-of-age anthem that summer was "Flashdance . . . What a Feeling." The only albums I'd listen to were Bruce Springsteen's "Greetings from Asbury Park" and the first Madonna LP. I played them nonstop. I was obsessed. I would hit the park with my auto-reverse Aiwa Walkman and play that same audio cassette every day. This music became the soundtrack for my athletic conversion. I pounded these songs into my head when I ran. These musicians became the architects of my adolescent athletic psyche that was solidifying by July.

Every workout I wore the same sun-faded Yankees cap, my favorite Boast tennis shirt with a cannabis leaf on it, my navy Choate athletic shorts with gold trim, and my Ray-Ban aviators. That was my uniform. The song "Holiday" kick-started every run. It was a celebration. "Blinded by the Light" made the rooster in my soul crow.

The Ray-Ban aviators that I had had since the eighth grade to hide my stoner eyes and were a key part of my Holden Caulfield character now became part of my athletic uniform. They made me feel like Chuck Yeager; I was obsessed with *The Right Stuff*. I rinsed the salt stuck between the gold rims and green glass after every run when I washed my uniform by hand and hung it to dry every day as I imagined a Spartan youth would have. The uniform stayed the same day in and day out, but beneath it I was transformed.

> *Deep down. I'm pretty superficial.*
> AVA GARDNER

In the beginning, I was highly motivated but it was primarily vanity driven. I would jog down to Times Square sometimes to look at the billboard of the Calvin Klein model leaning against a white obelisk. I had ripped the iconic image out of a *GQ* magazine and taped it to my wall. That photo inspired me to do more sit-ups and run harder, faster every day.

Then I'd go over to ogle the Atlas statue at Rockefeller Center and stand on the "630" engraved in the threshold behind the statue, which framed the spires of St. Patrick's Cathedral—a ritual I have to this day. I wanted his arms, his legs, and his abs—among other things. I wanted it all, and I got what I wanted, although I wasn't going to be on any billboards or carry the weight of the world. I made the most of what I had, and my body metamorphosed that summer. By August, I looked like a different person, but I still had a long way to go.

> *What I aspired to be, and was not comforts me.*
> ROBERT BROWNING

I am of the **"I'm OK, you're OK, but we can both still improve our lives"** school of thought—I believe we were all "sprung in completeness" and perfect just the way we are. You should never feel "less than" or a need to be perfect, but we must all still acknowledge that improvement is possible. And attempting to improve is a duty of being a human being.

> *We are all trying to get better—if you're standing still you're getting worse.*
>
> TIGER WOODS (BACK ON THE GOLF COURSE AT 6 A.M. TO
> PRACTICE THE MORNING AFTER WINNING A MAJOR.
> "I CAN'T BELIEVE IT. HE JUST WON YESTERDAY,"
> SAID AN ONLOOKER THREE HOURS LATER. "BELIEVE IT," SAID HIS COACH.)

The Metamorphosis
I Can Make You a Man

It is better to be beautiful than to be good. But it is better to be good than to be ugly.

OSCAR WILDE

When I started running in June 1983 my body was a toxic waste dump. I could run for about twelve minutes maximum. I was a weak, washed-out, drug-abusing teenager. From June to September, I went from being a cynical, messed-up kid to being an enthusiastic, ambitious go-getter. More impressive to me than having a new washboard stomach and strong, seventeen-year-old biceps was that my brain had been transformed. I was on fire. I could have been anyone I wanted. I felt unstoppable.

> *Life is 440 horsepower in a 2-cylinder engine.*
>
> HENRY MILLER

I walked with a new kind of peppy step and moved with intent. I had found the key to the universe inside some beads of sweat and tapped the biology of bliss. Most important, I learned that I could fill the God-sized hole I felt inside and that put me in control of my life. I had free will and the power to create a new reality—to do what I wanted with my life.

Running turned my life around. My confidence and self-esteem grew in tandem with my weekly mileage. At first I could only make it once around the reservoir, but by August I could run for more than an hour and do the whole outer loop. My learned helplessness and self-destruction waned; I had developed a sense of dignity. I went from being a straight-C student in high school to blazing through college in three years. I had velocity.

> *If they can make penicillin out of moldy bread, they can surely make something out of you.*
>
> MUHAMMAD ALI

It was a conversion experience. When I smell smells from that period, I go back to that time—Polo cologne and yellow Dial soap do it to me every time. Any familiar song from that era that isn't overplayed today will give me an instant flashback. I can feel how powerful that transformation was in every cell of my body. I am reminded of being seventeen again and again on a cellular level when these sensations catch my cerebellum off guard. And there is power to feel young again in these things.

I'm envious now of anyone who has yet to feel the shift in their neurons for the first time through sport, the virgins yet to have their athletic conversion. When you feel the connection between sweat and the biology of bliss in your synapses for the first time, it is like being born again. Exercise gives you the courage and tenacity to take life by the horns and say, yes—I can.

> *For me there's no terror. Only joy. Nothing focuses the mind like 750 horsepower at your foot and a license to use it. Nothing else demands that level of concentration. Or commitment . . . You're the force that makes it work. Without the driver, a racing car is just like a tool, dumb as a hammer. The driver transforms it into kinetic art, makes it waltz with physics. And the dance makes the spirits soar.*
>
> PATRICK BEDARD (NASCAR DRIVER)

IT'S NOT ROCKET SCIENCE
. . . OR BRAIN SURGERY

> *We're all in charge of where we choose to steer our own rockets. It's your life. One rocket, one astronaut.*
>
> RICHARD BERGLAND (NEUROSURGEON)

My neurosurgeon father made me think about the changes that breaking a sweat created in the architecture of my mind, the electrical currents and the chemicals flooding my brain. He spent his life researching the effects of pain and pleasure on the levels of hormones and endorphin in sheep, and I grew up questioning him about his work. His credo and scientific interests shaped me. I grew up with a three-pound, life-sized, rubber brain on my night table that I would bounce around like a superball. There were poster-sized photographs of twisted brain images—Purkinje cells, cerebellums, and microtubules—my dad's three obsessions, which he had photographed with an electron microscope and hung like modern abstract art in the family study. The brain was in my head in more ways than one . . . always.

Dad wanted very badly for his only son to be an international tennis champion, to become the next Björn Borg. He had gotten from Glendive, Montana, to New York on his tennis, and now he wanted me to carry the torch. He poured his hopes into me, and I started playing as soon as I could hold a racket. My dad was always fascinated with the Purkinje cells of the cerebellum, and their ability to hold muscle memory. When I was a kid practicing tennis every day, his words echoed in my mind: "Carve the grooves into the cerebellum, Chris. Think about hammering and forging your muscle memory with every stroke."

My greatest point is my persistence. I never give up in a match. However down I am, I fight until the last ball. My list of matches shows that I have turned a great many so-called irretrievable defeats into victories.

BJÖRN BORG

My whole childhood was devoted to trying to become the next Björn Borg. I had posters on my wall of him—I dressed like him in Fila sweatsuits, used a Donnay racket, and wore headbands to look like him.

I worked really hard to sweat and chase the ball to stir up lots of clay dust onto my calves. I wore that dirt like a badge of honor and would wait till late in the day to wash it off. I was very driven and extremely competitive. I put a tremendous amount of pressure on myself to succeed from a very young age. I wanted my father to be proud of me. I wanted to win every match. Being less than the best didn't seem like an option. My drive was inhuman, I felt the way Chris Evert once described herself: "When I was younger, I was a robot. Wind her up and she plays tennis." It wasn't until I had a meltdown in my later teens that I saw the other side of human passion and athleticism, and realized winning isn't everything. Part of my coming of age as a teenager was learning to have my sports drive come from a more human place, and learning to let it go and relax but still push myself really hard.

SWEAT AND BRAIN SCIENCE
DRIP, DRIP, DRIP INTO BLISS

You have to sweat, and roll up your sleeves and plunge both hands into life up to the elbows.

JEAN ANOUILH (FRENCH DRAMATIST)

Sweating makes me feel euphoric, and because of this exercise is never drudgery. Sweat is pleasurable, and it does more than take away my pain. Sweat is synonymous with ecstasy.

Once I made the connection that Sweat=Bliss, my objective became to explore this connection scientifically. I needed to be able to tap this bliss on demand. As a teenager I had spent years tweaking the perfect blend of mind-altering substances that would completely anesthetize my brain without quite killing me. Ingesting enough exogenous substances to numb myself was easy. But they made me depressed and hollow inside. With exercise, I knew I needed to train my body to produce and pump as much of this newly discovered life-giving elixir through my brain as possible, endogenously. These self-made molecules made me happy and feel so alive, so pure. But this brew was a little trickier and required some work to figure out.

I made myself a human lab rat in my own exercise-induced experiments on pain, pleasure, and ecstasies. When working out, I would periodically get orgasmic waves of sublime rapture, which made the back of my eyes wet, that I now call superfluidity. I wanted to isolate what was going on inside my brain as my state of mind changed. What triggered the changes? What were the stages? How could I be sure to re-create the optimum brain chemistry on demand?

I needed to come up with names and labels so that I could create these feelings systematically and then "bottle it" to share with other people. I started to do research on brain science and to talk to my dad for confirmation, all the while fine-tuning my athletic process just as a scientist would monitor an experiment with a system of controls. The more time I spent running in a petri dish (aka the treadmill of a gym), the more time I would have to isolate what worked and what didn't through trial and error. This became my life's work. Becoming an ultra-endurance athlete was in many ways an excuse to make this exploration seem like a career with a tangible purpose.

Buddha focused on the psychology and biology of pain and pleasure, too. There is an escape from suffering. The escape is to a place called nirvana, which is a place within. Nirvana is a state of mind in which you are released from fear and desire, but its roots are biologically triggered by meditation and other practices. Athletics can achieve the same effect. The essence of spirituality comes from the union of biology and the soul, or as I see it, as a union of cerebellum and cerebrum. When the human and the animal in us unites with "the other," you have Nirvana. Thomas Mann said that mankind is the noblest work. I agree.

I learned firsthand as a teenager that I could wash away my sadness with sweat and find a tranquil but elated state of Nirvana inside my head, even amid the turmoil of life. It is a state that you, too, will discover for yourself inside the athletic process when you sweat.

PHYSICALITY IS THE PATHWAY TO PEACE
SWEAT WILL BREAK YOU FREE

If you ache to break out and feel free—sweat will deliver you there. It doesn't matter what you do to make it happen. It's a simple neurochemical phenomenon—analgesics flood your brain in response to sweat and make you feel harmonious, centered, and euphoric.

The sweat—great slithering streams of it—pours down you. It runs down your legs, down the leg that is pedaling the sostenuto pedal, down the other leg. It oozes out all over your chest, flows down the binding around your middle where your full-dress pants soak it up. It flows everywhere, down your arms, down your hands. You become afraid lest too much perspiration will wet your hands too much, make them slide on the black keys, which are too narrow; you are playing at about a hundred miles a minute. But somehow they don't. As long as they don't you know you're all right. You're going good, well-oiled like an engine. Not too much sweat, not too little. It's only when you suddenly stop perspiring that your forearms go dull.

GEORGE ANTHEIL (CONCERT PIANIST)

NEW! IMPROVED! FALSE CLAIMS!
EAT MORE, EXERCISE LESS, AND LOSE WEIGHT

In this age, which believes that there is a short cut to everything, the greatest lesson to be learned is that the most difficult way is, in the long run, the easiest.

HENRY MILLER

Exercise fads will come and go. There will always be a new infomercial for the latest powder, pill, or secret formula. There will always be a product claiming to have some revolutionary ingredients. Some new variations on classics are revolutionary. Pilates, stability ball, and agility all work on core strength and balance, and these are fantastic newcomers. There are countless pills, powders, and potions that imply that you won't have to work in order to get results—this is not possible.

There are no shortcuts when it comes to fitness. You have to make an investment and stay committed. Lifelong changes are a series of daily commitments strung together. You must recommit every day and stick with it for the long haul. Exercise is work, and sweat is the sign that you are working.

There are no shortcuts to a place worth going.

BEVERLY SILLS

There are few things as physically pleasurable and rewarding as sweat. Remember all things we need to do for survival are designed to make us feel good—like sleeping, eating, or having sex. Physical work is one of these things. You should think of exercise as something pleasurable that you want to do. Shift your perspective. Seek exercise, don't avoid it. Make breaking a sweat most days of the week a goal and feel it transform your life.

LACE 'EM UP (ODE TO THE LAZY DOG)

BY CHRISTOPHER BERGLAND

Water and salt mix.
Add glimmer and slip.
A nosetip drip, hits a lip.
Beads and streams from every pore.
Forms a 'V' from groin to neck.
Dark wet weight, on a cotton shirt.
Runs down the spine, cools the mind.

DON QUIXOTE IN SNEAKERS
MY LIFE AS AN IRON MAN

The shoe that fits one person pinches another; there is no recipe for living that suits all cases. Each of us carries his own unique life form—which cannot be used by another. Be your own person—live your own life—you are unique, one of a kind—the world needs you—you have many choices—you can be many things.

CARL JUNG

I've had some terrific life experiences through sports and I've had some terrifying ones, too. I look back at my athletic stories here to bring you inside the only athlete's mind I really know—my own. I hope bringing you inside my athletic process will demystify the achievements in a way that makes you feel that you can go for it with anything in your life, too. The stories I am about to tell are geared to shorten your learning curve, not just to recap my race résumé.

Athletics has done more for my life than any other single force. I would have never imagined the places I'd go when I laced up my clunky gunboat sneakers for my first jog in 1983. Little did I know that sports would take me to almost every continent on the planet. Through sport I have pushed my body to the point that reality often became blurry, but in those hallucinations and visions I unraveled some mysteries. My goal here is to take those adventures and insights and show you how to use them right here, right now, in ways that can improve your day-to-day life.

*I've never been a very passive person. Physicality, feeling strong,
feeling empowered was my ticket out of middle-class Midwest culture. So I equate movement and strength with freedom.*

MADONNA

In this section, I will look back at some highlights from my athletic career, the roads I've traveled, people I've met, and insights I've gained. My
racing experience is extensive. As an athlete, I've had much success, and a
few failures . . . I had one DNF (did not finish) at Badwater in 2004, which
was the only time I ever had to quit an ultra. My body completely shut
down. The event was caught on vivid HDTV film in *Life in Death Valley* on
PBS, and on *60 Minutes* on CBS. It's always humbling to have your physical
meltdowns broadcast on national TV.

*Whenever I was upset by something in the papers, Jack always told
me to be more tolerant, like a horse flicking away flies in the summer.*

JACKIE KENNEDY

I have run coaching programs in New York City, worked at Chelsea
Piers Sports Center, and conducted workshops and seminars on *The Athlete's Way* in affiliation with my sponsor Kiehl's Since 1851, who have been
loyal and devoted to me since the late 1990s. I owe the owners of Kiehl's,
Jami Morse and former Olympic skier Klaus von Heidegger. Kiehl's literally
silk-screened their trademark "wings" on my back and sent me off to the
races—the emotional and financial support of everyone at Kiehl's allowed
me the resources to begin racing internationally.

Kiehl's has always supported adventure sports and pursuits that foster
human potential, like an Everest ascent in 1988. In 2003, I proposed that the
company get involved by providing athletes at Badwater ultramarathon
with skin-care products to protect them from the elements. In their charac-
teristically benevolent fashion, Kiehl's became the title sponsor of the entire
race and have been ever since.

Praise the bridge that carried you over.

GEORGE COLMAN

The Kiehl mottos are "Fun in the Fast Lane" and "Love what you do,
pour your heart into it and you will be rewarded." Both were coined by

Jami's father, Aaron Morse, and have been mantras for me as an employee and a sponsored athlete. Jami and Klaus inspired me to be my absolute best and are both mentors to me.

Without the financial support of Kiehl's I would have never had a flexible enough work schedule to train for ultra-racing, keep a roof over my head, food on the table, and still have the funds to actually get myself to the starting line. For this I am eternally grateful.

BRINGING THE PLAYING FIELD BACK TO LIFE
PASSION, PERSEVERANCE, PRIDE . . . PROVE IT

Be the exception to the rule.
SUSAN DELL

In early 2006, Lee Silverman hired me as the store manager of JackRabbit Sports, a specialty sporting goods store he was opening in Manhattan. By mid-2007, JackRabbit was up and running successfully and I felt the need to move on. Within a few weeks of resigning, my path crossed with Susan Dell, accomplished athlete and clothing designer. She was looking for someone to help launch a women's performance athletic clothing line and hired me as a consultant.

Susan Dell is the driving force behind the Michael and Susan Dell Foundation. With an endowment of more than $1 billion dollars, the Foundation has committed over $300 million to children's and community initiatives to date. Combating the childhood obesity epidemic is a top priority for Susan, who sits on the President's Council for Physical Fitness and has four children. She understands the power of physicality to transform lives, and is a role model to me. I have learned so much about loyalty, integrity, and giving back by knowing Susan.

In 2007 I also had a baby girl, Mirabel, with Bo Arlander, a triathlete friend of mine. My father passed away unexpectedly three weeks after the birth of our daughter. I was grateful that my father got to see the birth of his granddaughter and the publication of *The Athlete's Way* in hardcover. My priorities are different now. First and foremost, I want to be a good dad. I want to be present. Second, I want to take my life into my hands and use it in the best way I possibly can. I realize now that it's not "there" I'm trying to get to—it's here—and probably was all along.

THE ROMANCE AND ADVENTURE
SUCKING THE MARROW OF LIFE

I wanted to live deep and suck out all the marrow of life, to live so sturdily and Spartan-like as to put to rout all that was not life, to cut a broad swath and shave close, to drive life into a corner, and re-duce it to its lowest terms, and, if it proved to be mean, why then to get the whole and genuine meanness of it, and publish its meanness to the world; or if it were sublime, to know it by experience, and be able to give a true account of it in my next excursion.

HENRY DAVID THOREAU (*WALDEN*)

To me sport has always been about exploring human potential. Being an ath-lete is about the tightrope of living close to the bone while pushing against my own limits—in the struggle and ecstasy of this high-wire act. Tackling tem-pests, slaying dragons, and exploring new territories turns me on more than winning and filling up more milk crates with trophies to collect dust.

A gold medal doesn't make you happy the rest of your life. It doesn't wash the kitchen floor and it doesn't change the children's diapers.

CAROL HEISS (OLYMPIC GOLD MEDALIST)

Ultra-racing, for me, was all about human yearning and the quest. In sport, I found a way to tap human passion to feel more alive and connected to myself. The deeper I pushed into my own biology, the more something opened up that connected me to the outside world, to other human beings, and to my cellular nature. I could push myself hard, because I liked going deeper. It took me higher, and the struggle made me feel alive. If I could peel back all the layers and expose a raw nerve, I knew I'd succeed, because I felt alive again. That was my winning formula. I bring these methods to you, so that you can apply them to whatever you do—you can bring the same passion to a thirty-minute treadmill run and feel the achievement I do when racing, if you use your imagination.

If men cease to believe that they will one day become gods then they will surely become worms.

HENRY MILLER

I have always pushed myself to the limit, and I had brain science on my side. The harder I worked, the more analgesics I released and the deeper I got into my cerebellum and my unconscious mind. I could seat myself in my cerebellum in a way that I felt no pain, but I was not numb. It was completely sublime, and I felt completely connected. There is a place I go in my brain when I work out that is a million miles away from the day-to-day life on the street. It is a feeling of being completely absorbed and in the moment. I will teach you how to create flow and get to that place inside yourself, too.

> *What lies behind us and what lies before us are small matters compared to what lies within us.*
>
> RALPH WALDO EMERSON

Teaching you how to create flow when you exercise is one of the most important and fundamental lessons of this book. I have spent decades isolating how to create flow and will teach you these ways.

The term *flow* was introduced in 1974 by Mihaly Csikszentmihalyi (pronounced Chik-sent-me-high) of the University of Chicago. Csikszentmihalyi defines flow as the inherently enjoyable feelings that occur when there is a near-perfect matchup between a person's capabilities and the demands of the situation. He writes, "When the information that keeps coming into awareness is congruent with goals, psychic energy flows effortlessly. There is no need to worry and no reason to question one's adequacy. But whenever one stops to think about oneself, the evidence is encouraging. You are doing all right." In order to appreciate flow there needs to be some personalized feedback—which I will explain how to interpret specifically in chapter 6 on cardio.

PILGRIMAGE
HAWAII IRONMAN

> *Round the cape of a sudden came the sea, and the sun looked over the mountain's rim, and straight was a path of gold for him, and the need of a world of men for me.*
>
> ROBERT BROWNING (PARTING AT MORNING)

I did my first organized athletic event when I was twenty-two. In 1988 I entered the Fifth Avenue Mile. I tried racing because my good friend and coach Jonathan Cane urged me to. He had seen me running on a treadmill at the Printing House Gym overlooking the Hudson River for an hour every day at 10+ mph and thought I'd do well. So he took me under his wing and coached me that fall. I ran the mile race in 4:17. In doing so, I realized I actually had the potential Jonathan had seen in me. The rest of that year I entered every 5 and 10K in the park—and did well. I was hooked and willing to work as hard as I could to be the best that I could.

> You don't run twenty-six miles at five minutes on good looks and a secret recipe.
>
> FRANK SHORTER

From there I went on to do marathons, which remain the most grueling distance to do fast. Running a marathon well is the most brutal experience. Full throttle for 26.2 hurts more than anything I've ever done. I was a relatively fast marathoner, finishing my fastest in less than two hours and forty minutes. I would finish in the top percentile of smaller marathons, but at the international level I was very mediocre. But my top priority as an athlete was never about dedicating years of training to shave off a few minutes or seconds from a race I'd already done. I always sought new challenges and looked for different ways to push against my own limits. There was no fear in continuing to do marathons. At a certain point, it felt masturbatory.

I decided to start biking and doing "Duathlons," which require you to run-bike-run. Even though I didn't own a bike. But even on a loaner bike I had better success right out of the gate winning races as a duathlete. I would finish in the top percentile as both a cyclist and a runner, which equated to a few victories in the local racing series. I developed a love for cycling, which unlike running required more equipment and some disposable income. My coach lent me a bike for races, but I needed to buy my own eventually so that I could train outside.

I was waiting tables at the time, and prided myself on being financially independent, even if it meant making just enough money to keep a roof over my head and living on rice and beans. Ed Tedeschi, an advertising executive, was also an avid cyclist and saw some potential in my nightly Life-Cycle rides at the Printing House Gym. He became a generous benefactor. He'd let me stay at his house in Connecticut before races and sold me my first racing bike, a classic steel-framed Bottecchia with Campagnola parts, for $250 dollars, even though it was worth five times that. Ed played a pivotal role in nurturing what became a love for the thrill of bicycle riding out of doors.

But I started to get bored with the run-bike-run format. I needed new challenges. I decided to do a triathlon. The problem was, I didn't know how to swim. So, in 1992 I decided to teach myself to swim, I was twenty-six. Yes, you can teach an old dog new tricks. I joined Asphalt Green near my father's apartment on East End Avenue and hooked up with Phyllis Springer. She taught me how to swim and coached me in the water so that I could become a triathlete.

> Big shots are little shots who keep shooting.
> CHRISTOPHER MORLEY

I started entering local, short-distance triathlons and began to feel like a member of the New York athletic community. I made great friends. I was content with the local races and the sense of camaraderie until one snowy day in February 1993 when I saw the Hawaii Ironman on TV. They broadcast Patti O'Brien, a legend in New York circles whom I had never met. She worked at *Rolling Stone*. The show followed her around Manhattan training for Ironman and then during the race in Kona.

I decided that day that I was going to go to Hawaii. "Patti O" was a demigod to me. I taped the Ironman broadcast and watched her piece again and again—sometimes in slow motion. I finally met her later that spring. Patti was everything I aspired to be—hard working, fun loving, gregarious, competitive, free thinking—and an incredible athlete.

Patti and I became friends over the summer. I would go to her house on the Jersey Shore, and we would train together. She shared all the information she had about doing Ironman and was a mentor to me. I would sleep in the guest room with pictures of her crossing the finish line in Kona and fall asleep dreaming of crossing that line, too. I wanted nothing more than to have that life experience. It took me a few years to build up my base to be in Ironman shape, but I got there eventually.

> There is no such thing as a natural born pilot.
> CHUCK YEAGER

For two solid years I lived, breathed, and slept the Kona Ironman. I had pictures of all the Ironman greats—Mark Allen, Dave Scott, Paula

Newby–Fraser, Scott Molina—on my fridge. I made endless mixed tapes of songs that reminded me of Hawaii, volcanoes, and lava fields. I poured everything into that race. When I finally made it to Ironman Hawaii for the first time, it was like reaching Mecca. I had imagined being there with all the landmarks: A'lli Drive, the lava fields, the Kona Bay, the energy lab, the pit, the starting line by the Body Glove boat . . . for years. To have that fantasy become a crystalline reality was a dream come true, and kind of surreal. Having dreams become reality is weird—the romance of fantasy can be much more enticing.

Nothing was as thrilling to me as starting and finishing that race the first time. Returning every year since as a competitor or spectator is an annual pilgrimage. I know the course like the back of my hand. The smell of plumeria trees in the pockets along the race course is something I look forward to experiencing every year. That smell is deeply encoded in my cerebellar Kona memory box, and now I know when to breathe in through my nose to soak it in to reinforce that association.

During the last ten years I have become part of the international triathlon community and have gotten to know some of the legends of the sport that I idolized. The host cities of the races become like Olympic Villages. Being surrounded by like-minded people from around the world, hanging out for a few days together in a beautiful place before the race, and then going together through an incredible experience on race day makes bonding inevitable. I feed on the life force of other athletes; the universal traits and individuality in every athlete are amazing to witness. To rub against them in a race is the best combination of competition and camaraderie—thrashing in the water, hammering out on the bike, and pounding out the run, side by side. I have made great allies in the final miles of Ironman races, when all are stripped bare to the bone and bond human to human in a primal way.

One doesn't discover new lands without consenting to lose sight of the shore for a very long time.

ANDRÉ GIDE (FRENCH AUTHOR AND NOBEL PRIZE WINNER)

I hooked up with another highly motivated and passionate New Yorker named Bo Arlander, who wanted to reach for the stars, and together we have done Ironman races all over the world. Our return to Kona every October has become an annual ritual, whether racing myself, or just going to the

big island of Hawaii to cheer people on. It's all the same. As comrades and
competitors, Bo and I have a habit of giving each other a high five on the
Queen K Highway and saying "same time next year." In a shrewd way, we
both knew if the other was having a good day based on where our paths
crossed on the Queen K—but that didn't really matter. We were there. That
simple high five has been a motivator to get back there time and time
again—wanting to be out of the energy lab and back up on the Queen K
heading back into town before we passed was fuel to my fire to go faster
through the entire race. It was, in many ways, the need for human contact
that pushed me back to Kona year after year.

*There is nothing like returning to a place that remains unchanged to
find the ways in which you yourself have altered.*

NELSON MANDELA

As much as I love Kona, the Ironman distance itself became less challenging eventually. Getting through the race became like a day at the office.
After doing that race a couple of times, there was no mystery there. I could
do it by rote; there was a "been there, done that" feeling. I needed more
challenges.

In 1998, I tackled the Double Iron Man distance (4.8-mile swim, 224-
mile bike, 52.4-run) at the urging of my friend Scott Willett, who ran the
aquatics department at New York University. Scott, a legend in the Manhattan triathlon community, has been another mentor to me all along. He is the
most incredible swimmer I've ever seen. A human dolphin. He had done
Kona, too, and that race had lost its mystique to him as well. We were both
looking for some double trouble. So we jumped out of the frying pan and
into the fire for a scorching hot, humid Double Iron Man race in Virginia
Beach.

*Do not anticipate trouble, or worry about what may never happen.
Keep in the sunlight.*

BENJAMIN FRANKLIN

It was a grueling race, but I was hooked on the ultra distances and the
camaraderie of doing a race with a support crew. We worked as a team, riding out the highs and lows and staying up all night to get the athlete across
the finish line. Renee and Sandy, my sisters, and my stepmom, Elizabeth,

have crewed for me at most races, along with another mentor, soul mate, and role model, my loyal friend Donald Capoccia.

The high-stakes environment of an ultra creates a survival mode in which the real world dissolves. You become sleep deprived and punchy, so there's a lot of laughter and goofing around, even though it feels dire at times. I have learned great lessons about individualism, collectivism, and teamwork from doing ultra races. The volunteers at Ironman races pull you through always, but it's easy to take them for granted. In an ultra you have someone there handing you Gatorade for over twenty-four hours straight, sometimes even wiping diarrhea from your thighs. That makes it a bonding experience. I have learned many lessons about optimistic thinking, human compassion, and solidarity doing ultras.

> *If you believe that feeling bad or worrying long enough will change a past or future event, then you are residing on another planet with a different reality system.*
>
> WILLIAM JAMES

THE TRIPLE IRONMAN
THRICE-IN-A-LIFETIME CHANCE

> *How to hit home runs: I swing as hard as I can, and I try to swing right through the ball. . . . The harder you grip the bat, the more you can swing it through the ball, and the farther the ball will go. I swing big, with everything I've got. I hit big or I miss big. I like to live as big as I can.*
>
> BABE RUTH

I've had only one perfect race in my life. Ironically, I went to the starting line feeling worse than I have before any other race. There is a lesson there. The race was my first Triple Iron Man, which is a 7.2-mile swim, 336-mile bike, and 78.6-mile run done nonstop. I remember the day I got the announcement in the mail that they were bringing "The Triple" to the United States for the first time. I looked at the application in the elevator and thought, "That's insane, it can't be done." By the time I had unlocked the door to my apartment upstairs, I was in. I had to try this race. It made my heart hammer with excitement. My decision to do any race always starts with a certain feeling in my gut. I decided between the elevator door and my apartment that I was going to do The Triple.

I had done about a dozen regular Ironman races by that point—and a Double Iron Man. The Triple became the next challenge, another holy grail to me. Could I go that far? For me The Triple offered the ultimate epic adventure in the sport of triathlon because you had to do three Ironman races back-to-back without stopping, or without sleeping. That made it exciting and mysterious to me. I had to try it just to see what it felt like to go that far and be that far gone.

There are only two options regarding commitment. You're either IN or you're OUT. There's no such thing as life in-between.

PAT RILEY

The Triple was being hosted by Odyssey Adventure Racing. Don and Dawn Mann were the race directors. We had met at the Double Iron race they also put on, and had become friends. We hung out the night before The Triple and reminisced about past races and mutual friends. I had a cold coming on and made a vat of ginger tea, hoping it might clear my nasal passages, kill some bugs, and help me sleep. It didn't work. I tossed and turned all night in a big puddle of sweat and woke up feeling bad—achy, stuffed up, congested.

I remember sitting on the sea wall and listening to my anthem, which for that race was "If You See a Chance Take It." I said to myself in a coaching, third-person voice, "The essence of life is in the struggle, Chris. You've lived through other things; you'll live through this."

"But I feel like shit," was my gut response.

Dolendi modus, timendi non item.
(To suffering there is a limit; to fearing, none.)

SIR FRANCIS BACON

I had actually never felt so bad before a race in my entire life, and here it was, the biggest challenge I had to date. As always, Donald Capoccia, my sister Sandy, and stepmom, Elizabeth were there to be on my support crew, and I didn't want to let them down. We'd rented a huge RV, loaded it with food, and everyone was on board for the next forty-eight hours to lend a hand. I was supposed to be the star of the show. But it didn't seem like that was going to happen.

When you reach for the stars, you may not quite get them, but you won't come up with a handful of mud, either.

LEO BURNETT

As I watched the sun come up, I did my usual deep breathing, listened to all my anthems, visualized the race, put on some sunscreen, and said my prerace mantra, "Don't fuck up," about a hundred times. I walked around like a cat, stepping lightly but precisely, making my arches very high. I put on my wetsuit and got in the water for the swim; the gun went off and the race was on.

Don't fuck up.

RICHARD BERGLAND (BEFORE EVERY NEUROSURGICAL OPERATION)
CHRISTOPHER BERGLAND (AT THE STARTING LINE OF EVERY RACE)

I felt so congested and stuffed up that I was kind of numb to the feeling of my muscles pulling away from my bones as I swam. The water always feels good against my skin and I lose myself in the bubbles. The time goes fast when I am so in the moment like that. If I felt like slowing down, I did my usual trick of pretending that I was a shipwrecked castaway swimming toward an island with sharks chasing me and imagined John Williams's *Jaws* music in the background. Or I pretended that I was in a Herb Ritts video with Tony Ward, and that I had a dolphin tail while humming "Cherish." Either way, I kicked it up a notch and finished the 7.2-mile swim in about three and half hours.

After the swim, I threw on some bike shorts, shoes, and a helmet and got straight on the bike. Three hundred and thirty-six miles is a long way to bike. Whenever I drive more than 300 miles and watch the odometer, I am baffled that I could propel myself that far on a bike with just a few Powerbars, turkey sandwiches, and human will.

It's like driving a car at night. You never see further than your head-lights, but you can make the whole journey that way.

E. L. DOCTOROW

About 275 miles into the bike ride, I finally felt the cold I had break. It was as if my cells turned it off. It was gone in the middle of the night with only sixty miles to go. I was on the bike nonstop for about twenty-one hours, with only one three-minute Port-O-Potty break. I got off the bike about twenty-five hours after I had started the swim and headed off to run the three back-to-back marathons. It was sunrise of the second day, and beautiful out. I was on fire on the run. I felt like Apollo was pulling me. I floated the whole way. It was a very flat course—out and back, a mile in each direction—thirty-nine round trips that went quickly. I finished the 78.6-mile run in just over thirteen hours. All told the three nonstop Ironman races took me thirty-eight hours and forty-six minutes, and I finished in first place. It was the hardest challenge of my life, something I thought I could never do. But I did it. There was some emancipation from self-doubt in achieving that goal.

> *When I found that I had crossed that line I looked at my hands to see if I was the same person. There was such a glory over everything.*
> HARRIET TUBMAN (ON HER FIRST ESCAPE FROM SLAVERY)

I went back and did that race two more times and won it again each year. I am proud of having won the Triple Iron Man three times—that was the hat trick—but as with all my races, in a weird way I feel like somebody else did it. And who really cares? My athletic alter ego is in many ways a different person from the shadow of myself I see on the sidewalk, or the reflection I catch a glance of in a storefront window when I'm walking around in street clothes. But it's beyond ego. There is also an outside force that propels you through those races. It really is more about that force than my skin and bones. It is my ability to open up and channel that source that allows me to win races. I am just a conduit for it.

I especially felt this source of power when I finished the race in under thirty-nine hours. It was an ecstatic experience because I felt I was being pulled through the entire race by an invisible string attached to my sternum. All I had to do was keep tethered to that and nothing could stop me. Roger Bannister, the first person to break the four-minute mile, has often described the superfluid experience of tapping this source. The sensation happens at points during every race for me, but in my first Triple it wasn't really episodic. It went on for almost the entire thirty-eight hours and forty-six minutes. That is what made it a perfect race. I was tapped into an unknown, but very familiar energy source the whole time. When you run out of self-power and plug into another energy source as an athlete, you can't avoid believing in some quantum God.

Through sport you realize that there is a source, or a force that seems to connect you to something outside yourself that is also within. When you connect to that energy you tap a source of strength that feels like a quantum jump. Your energy goes from feeling like it is coming from within, to feeling like it is coming from without. It feels infinite and sublime. William Blake touched on the clarity of this feeling one can experience through sport when he said: "If the doors of perception were cleaned man would see everything as it is, infinite."

The word "Belief" is a difficult thing for me. I don't "BELIEVE." I must have a reason for a certain hypothesis. Whither I "KNOW" a thing, and then I know it—I don't need to believe it.

CARL JUNG

Although *The Athlete's Way* is secular, there is a spiritual foundation to my philosophy that touches on ideas of quantum mechanics. David Bohm, a London quantum physicist, believed that beneath the world of matter lies a vast and unobserved realm of energy governed by the laws of quantum physics. This unseen realm in Bohm's description was called the "Enfolded Order." In the book *The Three-Pound Universe*, Bohm explained, "Each individual manifests the consciousness of mankind; matter is like a small ripple on this tremendous ocean of energy."

God bless the roots! Body and soul are one.
Deep in their roots, all flowers keep their light.

THEODORE ROETHKE

Bohm was fascinated with Hindu mysticism and struck by the similarities between the revelations of modern physics and ancient Eastern philosophies. Both suggest that the observable universe, from subatomic particles to trees and planets and galaxies, is defined only by interactions with or connections to some form of consciousness.

When scientists see subatomic particles they are a trace on the screen. There is no there, there. That energy you feel in moments of superfluidity is quantum; it is everywhere at once and it is both a particle and a wave, or a "wavicle." It is nonlocal and contemporaneous.

"One can't believe impossible things." "I daresay you haven't had much practice," said the Queen. "When I was your age, I always

*did it for half an hour a day. Why sometimes I've believed as many
as six impossible things before breakfast."*

LEWIS CARROLL (THROUGH THE LOOKING GLASS)

As an electron's energy level changes it can behave like a particle with
physical substance—or it can behave like a wave, which is energy. The athletic experience of feeling this shift of energy from being tangible, linked to
glycogen stores and ATP, to being ethereal or from the source, is elusive and
episodic. But experiencing the ecstasy of that convergence is what makes
sport a religious experience.

THE KIEHL'S BADWATER ULTRAMARATHON
GRAPES OF WRATH

A cowboy is a man with guts and a horse.

WILL JAMES

Badwater is the most mind-boggling race on the planet. I heard about it one
day and within minutes knew I had to do it. Running the race involves 135
miles on foot through Death Valley in 130-degree temperatures from the
lowest to the highest point in the contingent United States in two 5,000-foot
climbs. It is the most challenging race I've ever done. I lived and breathed
Badwater for months prior to even being accepted to join the few lucky ones
at the starting line 282 feet below sea level. I dissected *New York Times* reporter Kirk Johnson's firsthand account of the race in the book *To the Edge*
and made endless CDs of songs from the West that reminded me of the
desert, of being a cowboy, and "Sweet Baby James."

I listened to "The Pretender" by Jackson Browne a lot, too, as part of my
preparation. The album felt like Southern California and the deserts east of
Los Angeles to me. Jon Landau, Patrick Leonard, and Peter Asher are record
producers whose sound captures the feeling of the desert and the romance of
sport for me. I used their albums, and Shep Pettibone remixes, as a training
tool for Badwater. I would slow their vinyl LPs and 12" dance remixes down a
few RPMs on the turntable and rip them to digital at a slower speed so I could
play them on my iPod. In analog, and slowed down, I could deconstruct the
production and feel myself slip into the grooves between the vinyl pressing.
I'd listen to the bits of each song that felt like a pinhole to another place again
and again, and slide through the hole in the garden wall each and every time.

Hitch your wagon to a star.
RALPH WALDO EMERSON

The afternoon I got my official acceptance letter to do Badwater, I put a blackout blind up in my bedroom and spent the next two solid days in the pitch black, on a ladder, with a miner's light on my head. I wanted to paint my bedroom ceiling with a galaxy of pin-sized microscopic glow-in-the-dark stars, including the Milky Way. To make it look real I needed thousands of slightly different-sized dots, so I used an actual safety pin with a varying amount of glow-in-the-dark paint on the end. "Every job needs a fanatic," Dad always said.

I wanted to be able to visualize the night sky atop Townes Passe, which Johnson described in his book, every night before I fell asleep. I wanted to be completely prepared mentally for the race. I would lie in bed every night staring at the blanket of stars and imagine being in Death Valley—while listening to the slowed-down Badwater "Promised Land" anthems I had compiled.

I dreamed of these places during my REM sleep phase every night. Even in Manhattan I was able to precreate state-dependent memories of a place I'd never been that would make me feel at home, and not scared, when I got there. It worked. Years later, the ceiling still glows and takes me there every night before bed, and makes me sleep well and wake feeling serene to face the workaday world, and the rat race I face daily out on the street these days. The universe of stars on my bedroom ceiling reminds me of the places I've been, the lives I've lived, and the people I've been—and to be honest, how many times I've almost died. Going from anticipatory fantasy to experience to serenity and back to reminiscent fantasy is a nice circle.

I kept *The Grapes of Wrath* on my nightstand and read passages from it every night before bed, romanticizing the journey west to a promised land. Heading west was the opposite of my dad's American dream, the one I grew up hearing about. He headed straight for the East Coast. I was striving to break free. I needed to reduce myself to a base level, and to find a core source of strength by making myself completely and utterly powerless by getting away from the East Coast, which is a very safe place for me.

Courage is the art of being the only one who knows you're scared to death.
HAROLD WILSON

I have a five-foot-high poster of Route 66 taken by Andreas Feininger in 1953 for *Life* magazine hanging in my living room. I would dive into it daily as part of training for Badwater. The "last chance Texaco" imagery and composition of the photo summed up the dust bowl of Badwater in a twilight zone way for me every afternoon on the couch. I would wring myself out there after sweaty runs or hour-long stretches in the 160-degree sauna doing heat training, and lose myself in the poster. Training for Badwater fried my up brain but made the imagination in my down brain run wild. Using your imagination and being creative in sports makes the physical pain easy to deal with, because it becomes entertaining. You can choose your perspective.

Courage is being scared to death—but saddling up anyway.
                                                              JOHN WAYNE

Death Valley in July is the most memorable landscape in which I have ever competed. It is a spectacular place. But Badwater will always remind me of Dante's Inferno, too. It's like being on Mars without a space suit. I was secretly happy on July 22 and 23, 2003, when I first did the race, that the thermometer reached record-high temperatures for those days since they had started keeping records in the nineteenth century. I wanted the race to live up to my expectations and prove to be the real McCoy. I wanted it to be a doozy, because that would make it more of an adventure—and more fun.

Regardless of a few extra degrees of mercury inside the thermometer, Death Valley in July is always hot. It is always a grueling climate and terrain. It is called "the world's toughest footrace" for good reason. I went into the race fearlessly the first year, but got slam-dunked with heat stroke and kidney stuff at about mile 110. I found myself a greenish blue shade of pale in the back of a white van—shaking, puking, shitting myself—with sheets held up by my sisters to block the ESPN camera. Ice cold in Owens Valley— Rigormortus Rex and looking like a cadaver with twenty-six miles to go.

Yea, though I walk through the valley of the shadow of death, I will fear no evil.
                                                              PSALM 23

Somehow, with the support of my crew, I pulled it together and basically crawled up Mount Whitney like a "little ole ant" on bloody elbows and skinned knees, humming "High Hopes" by Frank Sinatra. Because no matter what, even when you feel meek and weak, you hold it together, you get up the mountain, you reach the finish line, because that is the human way; that is the athlete's way.

I have made it up Mount Whitney twice, but both times, I did it only with the help of my family and friends on the support crew. The lessons I learned by being so close to complete and utter collapse and prevailing, with the help of others, are the best lessons for me as an athlete. That is the human condition.

An ant on the move does more than a dozing ox.
LAO TZU

As individuals we each have the potential to reach the summit, to rise above the sea of mediocrity that can be like quicksand and suck you in. Racing proved this for me. Bonding with other athletes like my good friends Monica Scholz and Dean Karnazes, as well as my support crew, always pulled me out of the quagmire and got me across the finish line.

I always sought the goal that was just outside my grasp and achieved it by plugging into the life force of the people around me, the powerful force of "the other," and the biology held in sweat and bliss. I listened to music and lost myself inside my own biology. That is how I have gotten through. We ultimately strive alone—but we prevail together.

Well if the earthquake happens, I've got my steel-toed shoes and some rope, and we'll get down a mountain.
STEVIE NICKS

Whenever I've done an ultra, I feel like a football being carried by my support crew to the finish line. I never did one of those races on my own. Unfortunately, ultra-athletic events inherently take place in the middle of nowhere. As a New Yorker, my dream was to showcase the ultra experience in downtown Manhattan. I decided to organize an ultra-distance race called the "Treadathalon: The Run for Life" a few blocks from my house. The contest required Herculean effort and was the most humbling athletic event of my career.

You can do more, you can always do more.
DAN MARINO

THE TREADATHALON: THE ROAD TO NOWHERE
RUNNING 154 MILES IN 24 HOURS

"You are a comet now. . . . Nothing can stop you."
LOUISE DEMIRJIAN (WORDS OF ENCOURAGEMENT
TO ME DURING THE TREADATHALON)

After a decade of exploring the outer reaches of human potential in far-off lands, I brought the world of endurance sports home in 2004. With the help of Abbie Schiller and Edger Huber of Kiehl's Since 1851, we organized a fundraiser and community event at our flagship store on Thirteenth Street and Third Avenue in Manhattan. I invited Dean "Ultramarathon Man" Karnazes to join me for a twenty-four-hour nonstop treadmill run.

We were raising money for YouthAIDS, and the race was called the "Run for Life." With the help of Tracey Budz of LifeFitness, I was able to have three brand-new 95ti top-of-the-line treadmills delivered to Kiehl's and set up in the window. I wanted the third treadmill so that local neighbors and friends could run with us, raise money for YouthAIDS, and experience firsthand for a few miles the camaraderie Dean and I were feeling. They became a link in the chain. They could run side by side with us and participate in an ultra event without having to do the whole thing or even leave New York. I hoped that the event would inspire onlookers and partakers to climb onboard a treadmill with a new perspective.

I hear and I forget, I see and I remember, I do and I understand.
JAPANESE PROVERB

I wanted to inspire people to realize that they could push against their limits, too, and achieve their goals. By seeing us run for twenty-four hours, and participating, maybe they would realize that the twenty-minute jog they were putting off was completely doable and didn't have to be a big deal. I think it worked. Lots of people tell me, "I thought of you the other day when I was running. I was dreading my run, but said if Bergland can run for 154 miles nonstop, I can surely get through a three-mile jog today—and I finished strong." Nothing makes me happier than to hear that.

The Treadathalon was a chance to celebrate community and sports while raising awareness and money for YouthAIDS, which does fantastic work to educate and prevent HIV transmission globally.

Trust yourself. Create the kind of self that you will be happy to live with all your life. Make the most of yourself by fanning the tiny, inner sparks of possibility into flames of achievement.

GOLDA MEIR

I was also trying to break a Guinness World Record. My nearest and dearest people volunteered as my support crew. Jonathan Cane, who got me started almost two decades earlier, was my official timekeeper. Nikki Haran, a soul mate, was in charge of keeping me fueled. My family was there too, of course. Throughout the event, people from my entire life came by and offered words of encouragement. It was a neighborhood block party. I sent a mass e-mail and people from all stages of my life popped up, which made it a reunion. They propelled me and pulled me through. Even when I couldn't see straight and flew off the back of the treadmill and hit a brick wall, they carried me on a pillow of goodwill.

About four weeks before the run, in an overzealous attempt to be ready, I had made a rookie mistake and was crippled, on bed rest for seven days, with a lumbar sprain caused by running at a much steeper incline (10 percent) than usual. Dr. Mark Klion, a fellow Ironman and sports orthopedist, played a pivotal role in getting me back in running form when I found myself unable to walk half a block.

Adversity causes some men to break; others to break records.

WILLIAM A. WARD

I was in peak form by race day, which I had scheduled for late April to coincide with the fiftieth anniversary of Roger Bannister's historic sub-four-minute-mile run. It would be a good time for people to watch outside. Fifty years ago, records were shorter and faster. The zeitgeist now seems to be longer and farther. Picking a date to coincide with what he did was my way of honoring his legacy; I also hoped to channel his legs. I was successful in breaking the record in the Guinness Book of Records that day by covering 153.76 miles in twenty-four hours. I did it by drawing visceral strength from all the love and support of my friends, family, neighbors, and coworkers.

You will do it. I know you will.

EDGAR HUBER OF KIEHL'S

(WORDS OF ENCOURAGEMENT FROM MY BOSS DURING THE TREADATHALON)

POLAR OPPOSITES CONVERGE
BANNISTER SUB-FOUR MINUTES

No longer conscious of my movement, I discovered a new unity with nature. I had found a new source of power and beauty, a source I never dreamed existed.

ROGER BANNISTER (ON BREAKING THE FOUR-MINUTE MILE)

On sabbatical at Oxford University in 1968, my dad converted the original treadmill on which Roger Bannister first broke the four-minute mile in an old fatigue lab in the basement of the anatomy and physiology building. My father's experiment put sheep on a treadmill to see what happen neurochemically when they trotted on it. (Dad said I crawled around on the floor of that lab as a two-year-old.) Roger Bannister, who studied neurology, too, has been a mentor of mine since I was a young kid. His description of breaking the four-minute mile remains to me the most well-articulated representation of what it feels like to push against your limits and break through to another place—through the pinhole—as a runner.

The lads ran their socks into the ground.

ALEX FERGUSON

Here is a recap of that historic event. What Bannister describes is what I call superfluidity—the athletic equivalent of feeling no friction or viscosity. When you experience it you will feel like you are laughing and crying at the same time. The backs of your eyes will feel wet—and have lots of slip—but you will feel sublime . . . and want to cling to that moment as long as you can.

When Roger Bannister decided to attempt the sub-four-minute mile outdoors, he chose to run on the same track on which he had run his first race at Oxford. He enlisted two other runners to set the pace—Chris Brasher and Chris Chataway. As Bannister describes that historic run:

There was a false start, and when the gun went off the second time, Brasher took the lead. I slipped in effortlessly behind him feeling tremendously full of running. My legs seemed to meet no resistance at all, as if propelled by some unknown force. Halfway through the mile, the time on the clock was at one minute and fifty-eight seconds. I was realizing so much that my mind seemed almost detached from

*my body. At three quarters of a mile the effort still seemed barely per-
ceptible; the time was three minutes .7 seconds, and now the crowd
was roaring. Somehow I had to run the last lap in 59 seconds.*

Just then Chataway took the lead, and held it until the beginning of the
backstretch. With 300 yards to go, Bannister passed him.
As Bannister described it,

*There was no pain, only a great unity of movement and aim. The
world seemed to stand still, or did not exist. The only reality was the
next 200 yards of track under my feet. I felt at that moment that it
was my chance to do one thing supremely well.*

Roger Bannister lunged across the finish line with about a .6 second to
spare in an effort that still ranks as a milestone in the history of track and
field. I have read that account many times, but each time I do it still stands
out as one of the most accurate descriptions of a feeling that is so hard to articulate. These moments of superfluid performance are like the Holy Grail
for an athlete; they should bring you back to your daily practice. This feeling is in your biology. With practice you can achieve superfluidity almost
every day.

THE LAND OF THE LOST
DINOSAUR MURAL ON THIRD AVENUE

*I want to stand as close to the edge as I can without going over. Out
on the edge you see all the kinds of things you can't see from the
center.*

                                                                KURT VONNEGUT

There is a green dinosaur mural painted on a building kitty-corner from
Kiehl's at Thirteenth Street and Third Avenue. This dinosaur became my
mascot for twenty-four hours when I ran in the Kiehl's window. As the sun
moved across the sky, the dinosaur became animated. In my cerebellum (my
reptilian brain) I was having an ongoing dialogue with that green dinosaur
mural on the wall across from me. I pass the mural every day on my way
home now, and pay homage. He became an ally to me during that event and
now his permanence amid all the construction is refreshing.

I felt terrific the first twenty-three hours, much as Roger Bannister described. I was so absorbed in running and connected to the people around me. At around 7 A.M., my brain shut down. Individuals became blobs of positive energy, but I couldn't distinguish between them. After twenty-three straight hours of running, it was just me and this dinosaur. When my brain shut down I was in Jurassic Park. The ephemeral athletic moment changed tumblers in my brain and opened to a surreal primeval world.

This city now doth, like a garment, wear the beauty of the morning; silent bare, ships, towers, domes, theatres and temples lie open unto the fields and to the sky; All bright and glittering in the smokeless air.
                                          WILLIAM WORDSWORTH

I remember the angle of the light that morning. I felt the energy of a sea of people carrying me, not their individual personalities. It was just a massive kaleidoscope of colors, yet I was still running. I lost all sense of time and space and could only take in scattered bits of outside stimuli, sounds and impulses of energy from the crowd. Not even music penetrated. Nothing was being processed by my conscious brain. It was like a deep sleeping dream. I was outside my body, but there was no conscious fear. I imagine that is what it must feel like to die. It was an extraordinary experience. I don't regret it, but also would never in a million years subject myself to it again.

The deep shines with the deep.
A deeper sky utters the sky.
These words waver
Between sky and sky.

To know
Meaning to celebrate:
Meaning
To become "in some way"
Another; to come
To a becoming:
To have come well.
                    HENRY RAGO (FROM "THE KNOWLEDGE OF LIGHT")

From about 7 A.M., twenty-three hours into the run, till the end, I don't really remember anything, but I ran for another hour at seven miles per hour and had no idea where I was, what direction I was facing, what time of day it was, who *I* was. My ego was gone. I was blacked out, but I was running. That is what amazes me. I was able to keep running from so many years of conditioning laid down in the purkinje cells of my cerebellum. The innate collective unconscious muscle memory of running stored in my cerebellum for millions of years allowed me to run without a fully functional cerebrum. I put one foot in front of the other in a purely instinctive way.

It ain't over till it's over.

YOGI BERRA

It was surreal to watch myself on the NY-1 news loop on the TV at the ICU later that morning, witnessing something I had no recollection of. I was catheterized and on the verge of kidney failure with CPK levels of 176,700 "international units" per liter (normal is 24 to 195 IU/L). CPK is a by-product of muscle breakdown and is a gloppy and viscous fluid that blocks the filtering screens of the kidneys. My CK-MB, an enzyme that measures heart muscle breakdown with a normal range of 0 to 34.4 ng/ml was at 770 "nanograms" per milliliter.

The saddest lesson I learned from the post-treadathalon blood work was that, in an attempt to squeeze every ounce of passion from my body, my heart had begun to eat itself. That sucked. My own desire to suck the marrow out of life would eventually cause me to self-destruct. I made a vow in the ICU that I would never push my body to the limit again.

Also, I realized that with the need-achievement brain chip that I have, when my dreams come true it means I need to raise the bar. I would always feel the need to bite off more than I could chew. For me there was now no place further to go as an athlete. I could never turn back and experience shorter races with the same sense of passion and adventure I once had. There was a loss of innocence that couldn't be undone. I had to move on to something else.

The treadmill record was the perfect bookend to my life as an ultra-endurance athlete, because it closed a chapter. I'll be the first to admit that because it is a Guinness World record, it was in many ways my crowning achievement, but it was also inane in many ways, as so many of those records are. The treadathalon was the last time I will ever take my body to the point of obliteration. I proved once and for all that I had enough mental toughness to kill myself. I had pushed the quest for adventure to a point of self-destruction. It was a turning point for me as an ultra runner. I had nothing else to prove. I needed to bring my knowledge and life experience back to the real world.

> *All great deeds and all great thoughts have a ridiculous beginning. Great works are often born on a street corner or in a restaurant's revolving door.*
>
> ALBERT CAMUS

FROM ATHLETE TO AUTHOR
NEW CHALLENGE: SIMILAR SKILL SET

> *New ideas pass through three periods: 1) It can't be done. 2) It probably can be done, but it's not worth doing. 3) I knew it was a good idea all along!*
>
> ARTHUR C. CLARKE

I've always sought out the biggest challenges I could find. After decades of living a primarily cerebellar existence as an athlete, I decided to flip from down brain pursuits to something more intellectual, more up brain. I wanted to challenge myself cerebrally. Dad always said to me when I was training up to nine hours a day, "There's one muscle you're forgetting to flex, Chris, and that's your brain. It's going to shrink." He knew if I didn't use it I'd lose it, and I'd have rock-hard abs and a cranium full of mush. Even though I come from a family of brainiacs, I have never been particularly academic, and sitting still has always been tough for me.

> *If you wish to be a writer, write.*
>
> EPICTETUS

I knew writing a book was the most daunting task I could think of, so of course, I had to do it. I also knew I still needed to make my dad proud, and prove to him that I could do it. But I didn't want to do it just to say I'd gotten something published. I wanted to write a really comprehensive, entertaining, and inspiring book that could improve people's lives. I wanted to create something meaningful, and to do it well. So I made a commitment that I would plant myself firmly in a chair for a year, live in seclusion, cut back to a tonic level of fitness (three hours a week), and see what happened. I transferred all my focus and determination into researching and crafting this book for that entire time. It was intense.

It's hard to beat a person who never gives up.
BABE RUTH

My stamina and ability to focus came in handy. Most days I spent about fourteen hours straight researching and writing. I took few, if any breaks. I often forgot to eat and didn't really sleep. It was more exhausting than sport. Thinking hurts more than running to me. After eight months of writing I looked up from my computer and realized I had whittled away to nothing, but had written more than four thousand pages. I had become so completely absorbed—I lost myself. It was a superfluid and sublime experience but now I had overdone it again and had a big mess on my hands.

With sort of a mental squint.
LEWIS CARROLL

Just as my heart had started to eat itself during the treadathalon, my desire to say everything I could possibly say in one shot meant that I had a manuscript almost three feet high. I needed to cut it down a lot. And I did not want to fuck up. So I battened down the hatches and just started reeling it in—just like I would at the end of a race. I became very patient and mostly a diligent taskmaster. The creative work was done and I couldn't run free. Now I just had to pull it off and not fumble, choke, or drop the ball.

I will try to cram these paragraphs full of facts and give them a weight and shape no greater than that of a cloud of butterflies.
BRENDAN GILL

I knew that to see this through to the finish line I would need support, just like in a race. That is when my editor, Diane Reverand, came to my rescue. She became like my support crew in an ultra-endurance race, giving me advice, strategizing, nurturing, and pushing me harder to be the best I could be as a writer. She was a tough coach, and I appreciated that. There was no compromising. What made Diane the ideal editor for this project was that she applied the athletic mind-set to everything she did—and always had. Diane understood *The Athlete's Way* because she had lived her life that way. She understood everything I was trying to say—and helped me say it better.

> *You don't concentrate on risks. You concentrate on results. No risk is too great to prevent the necessary job from getting done.*
>
> CHUCK YEAGER

The greatest thing for me about my conversion experience of becoming a writer is that it was very similar to becoming an athlete. I believe that anyone can become an athlete. The fact that I was able to become a writer was proof of neuroplasticity and transformation through hard work, persistance, and dedication. If I can make an author out of myself, you can make an athlete out of yourself.

I went from being a mediocre typist and wordsmith to learning how to actually type really fast and use words well enough to articulate my thoughts. I still have a long way to go, but have crafted a book. I didn't want my book to be just another humdrum cookie-cutter fitness book. I wanted to create something original. I wanted the book to be fun to read, educational, inspiring, and revolutionary to some degree. A daunting task for a rookie, but I gave it the real college try. I did the absolute best I could and took some risks. So I'm proud of it.

A HUMAN BEING, BEING AN ATHLETE
WE'RE ALL IN THE SAME BOAT

> *I did not wish to take a cabin passage, but rather to go before the mast and on the deck of the world, for there I could best see the moonlight amid the mountain. I do not wish to go below now. Only that day dawns to which we are awake. There is more day to dawn. The sun is but a morning star.*
>
> HENRY DAVID THOREAU (*WALDEN: CONCLUSION*)

Whether you are walking briskly around the block, riding an elliptical trainer, or jogging on a treadmill, you can apply the principles of *The Athlete's Way* to your workout. I refer to an athlete in this book as anyone who exercises regularly with intent. *The Athlete's Way* is the process by which you go about doing what *you* do.

The Athlete's Way is about adopting the character traits of an athlete and applying them to your daily pursuits—regardless of how athletic you are. I never considered myself a "runner" and still don't. Whether you hate to work out or you love it, you can apply the ideals of this program in a way that fits your lifestyle and will change your life. Success in this program is getting to a point at which exercise becomes something that you seek and will enjoy for the rest of your life.

> *People of mediocre ability sometimes achieve outstanding success because they don't know when to quit. Most men succeed because they are determined to. Persevere and get it done.*
>
> GEORGE E. ALLEN

Whether you are just trying to squeeze in twenty minutes a day walking in the neighborhood or training for an Ironman, this book will help you achieve your goals.

The key is:

- *finding your tonic level of exertion between boredom and being overwhelmed*

- *creating a state of fluid performance, aka flow*

- *setting goals that are challenging, but achievable*

- *achieving goals consistently*

This is what athletes do intuitively, and why they seek exercise. The ultimate objective is to transform you into a person who loves exercise. The program is not complicated, but it is complete. As an interdisciplinary approach to self-improvement, it leaves no rock unturned.

THE ATHLETIC PARADOX: EAT OR BE EATEN
THE HUNGRY AND THE HUNTED

Don't look back, something might be gaining on you.
SATCHEL PAIGE

The juggling act of contrasting motivations is part of what I call *the athletic paradox*. Learning to balance cutthroat competition and a desire to win with sportsmanlike behavior makes *the athlete's way* a physical and ethical balancing act you master over time. As Spike Lee said, "Do the right thing." Be a good sport, play fair, never cheat, and be gracious whether you win or lose. But always try to win—not for a trophy but because that mind-set of victory is synonymous with giving your best effort, and never, ever dogging it. Learn to balance competition and camaraderie in order to bring out the full potential in yourself and those around you.

I play to win, whether during practice or a real game. And I will not let anything get in the way of me and my competitive enthusiasm to win.

MICHAEL JORDAN

Although this book is not just for people who are planning to do races, I encourage you to sign up for a local race regardless of your skill level. If nothing else, do it for the community building and camaraderie of the experience. Racing is a great way to tap the romance of sports and the paradox of feeling bonded, and free. If you need an album to listen to that is about the power of breaking out of your own skin when you run—or race—check out "Born to Run" by Bruce Springsteen. Lots of clues there. "Jungleland" especially, sums it up for me.

After decades of racing, the best advice I have to anyone competing in a race, or in life—is to use the people around you to maximize your performance. If you are the leader of the pack, imagine a herd of a thousand buffalo behind you. If you are like 99.99 percent of the people in the race, think about the buffalos because they are behind you, too, but focus on the person by your side—or right in front of you. Latch on to that person like a ladder rung and use him or her to advance. I think of playing Pac-Man and eating people up (in a nice way). I literally tilt my head down and fix on an athlete in front of me. Or I glom onto a specific detail on an article of clothing, or part of the person's body, and hold on to it really tightly mentally. It becomes a pinhole.

I also use the nature around me as inspiration—the light, trees, landscapes, and smells. I lose myself in the landscape and the rhythmic sounds of breathing and splashing, bike gears shifting, or footsteps hitting pavement. Try to lose yourself in these things, too, when you train or race.

But mostly I try to bond with other athletes—to other human beings—in a friendly way in any race, and make spoken or unspoken connections with them out on the course. Remember to stay in the present tense. Don't dwell on past mistakes, or how far you have to go. Think right here, right now. But don't think too much.

Whether you have one mile left or a hundred, focus on the present millisecond and say, **"Right here, right now, I am doing the best I can."** Ask yourself if quitting is a matter of **can't or won't.** If it's "won't," finish because it hurts, you have no choice. You have to keep going.

This should be your only measure of success. How you perform in that moment, inside your own game, but always mindful of the bigger picture. If you are doing the best you can and doing the right thing in every second of every minute, you can't go wrong. But don't expect to sustain that level of excellence all the time. That is humanly impossible. Choose your battles wisely—and give yourself plenty of time to decompress and regroup before heading back into battle. You can't give 110 percent a 100 percent of the time or you will burn out. But you can always try—just know when to pull in the reins.

> *I did everything I could every day of my life.*
> **LOUISE BOURGEOIS** (FRENCH-BORN AMERICAN ARTIST)

The most valuable lesson that I've learned about the athlete's way is that it isn't just about the outcome, it really is about what happens along the way. The trick is to set goals and achieve them, but to take it down a thousand. To keep the bar high but stay very relaxed. You need to demand the most of yourself, but cut yourself some slack. Don't be a control freak, or try to be perfect—but still try to be the best you can. This is that tightrope walk of the athletic paradox.

With that said, it is still the hard line my father used to ensure he did the best he could for every patient that echoes in my head as an athlete and life. The maxim that sums up the secret code to achieving excellence is best summed up by learning to breathe deeply, relax, and say, "Don't fuck up" to yourself before you face any challenge that really matters.

CHAPTER TWO

SWEAT AND THE PURSUIT OF HAPPINESS

Jump.

JOSEPH CAMPBELL

In order to get started with this program and begin transforming your body, mind, and brain, you need to be working out. As we all know, getting started with an exercise regimen is by far the most difficult phase of the process. A disheartening aspect of making a resolution to start exercising is that the odds are not in your favor. Most people who vow to get started and stick with an exercise program fail. Make this time different.

You have probably tried to start an exercise program before and have fallen off the wagon. After repeated attempts to change old patterns of behavior with no success, most people tend to give up and fall back into the same old rut. Don't do it! *The Athlete's Way* offers new hope that it is possible to change. You can slay this dragon once and for all.

By adopting the optimistic and resilient disposition of the athletic mind-set, you will not only learn to enjoy exercise, but your brain will also ultimately be reshaped to live a happier, healthier life. Again, this book is aimed at long-term changes, not short-term quick fixes. The key is that you have to be relentlessly consistent. Only you can do that for you, but this book will give you tools to stay motivated and inspired.

90 percent of success is showing up.

WOODY ALLEN

MAKE A VOW TO SUCCEED
THE FIRST DAYS WILL BE THE HARDEST DAYS

The secret to getting ahead is getting started. The secret of getting started is breaking your complex overwhelming tasks into small manageable tasks, and then starting on the first one.

MARK TWAIN

In order to muster the courage to get started, you always have to take a deep breath. Relax first. Think about the calm before the storm, like a cat about to pounce. Come up with a game plan and take the plunge. Always commit to finish what you start. Never quit. Lace up your sneakers and start today. Start now. Do something . . . do anything!

Remember to take it slow. You don't have to kill yourself—getting the blood moving should be your goal. A small time commitment will reap huge benefits. As little as twenty to thirty minutes most days of the week is all you need to be doing to see results. That's less than 3 percent of your waking day, and you'll feel better for the other 97 percent. Think about it. Be pragmatic. That is a great return on investment.

Just as the first few days are the hardest, the first few minutes of cardiovascular exercise are tough for everybody. I always remind clients of this when we start out on a jog together. The first five minutes are always hard. The key is to ease into it. The shift from being sedentary to moving is a shock to the system. It takes a few minutes for your aerobic system to click on and about seven to eight minutes for the blissful neurochemicals, cannabinoids, and endorphins to kick in. Don't think there's something wrong with you if you don't hit the ground running and feeling like Captain Fantastic. Everyone takes a few minutes to warm up.

Eventually every person who exercises regularly gets to a point where he or she can't *not* do it. Athletes don't necessarily have more discipline or willpower than other people. Instead, the athletic process gives them immense pleasure. Even during blistering hot summer runs or freezing cold pre-sunrise swims, I exercise because of the pleasure principle. Consistent exercise ultimately becomes about maintaining a certain level of balanced bliss. When you work out regularly, you feel a little off on days you don't work your body. One of the results of sticking with *The Athlete's Way* program for eight weeks is that at the end your body and mind will create such a strong correlation between moving and feeling good that you won't be able not to do it.

DIE OLD, STAY PRETTY
SOME REASONS TO EXERCISE

How badly do you want it?

GEORGE E. ALLEN

Below are some reasons regarding disease prevention and premature death that will motivate you to get started and stick with it. Vanity isn't on this list, but it is a prime motivator for all of us. That's OK. But more important, your chances of succumbing to top causes of death can be lessened by cardiovascular exercise, strength training, stress reduction, and better nutrition. More than half of the ten leading causes of death are directly linked to lifestyle. Regular exercise will not only make you live longer, but will also improve the quality of your life.

TEN LEADING CAUSES OF DEATH IN THE UNITED STATES
(IN PERCENTAGE OF DEATHS)

1. Heart Disease 31.4

2. Cancer 23.3

3. Stroke 6.9

4. Chronic Lung Disease 4.7

5. Accident 4.1

6. Pneumonia 3.7

7. Diabetes 2.7

8. Suicide 1.3

9. Kidney Disease 1.1

10. Liver Disease 1.1

DO YOU WANT TO LIVE LONGER AND BETTER? EAT LESS, MOVE MORE, TEND, AND BEFRIEND

You should never give up too soon. You can always get one more spoonful of juice out of a grapefruit.

MILT WEISS

The secret to longevity is simple. Since the 1970s people like René Dubos of Rockefeller University and Alexander Leaf of Harvard Medical School have studied the secrets to living a long and prosperous life that are at the core of *The Athlete's Way*.

THE FOUR SECRETS TO LONGEVITY

- *Energy-balanced diet (do not consume more energy than you exert)*
- *Physical activity*
- *Close-knit human bonds*
- *A sense of purpose*

We are in an energy crisis—the ratio of available energy in our gas tanks and the surplus of energy stored on our hips doesn't match up. By one estimate, the American airline industry spent $300 million in added fuel costs in 2004 to lug around the extra ten pounds that each American weighs today compared to twenty years ago. A core tenet of *The Athlete's Way* is to seek transportation alternatives and use your own energy to commute.

I urge you to decide today to make changes in your consumption and expenditure. Create an energy balance and try to conserve fuel. The other three secrets to longevity: physical activity, close-knit human bonds, and a sense of purpose will be expanded on throughout this book. In the meantime, think about ways that you can maximize each of these in your daily life.

THE HEART DISEASE AND DIABETES REMEDY
TAKE ACCOUNTABILITY: EAT LESS, EXERCISE MORE, AND DE-STRESS

What is good? All that heightens the feeling of power in man, the will to power, power itself. What is bad? All that is born of weakness. What is happiness? The feeling that power is growing, that resistance is overcome.

FRIEDRICH NIETZSCHE

Some things that influence the development of heart disease, diabetes, or stroke are out of your control. In perhaps 5 to 10 percent of the population, genetic factors are so dominant that heart disease develops regardless of any protective factors. For most of us, what we eat and how we exercise may interact with a mild genetic predisposition for heart disease and diabetes.

You can change or control most of the conditions that hasten the development of heart disease, including high blood pressure, high blood sugar, physical inactivity, obesity, and high cholesterol by becoming physically active. The best ways to address these are through your diet and exercise. If you smoke, quit. As the Framingham Heart Study suggests, it's best to look at heart disease as a forest before focusing too much on the single tree of cholesterol reduction.

Exercise is proving to be the most important single factor. Researchers have found that exercising may do more to ward off death from heart disease than just cutting calories, says Jing Fang, M.D., and her colleagues at the Albert Einstein College of Medicine in the Bronx, New York. "The fact is that those who both exercised more and ate more nevertheless had low cardiovascular mortality," says Fang. Expending energy through physical activity may be the key to cutting the risks of heart disease and living a longer, more healthful life, she says.

WHAT IS YOUR CREDO?
CREATING A SYSTEM OF BELIEF

Life loves to be taken by the lapel and told: "I'm with you, kid. Let's go."

MAYA ANGELOU

The Athlete's Way is as much about mind-set as it is about physical exercise. This chapter begins to teach you how that feedback loop works by looking at psychological sources of inspiration that will result in better physical performance. The single most important aspect of learning to think like an athlete is to make a decision to believe that breaking a sweat every day is going to feel good.

Make the affirmation right now that you will commit to eight weeks of exercise most days of the week beginning—not tomorrow—but today. Decide that you are going to enjoy the process, because exercise makes all human beings feel good. Start believing that Sweat=Bliss, and it will become something you seek and don't avoid.

If you think you can, you can. If you think you can't, you're right.

MARY KAY ASH

Even if you have never viewed exercise as an agreeable experience, decide today that you will begin to take that view. Millions of exercise lovers can't all be wrong. Don't believe the myth that only other people are capable of experiencing runner's high or athletic bliss. This is not at all the case. Biology is universal. I am going to prove to you that you can become an athlete who loves to exercise, but you have to trust that and begin believing it now.

Champions aren't made in gyms. Champions are made from something they have deep inside them—a desire, a dream, a vision. It's the repetition of affirmations that leads to belief. And once that belief becomes a deep conviction, things begin to happen.

MUHAMMAD ALI

Remember, the same anandamide that flows through you flows through all athletes. You just have to get it pumping. I will teach you how to create that flow by finding your personal tonic level. Exercise is not something painful to be avoided, but something pleasurable that you should seek. I can tell you this a million times, but you need to discover this for yourself, experience it firsthand, and make it yours.

MIND-SET IS NOT FIXED
YOU CAN REINVENT YOURSELF

The first step towards getting somewhere is to decide that you are not going to stay where you are.

JOHN PIERPONT MORGAN

Scientists thought for centuries that the neural connections in our brain were fixed at birth. They now know that the neural connections of the brain are constantly being reshaped. The infrastructure is most impressionable from infancy to our early twenties. The degree of nurturing and safety that a child feels greatly influences the way his brain is wired. Drug use has been shown to carve grooves along specific neural channels that can become welded together and difficult to undo as adults, but it can be corrected. Even though the brain is very resilient and pliable, don't abuse the generous biological design by bombarding it with exogenous sources for pleasure.

An eight-month-old baby has twice as many neurons (200 billion) as a five-year-old child. The planned extinction of half of these neurons happens as the toddler's brain is fine-tuned for its particular environment. The brain is shaped specifically to adapt and survive in the circumstances it inhabits in order to survive. The brain is designed to become what it needs to be. It begins as a tabula rasa—a clean slate—with billions of potential connections to be made. The infant brain is neural plasticity at its purest. As a baby grows, billions of neurons are shaped by every sight, sound, taste, smell, and touch that baby experiences. Specific neurons and their connection to others are strengthened, while those that are not regularly activated are starved of nutrients and oxygen, grow weak, and die.

At this crucial early stage of development, blindfolding a baby would kill off its optic nerves and blind the child for life; a child wearing earplugs would become deaf. The nerve cells that are not used become superfluous and die. The brain is efficient; it trims the fat and streamlines the connections that work. Such brain sculpting occurs in all animals, including insects. This shaping continues throughout our lives as we continue to grow and evolve. New connections are made, others weaken.

Begin to be now what you will be hereafter.

WILLIAM JAMES

Since neurons follow the use-it-or-lose-it principle throughout your entire life, your job is to stay positive and active. Those neural nets will be strengthened and pleached, twisted together like vines, while pessimism, helplessness, and rejection sensitivity and their corresponding neural nets will become weaker. Visualize snipping the connections with gardening shears like Edward Scissorhands, making bunny rabbits and horse sculptures out of a hedge. Consider your brain a sculpture that you work at every day. Snip away the negativity. Let positivity run wild. This is an image that you should remember as you go about changing and reshaping your mind-set.

Go often to the house of thy friend; for weeds soon choke up the unused path, and don't let your sorrow come higher than your knees.

SCANDINAVIAN PROVERB

The neural pathways along which thoughts travel in your brain can be compared with a path through the woods. As hikers take the same route through the woods, they create a path. The more feet that travel this path, the more deeply worn it becomes and the easier it is to follow. The same goes for neural connections of our memories and behavior. The more we repeat thoughts or actions, the more deeply they are etched in our neural pathways. Likewise, the less we engage them, the sooner they atrophy. Learning depends on the plasticity of the circuits in the brain, the ability of the neurons to make lasting changes in the efficiency of their synaptic transmission.

You cannot play with the animal in you without becoming wholly animal, play with falsehood without forfeiting your right to truth, play with cruelty without losing your sensitivity of mind. He who wants to keep his garden tidy doesn't reserve a plot for the weeds.

DAG HAMMARSKJÖLD (FORMER UNITED NATIONS SECRETARY-GENERAL)

Your brain could also be viewed as a garden. Your thoughts and actions water and fertilize the neurons associated with that state of being. Whatever mind-set or habit you engage makes those neurons blossom. Likewise, disengaging them causes them to atrophy. What you think matters. A thought reinforces an *engram* (neural network), which reinforces a mind-set, which reinforces a habit, which reinforces your character. The neuroplastic reinforcement of a neural network through repetition nourishes that endeavor, which is why practice makes perfect.

The neurons are reshaped, hammered, and forged through practice, and that practice is hardwired nightly when you dream. Your cerebellum hones fine-tuned motor skills during the day, and these skills are reshaped during your sleep. The dream weaver makes the novice and pro athlete an artisan of brain sculpture, primarily during the REM (rapid eye movement) phase of sleep when we dream most. Dreaming transfers learning to long-term memory storage regardless of your level of ability; everybody improves with practice.

It takes time for the chemical signals at the junction between cells (the synapses) to take place. Learning and memory occur during the day, but researchers believe synaptic changes are solidified at night when we sleep and dream. The brain needs some downtime to hardwire changes made in the wake cycle spent transporting chemical messengers and biochemical changes associated with the new connection between cells. This is one reason why sleep is so important. During rest, the brain keeps working. On an EEG the up brain appears to wake up during REM, as the down brain goes off-line and puts your body into a paralyzed state so it can transfer its wealth of information up north.

One of the keys to creating flow in sport is using the vestibulo-ocular reflex (VOR), which is the ability of your eyes to lock on a target and move your head; it is a cerebellar reflex. In a sport like tennis, Ping-Pong, or baseball, the VOR allows you to keep your eye on the ball and swing a racket, paddle, or bat to hit it in the sweet spot with laserlike focus. In sports of repetitive motion like running, biking, or riding the elliptical trainer I've found that if I lock on to a target, like the red "power on" light on the TV in front of me, and move my head back and forth and relax the tonus in my throat by sticking my tongue out a little bit, I will go into a trance.

I stumbled upon the link between VOR and trancelike states through hours of treadmill running and the time I spent chanting in ashrams when I meditated in college. Later, in researching REM sleep, I learned that when the tonis in the throat is lost, the tongue relaxes. The body is paralyzed and the eyes dart back and forth as we dream. The most likely reason for this is so that we don't act out, or talk in our sleep during our deepest dream states. It became clear to me that creating a dreamlike default state of flow through sport was linked to VOR, too. It was really REM in reverse. This is my original hypothesis. My father thinks it makes sense, but other scientists have yet to explore this theory.

My educated guess is that the cerebellum is the hinge, or the pinhole, to all dreams, both day and night dreams. Behind the veil of sleep, with the cerebellum "off"—there is tons of slip behind your eyes and you slide into a dreamscape—or you could create that same slip when you are awake by consciously activating the VOR in the cerebellum—you turn the down brain "on" and the cerebrum goes off line. Sleep and consciousness are polar opposites. By fixing your eyes on a target, the hinge of the cerebellum would let you slide through the pinhole into a trance by shutting down the up brain.

In moments of superfluidity, the backs of my eyes always get really wet—like I'm going to cry. I think this state can be considered "tears of joy." The next time you feel a surge of water hit the backs of your eyes when you are overflowing with joy, take inventory and realize that whatever lined up in that moment holds the keys to the secret gate. That water is a sign that you are lubed up and sliding into a state of superfluidity.

SHED YOUR SKIN
A FRESH START AFTER EVERY SWEAT

If there is no struggle, there is no progress.
FREDERICK DOUGLASS

Sports can be a daily metamorphosis. Athletes crave exercise. Everyone who sticks with a regular exercise program does so, because at the end of the day, they have learned it makes them feel good. Athletes are driven to exercise not because of superhuman willpower and discipline, but because a switch in their head has been turned on. They have seen the light and associate exercise with pleasure. This is what keeps them coming back for more.

Exercise gives you a chance to be renewed every day. Every time you exercise, you are given proof that it makes you happy by the mood shift that takes place before and after each workout. Anytime you break a sweat for at least twenty minutes you are guaranteed a fresh start on the day. Begin to take note of your mood, attitude, and perspective before a workout and when you're done.

Visualize the best, anticipate the best, believe in the best—and you will usually get the best.
GIL ATKINSON

The mandate for the first eight weeks is to write these observations down in a training log or workbook. The best way to prove to yourself that exercise makes you happy will be to see those numbers in black and white. Take inventory before exercising or going in to the gym—and then compare that mood to how you feel when you're finished or as you walk out the door. I call it the in-out survey. The rating scale should be –5 (stressed/cranky) to +5 (calm/elated). Staying north of zero is the goal every day. Get in the habit of introspection. Say, "OK, I am heading into this workout at a +1 to-day . . . let's go to a +4."

COMMIT TO FIFTY-SIX DAYS
GIVE IT EIGHT WEEKS AND YOU ARE HOME FREE

It is the "follow through" that makes the great difference between ultimate success and failure, because it is so easy to stop.

CHARLES F. KETTERING
(INVENTOR OF ALL LIGHTING AND IGNITION FOR EARLY AMERICAN AUTOMOBILES)

It is going to take about two to four weeks to reshape your neurons—and to form new habits. If you can commit to *The Athlete's Way* program for eight weeks, you will be home free. Do whatever it takes to make yourself stay committed. Start the program with a buddy, sign up with a trainer, have a friend, coworker, partner, or a parent become a sponsor to chart your progress. Surround yourself with reminders—calendars, pictures on the fridge, an elastic band on your wrist, a rubber-band ball. Use training partners, uniforms, minute-minder timers, anthems. Do whatever it takes to stay committed for at least fifty-six days. This book will be there to guide you throughout the process.

You have to find it. No one else can find it for you.

BJÖRN BORG

The most benefit will be reaped if you read this book while working out. Drip sweat onto the book holder of your stationary equipment. That way you can begin to draw parallels to the advice given here as it plays out in your day-to-day life. A lot of the learning is going to be state dependent, meaning that you learn it inside the athletic process. In order to extract it for day-to-day use, you need to identify it by giving it a name. You should get in the habit of keeping a journal or note cards handy to jot down insights immediately after working out.

BACK IN THE SADDLE
STATE-DEPENDENT MEMORY

Things are in the saddle, and ride mankind.

RALPH WALDO EMERSON

We all know our jobs like the backs of our hands. If you go on vacation for a month, within hours of being back at work it seems like you never left. This is called state-dependent memory. At my job for Kiehl's I wore a white lab coat. The minute I put the lab coat and my wing pin on, I would click into that state-dependent memory and could train others about ingredients and their functions almost on autopilot. If you ask me to do the same when I'm not in my workout uniform, it won't happen so automatically. We remember things we learn from the environment in which we learn them. As you explore your athletic process, remember that your personal insights from inside the process are invaluable. Some insights might be what time of day you have the most energy. What songs inspire you—or that you don't like working out with music at all. But look at it as a chance to be clean of any technology and just lose yourself in your breathing and the sounds around you. You won't have access to them again until you're back in it, so take mental notes. I literally say, "Note to self:_____," and try to take at least three lessons out of every workout. I suggest you do the same. Flex your declarative memory when you exercise by making mental lists.

I wrote this book inside the athletic process. While exercising indoors I jotted down insights on salt-stained and smeared fluorescent note cards I kept on my coach's clipboard while I rode the stationary bike or stashed in the water bottle cage of the treadmill. While training outside I carried a Dictaphone in one hand, an iPod in the other, and took stream-of-consciousness dictation on what I was experiencing.

State-dependent memories are triggered when you are back in the same environment and mind-set. This book will make sense when you are working out, because that is where the ideas originated. Some things you read here may seem odd when you read them sitting in your armchair, but when you are inside the athletic process, you will say, "Aha, now I get it." I encourage you to keep an eight-week training log and take notes on what happens inside the process.

Take notes immediately after you are done working out—review these note cards or notes before you go to bed at night or in weekly recaps. I have revelations during every workout. If I have no way to record them, I practice memorizing them. When you get back inside the process, trigger words, images, and ways of thinking will flood your mind. Try to remember these things and use them by writing them down.

THE EIGHT-WEEK WORKBOOK:
SIMPLICITY AND SINCERITY

Say it hot.

D. H. LAWRENCE

As you embark on your athletic immersion, the most important thing to do is to make a fifty-six-day commitment and to record your insights and progress in writing. Document it. You don't have to write a daily manifesto, but take notes. Be patient and consistent. The transformative process takes place at different rates for everyone. Personalize the program—make it your own. Research has shown that this is the only way that people actually make long-term changes. This book is high on insight and advice but low on dogma.

I would encourage you to follow the first week day by day and to do the program by rote for seven days. By establishing this seven-day program, any time you fall off the wagon, you can kick-start your program by deciding to reboot, by rebeginning the seven-day plan. I have found with clients that having a specific seven-day routine to start is good. During the following seven weeks, I encourage you to tailor the program.

Most changes may take a few weeks to click in, but with persistence you will have a transformation. The important thing is to invest time in sticking with the program for eight weeks and to keep a journal every day. Chart your progress by looking back in your journal every seventh day. Build momentum.

TOOLBOX SUPPLIES

Here are some helpful tools for the eight-week course.

- *Calendar*

- *Large journal for log keeping*

- *Package of note cards*

- *Package of rubber bands size #33*

- *Pens*

- *Binder clips*

- *Minute-minder timer (hourglass or actual timer)*

- *Small notepad for weight lifting/diet recall*

THE ATHLETE'S WAY *EIGHT-WEEK WORKBOOK*

- *MORNING CONTRACT AND EVENING REVIEW PAGES: Write down your objectives every morning and your accomplishments every night.*

- *RECORD TIME INVESTED: Keep tabs on how many minutes you exercise every day.*

- *CHART YOUR FLOW CHANNEL: Take note of the level of challenge that keeps you engaged and allows you to lose yourself in fluid, or super-fluid, performance.*

- *FIND A MENTOR: It could be a stranger, a celebrity, or a friend.*

- *CREATE AN ATHLETIC ALTER EGO: Use your imagination, clothing, smells, music (or anything else at your disposal) to reinforce the character of your ideal athletic self.*

- *TAG IT: Identify different mental states by giving them a name*

- *SONG WORK: Use anthems and soundtracks to punctuate the athletic process and energize you.*

- *THE PINHOLE: Look for the combination of circumstances that coalesce to allow you to slip into a state of superfluidity.*

- *RATE MOOD SHIFTS: Take emotional inventory about how you feel before and after a workout. Use a rating scale of −5 to +5. Zero is baseline—anything above is positive.*

- *ENERGY BALANCE: Keep tabs on calories in and calories out. Use more energy than you consume every day, and you'll never gain weight.*

THE SHERLOCK HOLMES APPROACH:
WHO, WHAT, WHERE, WHEN, AND WHY

Try to learn something about everything and everything about something.

THOMAS H. HUXLEY

When writing in your log, you need to cover the basic questions a reporter or detective would ask. Learn to observe and analyze. Take notes on the internal and external things that motivated or deflated you. The most important thing to do every day is to rate how you felt before and after the workout. Circle those numbers and look back to see the direct correlation between mood and movement. Be inquisitive and get to know yourself inside and out. Examine yourself and the process; stay curious. Ask who, what, where, when, and why.

- *Date*

- *Time*

- *Distance*

- *Exertion*

- *Internal insights (psychology)*

- *External observations (environment)*

- *Pattern breakers*

- *Positive reinforcers*

- *Derailers*

- *Trigger words*

- *Anthems*

- *Before/after (–5/+5)*

THE BASICS OF THE WORKBOOK (SAMPLE ENTRY)

- *WHEN: July 1. Total time: 28 minutes.*

- *WHERE: Did 2 laps around the Central Park Reservoir.*

- *WHAT: It was an easy run—but we ran faster near the end.*

- *WHO: I met Adam and we ran together.*

- *WHY: I needed to decompress after a hectic week at work.*

- *INTERNAL INSIGHTS: I had a lot of energy today—I was very wound up . . . my feet felt light. I realized the problem I was having at work with the inventory transfers. Made notes to myself the minute I walked in the door.*

- *EXTERNAL OBSERVATION: It was really humid today but the park was bustling. Lots of sweaty bodies. I love New York in the summertime.*

- *MOOD BEFORE/AFTER (-5/+5): –2 (high-strung) before, about +3 afterward.*

- *CALORIES IN/CALORIES OUT: I ate well today. I skipped dessert and just had mint tea after dinner, because I have a big race in two weeks and want to be lean.*

THE DAILY ROUTINE BECOMES A WAY OF LIFE:
RECOMMIT EVERY MORNING

Set a goal and don't quit until you attain it. When you do attain it, set another goal, and don't quit until you reach it. Never quit.

BEAR BRYANT

Lifelong changes are made one day at a time. Recommit every day. Do three things every morning.

1. Plan what you are going to do that day and visualize it—from beginning to end. Watch it like a movie.

2. Jot down your goals for today on a note card (I like fluorescent ones). Stick this card in your purse or a pocket—carrying it with you is a reminder that it is your daily commitment contract. You can jot insights about the workout on the back of the card and save it at home and watch the stack grow. Review at night every once in awhile. These cards will remind you of your investment and your journey.

3. Put a new elastic band on your wrist every morning, or before a specific workout, as a positive reinforcer and to signify your commitment to a specific goal. On the first day you will tie this around itself to make a core for what will become a huge, bounceable rubber band ball. Every day you achieve your goal you will add the rubber band that you put on as you made a commitment to follow through on your goals. And you will watch the rubber-band ball grow. It will be a tangible reminder of your investment and achievement. And you can bounce it around.

> I don't measure a man's success by how high he climbs but how high he bounces when he hits the bottom.
>
> GEN. GEORGE S. PATTON

FEELING UNINSPIRED OR FULL OF DREAD?
TAKE THE BULL BY THE HORNS, RIGHT NOW

> Do not fear mistakes. You will know failure. Continue to reach out.
>
> BENJAMIN FRANKLIN

If at some point you fall off the exercise wagon, kick-start your program by beginning with week one again. Develop a ritual and routine. Surround yourself with music, images, and smells that remind you of the process so that you can get yourself motivated.

Make the workbook process a routine, but keep it fun. The act of recording your daily achievements will serve not only as a positive reinforcer but also as a way to keep tabs on your progress and what you are learning. Writing down your accomplishments should be something you look forward to. Seeing what you have achieved in black and white makes your work tangible. Looking back on it will help you see where you've been, what you've learned, and how to chart your course.

Sometimes you think of something and it is so light, so fleeting, that you don't have time to make an entry in your diary. Everything is so evanescent, but your drawings will serve as a crutch for your memory, otherwise what you were thinking will be lost.

LOUISE BOURGEOIS

You want to keep your workbook simple and keep it honest. In the past, I have had people create elaborate workbooks that actually end up taking time away from working out and living life. If you like to write a lot and have time to go into detail, go for it, but in general a few quick observations will suffice. Your workbook should take about five minutes a day. Find a notebook that you like—personalize it and make it *your* workbook. Your workbook should be a no-BS and judgment-free zone. Remember that you don't have to share it with anyone.

THE FIRST WEEK
JUMP TO IT

Leap . . . and the net will appear.

PROVERB

As you embark on this program you can structure your eight-week course chapter by chapter. Since everyone progresses at different rates; if there are parts of the prescriptive that seem more relevant to you, spend more time focusing on those.

DO THIS EVERY DAY

1. *Morning recommitment ceremony: Note card/elastic band*

2. *Something physical for at least twenty minutes*

3. *Make a pre- and postworkout "mood" entry (–5/+5).*

4. *Record observations and insights immediately after workout.*

5. *Replay the day's events before you go to bed.*

SEVEN DAYS TO THE ATHLETE'S WAY

Though I do not believe that a plant will spring up where no seed has been, I have great faith in a seed. Convince me that you have a seed there, and I am prepared to expect wonders.

HENRY DAVID THOREAU

Day One: Get Organized at Home

The first day of this program is about getting organized. Start by organizing your living space. Spend time organizing your external environment, taking inventory about the equipment you have. Organize your internal environment as well. Decide what your goals are. You want to come up with a game plan. Begin to strategize about how you will achieve your goals. Look at your patterns of behavior and think of role models. Tell someone that you are starting an eight-week program, find a buddy, decide where you'll work out.

- *Buy office supplies: journal, calendar, note cards, rubber bands, fridge magnets.*

- *Write down your long-term and short-term goals.*

- *Devise how you'll go about achieving them.*

- *Decide if you want to work out alone, in a group, or take a class.*

- *Organize your living space—clear a shelf for workout gear. Take inventory.*

- *Find a decompression spot in your house where you will stretch.*

- *Put a dream journal by your bed and begin keeping track of dream snippets.*

- *Read things before sleep knowing that you will learn them in your sleep and that they will shape your dreams.*

- *Buy some sunscreen, lotion, new soap, perfume/cologne (if you like smells, but be considerate of other people's noses . . . don't overdo it). Use this as olfactory encoding over the next eight weeks as you work out and choose specific smells to identify with the athletic process.*

Day Two: Organize Athletic Life

Today you want to get your sporting life in order. If you don't belong to a health club, look into joining a gym or community center if possible. Get the equipment you need to get started (refer to the equipment list at the end of this chapter). Think about a trigger in your environment that will mark the transition. I recommend beginning to put things on your fridge or dresser that remind you of who you'd like to be, where you've been, and where you're going.

- Find the place where you are going to work out—gym, health club, recreation center, basement, outdoors.

- Get the sporting goods equipment you need. Buy items based on your inventory. Keep it simple! Think: "This is my uniform." Don't waste a lot of money on useless stuff.

- Buy and start using your sports watch for every workout.

- Choose music and make some play lists—go for songs with strong emotional significance. Pick some anthems and create personal soundtracks.

- Start a shrine on your fridge of mentors, magnets, photos, cards, clippings, quotes.

Day Three: Nutrition, the Twenty-Four-Hour Diet Recall

Diet recall is a term nutritionists use for keeping an exact log of food and fluids a person consumes in a day. Today you are going to keep track of everything you eat during twenty-four hours and calculate how many calories you consumed and the unit sizes. Eat your normal unmonitored diet. This is not about eating less. I want you to establish how much you tend to consume each day on average. Then do some calculations based on your basal metabolic rate to make changes. We will talk more about nutrition in chapter 9.

Write down everything that passes your lips—all food and drink. Calculate your total caloric intake and educate yourself on portion sizes. Go online to www.theathletesway.com to find calorie counters and how to read nutrition labels. Keep an eye on food labels, and get to know how many calories you tend to consume. This is your only job for today. Be very fastidious about this. When the twenty-four hours are over, continue to keep tabs.

Recording your daily intake (time of day, foods, amounts, and emotions) in a food journal increases awareness. If you are an emotional eater who eats because of feeling states rather than hunger, you need to become more aware of your thoughts, feelings, and behavior patterns. It's harder to fool yourself about what you are eating and why when you see it written down in black and white. Writing it down can help you to identify trouble times, patterns, and situations. Keep an eye out for calorically packed beverages. Remember that smaller plates and smaller utensils will actually help to make you eat less. Eat slowly, chew your food, really taste it . . . and enjoy it.

Day Four: Aerobic Training Zones

The goal today is to find out your three basic training zones—easy, medium, and hard—and the external feedback (speed, heart rate, level . . .) surrounding each. You are going to be establishing your flow channel and tonic level. These two terms are the core of *The Athlete's Way*. Your flow channel is the range between boredom and being overwhelmed. The tonic level is that just-right spot that you fall into instinctively, Not too hard, not too easy. It is intuitive to know what this feels like. We will go into more detail about this in chapter 6 on cardio.

If you have a heart-rate monitor, take note of your heartbeats per minute in relation to the intensity/level and your perceived exertion (how hard *you* feel that you're working). The flow channel will be around 60 to 80 percent of maximum exertion. Get to know how you feel in each zone. What is your comfort cusp (when you start to feel like you are pushing too hard)? Identify the feeling of being at your tonic level. Whenever bored, increase the challenge. That took me ten years to figure out. Be patient. Trust yourself—no one else can find your tonic level. Follow your intuition, use common sense, and trust your gut. You'll find it for yourself.

- Familiarize yourself with equipment.

- Find a few options to mix it up.

- Familiarize yourself with levels of exertion.

- See what feedback you have available (heart rate, watts, cadence).

- *Find your flow channel.*

- *Get familiar with rating perceived exertion (how hard you're working).*

Day Five: Focus On Strength Training

Your focus today will be on strength training. If you are working out at a gym, get advice from a professional on staff there. Have them show you the ropes. First familiarize yourself with the machines or weights you will be using. Spend most of the time getting organized and deciding what your strength-training routine is going to be. You want to establish the number of plates or pounds of weights you can lift eight to twelve times. This is technically the repetition maximum. If you are working out at home and don't have access to a trainer, we will talk more about strength training in chapter 7. I'll teach you everything you need to know to get started.

- *Focus on establishing your strength-training routine.*

- *Decide what exercises (machines/free weights) and body parts you are going to work on.*

- *Use a workbook to record results.*

- *Establish the amount of weight you lift for each exercise.*

- *Buy weight gloves.*

- *Create a contiguity routine at the gym . . . but be adaptable. Don't wait around for machines.*

- *Go with the flow. Start your stopwatch and move quickly from exercise to exercise.*

Day Six: Flexibility and Balance

Today the focus is on flexibility and balance. To create a ritual, get a mat or a towel that you will use every time you stretch. Decide where you like to do these exercises and make it a routine. Clear a space and make it your stretch and balance area. Learn the sequences in this book—and make your own stick-man figure sketches to personalize it. We'll talk more about stretching in chapter 8.

- *Create a routine around stretching.*

- *Block out a special time to stretch.*

- *Stretch more after a workout, not before.*

- *Create a sequential routine.*

- *Assign a towel and mat.*

- *Practice balance work regularly.*

Day Seven: Time-trial Testing. Review and Regroup

Today you will establish benchmark testing. You'll also look back at the week and plan next week. During the program, you will add up your weekly cardio and strength-training times and record your body weight on this day every week. Then you can look back at the times to see your long-term trends and observe patterns. You can even chart the results in a graph if you are so inclined. It will be fun to look back at this a year from now and add up all your dedication.

It is also a day to do time-trial cardio testing. Choose a specific time or distance and exercise as intensely as possible. Whether you power walk or jog, consider this race day. Get psyched up. Do this test again every week or few weeks. This should be a day to check your progress and create a sense of eagerness, maybe even feel butterflies in your stomach.

If it's the first week, you will be establishing these baselines. For example, today you would time how long it takes you to go once around the reservoir or to stationary bike three miles. Next week, you would try to do it faster. Today is a day to rally the troops and push against your limits. Challenge yourself and break through to a higher ground.

- *Plan next week's workout block out on calendar. Recommit.*

- *Weekly minutes. Review minutes worked out and add them up.*

- *Weigh yourself.*

- *Regroup for the next week.*

The Five Stages of the Daily Athletic Process

Begin at the beginning and go on till you come to the end; then stop.

LEWIS CARROLL

Each workout needs to have a beginning, a middle, and an end. I have isolated five key stages to the athletic process: **anticipation, preparation, action, perspiration,** and **completion.**

Set clear-cut goals and finish what you start. Get in the habit of deciding before you start every workout exactly what the workout is going to entail. Before you begin, play the workout forward in your mind. Extract a few specific vignettes from the process. We will elaborate on this more in chapter 10. These five stages are one of those very simple ideas that took me decades to isolate.

You will use different mental skills and psychological angling to cope with each stage. I will expand on these stages later in the book. For now, as you read these stages, play them out in your mind as you would in your day-to-day life.

FIVE STAGES TO THE ATHLETE'S WAY DAILY WORKOUT PROCESS

1. ANTICIPATION: Come up with a game plan. Visualize it. Play it forward.

2. PREPARATION: Pack the gym bag, get to the gym, lace up sneakers.

3. ACTION: Go! This is the actual moment you clear your watch and push "start."

4. PERSPIRATION: This is the workout itself. Create flow. Lose yourself. Sweat!

5. COMPLETION: The finish line. You did it. Sense of achievement and reward.

THE ANATOMY OF ATHLETIC BLISS

It's good to be just plain happy; it's a little better to know that you're happy; but to understand that you're happy and to know why and

how . . . and still be happy, in the being and the knowing, well that
is beyond happiness, that is bliss.

HENRY MILLER

The pursuit of happiness is the prime motivating force in most people's lives. Athletes like to exercise because it makes them happy. If you are someone who thinks of exercise as a suffer-fest, a disagreeable, unpleasant experience to be avoided, the key is going to be for you to flip your perspective to associate physical activity with happiness. This is easier than it sounds. You will learn how to do that systematically in the pages that follow. Athletes consider working out to be rewarding and pleasurable, because they intuitively incorporate the four tenets of athletic bliss into every workout.

THE FOUR TENETS OF ATHLETIC BLISS

- *Presence of positive emotions*

- *Physical pleasure*

- *Meaning/significance*

- *Sense of achievement*

If you can make even one of these a part of your exercise experience, you will be on your way to enjoying working out.

The goal of every workout from beginning, to middle, to end is for you to figure out how to associate exercise with pleasurable experience on an intellectual and a gut level. All animals seek pleasure and avoid pain. This is called "The Law of Effect" or "The Pleasure Principle." The problem with the "no pain, no gain" motto is that it goes against the Pleasure Principle and sets up an instinctive aversion response to exercise. I say "no brain, no gain." Shift your perspective to see the absolute pleasure of breaking a sweat. Recondition yourself to seek exercise by realizing it feels good.

As you will learn later, you have a thinking brain that is going to come up with the positive psychological perspective and a nonthinking brain that is going to be reprogrammed to like exercise. The key is to figure out psychologically and behaviorally how to perceive every stage of the athletic process as being an agreeable experience. Bottom-up messages get sent from your animal brain as gut responses. You send top-down messages consciously. The goal is to have them match up. In order to do that, you need to start working out so that you can begin to take inventory on your mind-set, attitude, and behavior surrounding your exercise. By incorporating the four tenets, you will have a perfect match between the intuitive response and the mental skills you need to make exercise enjoyable.

In short, the presence of positive emotion results from a decision to have an optimistic, hopeful, and curious outlook. The physical pleasure comes from finding the flow channel, losing yourself, and being totally engaged, knowing that anandamide, dopamine, and endorphins are released as analgesics. Meaning/significance is very individual, and most creative. It could be anything from hearing your favorite song on shuffle mode at an ideal moment and noticing a perfect middle-C note or seventeenth chord, seeing your muse entering the pool deck and then swimming side by side, stroke for stroke with you, feeling a part of a sports community, the way the light is hitting the side of a skyscraper, having some time alone, smelling a tropical plumeria tree on a familiar road, sniffing wood burning outside on the route home, sensing gratitude for being healthy enough to move. These are mine. Last, the sense of achievement comes from accomplishing a goal and being able to say, "I did it," the hit of dopamine, and the boost of self-esteem and confidence.

PRESENCE OF POSITIVE EMOTIONS

I am still determined to be cheerful and happy, in whatever situation I may be; for I have also learned from experience that the greater part of our happiness or misery depends upon our dispositions, and not upon our circumstances.

MARTHA WASHINGTON (AMERICAN FIRST LADY)

Athletic performance requires a state of optimism to create peak physical output. To keep going when part of you really wants to give up or quit, athletes learn to create a resilient, positive outlook. An optimistic disposition gives athletes the most potent mental and physical energy needed to move. This daily practice required to get from point A to point B in a workout also reshapes your synaptic connections to the athletic mind-set. The daily practice of learning how to look on the bright side originates in your up brain in your frontal lobes and is sent to your emotional down brain via up-down processing.

Research has found that serotonin and other neurotransmitters released during exercise build more of this area and allows for more upbeat cross-talk from the frontal lobes to the down brain. In most cases, you choose to send an optimistic perspective to your emotional and unconscious down brain, which might think things are not so rosy.

Strengthening the neural networks associated with an optimistic state makes the brain reshape itself to be more likely to create the presence of positive emotions, which will exhibit themselves even when you're not working out. The emotions have been linked to thicker neuron growth in the frontal lobes, which can create a brighter perspective on reality.

Why should we think upon things that are lovely? Because thinking determines life. It is a common habit to blame life upon the environment. Environment modifies life but does not govern life. The soul is stronger than its surroundings.

WILLIAM JAMES

The secret to staying positive is learning to guide and sift your thoughts. The key to doing this is to create two bins, positive and negative good and bad. Every thought that you allow to enter your consciousness is labeled and put in an agreeable or a disagreeable bin depending on how it makes you feel.

Everyone knows the feeling when a negative thought takes hold and gets into a loop in your brain. As we will explore in more detail, this loop of thought is actually synchronized firing and locking together of specific neurons in your brain. You need to avoid engaging that frequency or thought by not locking on to it. Let it slip from your memory. The easiest way to do this is either to redirect the inner dialogue in your head or to let it go.

Inside the athletic process you are going to be sifting thoughts based on this rapid-fire gut decision either to hold it or to make it dissolve away. Guiding thoughts is much like swinging from vine to vine in the jungle. When I do Ironman races, I swing from positive thought to positive thought. I scan the horizon for any potential thought or vision bombarding me and attach only to things that hum of positive emotions and lock in to that thought. When that stops humming, I look for something else to latch on to. This neuronal choir is a group of neurons chanting in unison above the din of the crowd and could be seen on brain imaging technologies as a specific tapestry of neurons.

If a negative thought enters my mind, I make it very slippery. I imagine covering the neurons in Teflon and chicken fat. Happy thoughts are covered in Velcro and magnets and Superglue. They stick to my brain.

*That's my gift. I let that negativity roll off me like water off a duck's
back. If it's not positive, I didn't hear it. If you can overcome that,
fights are easy.*

GEORGE FOREMAN

When you see a positive thought on the horizon or entering consciousness, allow it to stick and know that you are holding an electrochemical
neural network together. Remember that the longer you hold on to a negative thought you are reinforcing a habit and strengthening a neural network. Any bad thoughts that creep in, zap them with your mental laser
guns or just let the thought roll like water off a duck's back with a deep
exhalation.

Once you identify thought entering your mind, you may want to go one
step deeper and open it up, dissect it to see if what's inside makes you feel
good or bad. Remember that only by attaching onto thoughts associated
with a controlled, safe, happy feeling will you create a state of flow and
carve the neural pathways that will support an optimistic, happy athletic
mind-set. In most situations, worrying or being negative is not productive.

Spending time thinking about things that are upsetting or hard is part
of human life. Don't live in a *Valley of the Dolls* medicated haze or repress
feelings. Habitually practicing learned optimism reshapes the brain and
causes the athletic mind-set to seep out into everyday life, which is why athletes tend to be happier, more optimistic, and more resilient than the average person.

Another great trick for improving your outlook on the world is wearing
tinted glasses. It sounds sophomoric, but studies have shown that there is
some truth to "rose tint my world." I have worn sunglasses for almost every
moment I've spent outside since I was a teenager. My eyes are blue and really
sensitive to the light. I learned years ago that it was the orange lenses that put
me in the best mood. When I train on gray days, they actually make the world
look brighter. I recommend polarized lenses to reduce glare and orange lenses
to help create the presence of positive emotions year-round.

PHYSICAL PLEASURE

If you eat a live toad first thing in the morning, nothing worse can happen the rest of the day.

UNKNOWN

Researchers are actively investigating the connection between neurochemical levels and feelings of happiness and euphoria during exercise. The focus recently is on the role of anandamide in creating relief from pain and anxiety as well as an overall feeling of well-being during sport. Anandamide may in fact be more responsible for the runner's high than endorphins. The five key neurochemicals identified as creating athletic bliss and feelings of pleasure when you sweat are: anandamide, dopamine, serotonin, adrenaline, and endorphin. We will discuss these in detail when we go inside the athlete's brain in chapter 3. Your job to creating physical pleasure is working out at a level of exertion that feels good, your tonic level.

The dopamine pathway is activated by goal-oriented behavior. Neuroresearchers have made progress differentiating the positive feeling of approaching a goal, which maps onto the dopamine system, and the sensory pleasure of enjoying something, which maps onto the opioid system. There is enough scientific and empirical proof to know that if you set up your workouts to include a goal and the proper level of intensity, you will trigger the release of both these molecules into your nervous system.

The tonic level, the point of perfect skill/challenge balance within your flow channel, feels the same for everybody, but we all have slightly different rates of exertion that produce this just-right feeling. Your job is to find your flow channel in order to feel physical pleasure. The easiest way to do that is to establish the perimeters of your flow channel by finding a point of physical exertion between boredom and being overwhelmed.

When work is a pleasure, life is a joy!
When work is a duty, life is slavery.
MAXIM GORKY

Most people either work out too hard or too easily and miss their flow channel altogether. With cardio training, this level of exertion has a rate of breathing that would allow you to speak a brief four- to six-word sentence and to be totally engaged/focused but not overwhelmed. If you are bored or impatient working out, increase exertion; if you are overwhelmed, decrease exertion. This is the simple rule for staying in the flow channel. The first thing to do is look for a level of challenge that matches your level of skill in a way that makes you feel engaged but not overwhelmed. Beyond that, you will learn to interpret the feedback associated with a tonic feeling, based on inner dialogue, breathing rate, perceived exertion, heart rate, and actual level of exertion (speed, watts, level).

Keep it simple and take note of the specific circumstances when you settle down into the clickity-clack of fluidity so that you can re-create it on demand. With practice, staying in the flow channel becomes like tuning a radio, and staying there becomes a nonthinking gut instinct. You can chug along like a rhythmic steam engine and completely lose yourself in what you're doing.

But remember, the physiological and technical levels of your ability are not set in stone. As your skills improve, the challenge level must be raised in order to sustain flow. Don't get stuck in a rut. Keep track mentally of specific levels of exertion and circumstances that produce a flow channel for every activity in your life. Learn to use your instincts to gauge your emotions and inner dialogue to stay in the flow channel by matching your level of challenge to your level of skill. As your level of ability increases challenge, watch your fitness improve.

MEANING/SIGNIFICANCE

The sun is shining—the sun is shining. That is the magic. The flowers are growing—the roots are stirring. That is the magic. Being alive is the magic-being strong is the magic . . . it's in every one of us.

FRANCES HODGSON BURNETT

The terms *meaning* and *significance* tend to make people think that something has to be hugely profound in order to matter. Sometimes that is true, but it doesn't have to be. Most of the time it is the absolute smallest things in life, those most easy to take for granted, that are the most meaningful and significant. Things like hot water coming out of the taps or the special hue of amber light that beams down the hall of my apartment at sunset for a few days in late August, every year when sunset hits the horizon on Fourteenth Street dead-on and signifies summer is over. The same is true in sport.

Anything that reminds you of the reason you're exercising or gives you a sense of purpose in the moment can have significance. Interpreting this for yourself is personal and private, but some generic examples include: feeling connected to God, your favorite song coming on the iPod at the perfect time, lowering cholesterol, or keeping you from smoking.

Some days you will be motivated purely by vanity or things that may seem insipid. Even if they are, so what? They are just as valid. Don't make any judgments about what gets you to the gym every day. If you are doing it, and loving it, that's all that matters.

I usually have about twenty different reasons for getting to the gym on a given day—anything from my slowing metabolism and shrinking muscle mass to concerns for overall health, from mood-energy balance to vanity. Having a muse is often the number one motivator for me.

Some days, sharing a lane with the swimmer whose form I admire, or who is just easy on the eyes, gets me in the pool, allows me to activate my imagination and some mirror cells by swimming side by side. "This is why I dove into this freezing water today," you might say as you see the person in your peripheral vision on the pool deck. It doesn't matter what the meaning is if it makes you appreciate that it is significant, and tag it.

The meaning and significance will be changing constantly, but you always have to make sure that it's there. In your workbook, keep tabs on what motivates you. Remember to give it a name and tag it. Whenever you identify something, jot it down on a note card or in your workbook. Get in the habit of doing this for the first eight weeks as part of your athlete's way immersion. This will give you a list of reasons to keep coming back. Record the thoughts and insights that remind you when you're working out why you are doing this. If you fall off the wagon, you can come back to this list. Keep it simple and honest. Don't use any judgments or think that the meaning/significance you find in something is embarrassing or trivial. The objective is to put your antennae up so you can find the things that inspire and motivate you. Attach yourself to whatever works wholeheartedly without judging it.

SENSE OF ACHIEVEMENT

You have to wonder at times what you're doing out there. Over the years, I've given myself a thousand reasons to keep running, but it always comes back to where it started. It comes down to self-satisfaction and a sense of achievement.

STEVE PREFONTAINE

Achieving goals and feeling rewarded is the best way to create positive reinforcement. Every time you accomplish a workout, there is a feeling of tremendous satisfaction and pride in being able to say "I did it." You need to make that sense of achievement the key driving force to following through with every workout and always finishing what you start. In doing so, you will trigger the dopamine pathway of goal-oriented behavior and create a double whammy of athletic bliss. On the flip side, you don't want to quit or bail on a workout if you can help it. You need to achieve your goals to carve the neural pathways associating exercise with happiness.

The trick is to choose your level of challenge carefully. You want to be right on the cusp of difficulty, the comfort cusp, on the upper end of the comfort zone. You gently nudge it. That is the key to flow and feeling accomplishment. Push against your limits and remain in the flow channel but always be able to achieve your goals.

> So cheat your landlord if you must, but do not try to shortchange the Muse. It cannot be done. You can't fake quality any more than you can fake a good meal.
>
> WILLIAM BURROUGHS

If you need to run a hundred miles or more to feel that you've achieved something, you may be setting yourself up for unhappiness. For most of us, a long walk with a good friend, a brisk twenty minutes on the treadmill, or an hour of splashing around in the pool, interrupting the laps with diving practice or learning acrobatic tricks, can provide a feeling of accomplishment. Decide for yourself. Set achievable, challenging goals, and then succeed at them. Once you accomplish your goals, celebrate yourself.

CHAPTER THREE

THE BRAIN SCIENCE OF SPORT

You have brains in your head. You have feet in your shoes.
You can steer yourself in any direction you choose.

DR. SEUSS

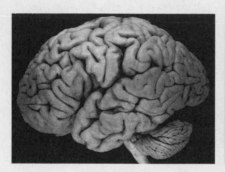 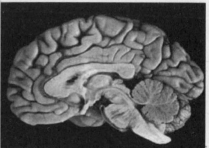

The average human brain weighs about three pounds.

The human cerebellum weighs about one-quarter of a pound.

The cerebellum is only 10 percent of the entire volume of the brain, but contains more than half of all of the neurons in the brain.

In 1504, Leonardo da Vinci produced wax castings of the human brain and coined the word cerebellum—Latin for "little brain."

The brain accounts for about 2 percent of the body's weight but uses 20 percent of the body's energy.

The human brain is about 85 percent water.

The electrical output of the brain is equal to that of a 20-watt lightbulb.

*T*he mind is what the brain does. The brain is the hardware; the mind is the software. Our mind is the pattern of neurons linking up inside the brain. This tapestry of neurons—not the brain itself—is what makes us what we are.

In this chapter we will explore brain science as it relates to the athletic process. I have divided the exploration of the brain into three basic categories: **architectural** (physical structure), **chemical** (molecules), and **electrical** function (neuron firing rates). In this chapter, I will outline the neuroscience behind athletic bliss. We will look at the architecture of the brain, focusing on the cerebrum and the cerebellum. Next, we will examine neurons, neuronal networks, and neurochemicals. All of this is important because exercise not only reshapes the brain through the physical experience itself, but also shapes the thoughts and mental signals used by athletes to achieve their daily fitness goals and strengthen the neural networks of the athletic mind-set of optimism and resilience in one's daily perspective. Neuroscience should become a prime motivating force to make changes in your life that you've been putting off. You can do it. You can change. Start today. Put on your sneakers and get your blood moving—exercise has the ability not only to transform your brain and your mind but also to transform your life.

Exercise literally makes your brain bigger. Just like weight lifting makes your muscles grow, flexing your brain and filling it with nutrients makes it bulk up. Two of the most important discoveries in neuroscience in the twenty-first century are that our brain can produce new brain cells and that existing neurons can become thicker, longer, and stronger. The growth of new neurons is called neurogenesis. Exercise causes new neurons to come into being, and older ones to become fortified.

Until recently, the commonly held belief was that we were born with all the neurons we would ever have and that part of the decline of aging was watching this finite number of brain cells dwindle. The fact that we can create new neurons and enlarge the ones we have is a huge discovery. Add neurogenesis to your list of reasons to exercise every day.

In addition to the basics of neuroscience this chapter will also deal with some cutting-edge discoveries about mirror neurons (observational learning), microtubules (intracellular delivery pipelines), Purkinje cells (key to muscle memory), and the cerebellum as the seat of the athletic brain and the subconscious mind.

PART ONE: BRAIN SCIENCE
BRAIN ARCHITECTURE

Baseball is ninety percent mental and the other half is physical.
YOGI BERRA

People often say that sports is all mental, but very few people delve into the brain science behind the athletic mind. This chapter will trace the roots of our athletic mind way back to the dawn of time and bring you into the twenty-first century using the latest brain imaging and scientific discoveries.

The reptilian brain, which includes our cerebellum today, first appeared in fish approximately 500 million years ago. It continued to develop in amphibians and reached its most advanced stage in reptiles roughly 250 million years ago. The cerebrum began its explosive expansion in primates, which led to the human mind, about two or three million years ago. Through this expansion our foreheads protruded and the genus *homo* emerged. Since all the structures of our brain serve a purpose and have proven their effectiveness over time, there was no reason for them to disappear. Instead, evolution favored a process of building additions, rather than rebuilding everything from scratch. Peak performance in sport comes from strengthening and using all parts of your brain.

As humans, we still have leftover reptilian functions at the base of our brain. You can envision your athletic brain as a reptilian brain and your thinking brain as a primate brain. After millions of years as a distinct species, *homo sapiens* still operates with a brain that is half reptilian, governed predominantly by instinct and not concepts of reason.

A mind stretched by a new idea never retracts to the same place.
UNKNOWN

The human brain can be viewed as an ancient city with a long history like Rome. Our brain has old sections down near the spine that would be like the aqueducts or the Colosseum. On top of that would be low-rise buildings and paved roadways. Then you would have modern architectural structures literally built on top of ancient foundations, communications lines with digital access and high-speed Internet, all leading to Prada and Apple computer shops sitting atop ancient mortar. This would be your prefrontal cortex. Just

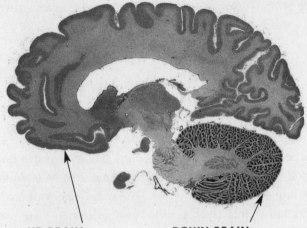

UP BRAIN	DOWN BRAIN
CEREBRUM	CEREBELLUM
Big brain	Little brain
Primate platform	Reptilian platform
Thinking (psychology)	Non-thinking (behavioral)
Cerebral	Cerebellar
Thinking and deciding	Doing and feeling
Rational	Emotional
Intellectual	Intuitive
Free will	Impulsive
Human	Animal
Declarative memory	Implicit muscle memory
MapQuest directions	Autopilot
Conscious memory	Unconscious memory
Strategic	Athletic
Voluntary movement	Proprioception
Lyrics	Music
Volition	Habit
Autobiographical self	Core self
Modern	Primitive
Superego	Id
Reality	Dream
Tip of the iceberg	Under the surface iceberg
Knowing	Knowing without knowing
Ethics/values	Cravings/urges
Sportsmanlike	Survival of the fittest
Top-down processing	Bottom-up processing

like any city with a history, these units coexist and interact with each other. Your brain operates the same way.

THE CEREBRUM—AKA GODZILLA
THE BIG BOSS

The cerebrum makes up 90 percent of brain volume. I refer to the cerebrum as Godzilla because it is so big and so strong. It is responsible for conscious thinking, declarative memory, language, volition, free will, planning, strategy, and voluntary muscle movement. The outer cortex of the cerebrum, only an eighth of an inch thick, is called gray matter. In the actual slice of a brain pictured on the previous page, the cortex is the darker ridge surrounding the cerebrum. All thinking occurs in the folded fissures of the cortex, which have the surface area of a pillowcase.

The cerebrum is divided down the middle by a fissure that creates a left and a right hemisphere. In the 1970s scientists believed that the left brain was a verbal-mathematical center and that the right brain was the visual-creative center. This view is not held by all neuroscientists anymore. *The Athlete's Way* presents a revolutionary new split-brain model, which is divided north-south, not east-west. This book brings you a new split-brain model called down brain, up brain, which I coined to update the left brain / right brain. Under this division the cerebellum is the down brain; the cerebrum is the up brain. The mid-brain is the connecting midway between these two brains.

THE CEREBELLUM—AKA MIGHTY MOUSE
THE LITTLE BRAIN WITH A BIG JOB

The cerebellum is the key to athletic performance; it is responsible for all co-ordinated movement, balance, body posture, muscle memory, implicit memory, and much, much more. Leonardo da Vinci gave the cerebellum, Latin for "little brain," its name, after he made wax castings of the brain in 1504. Da Vinci was one of the first people to realize that there was a mini brain tucked under the bigger cerebrum. Ancient and built on a reptilian platform, the cerebellum is a feeling and doing brain.

Although the cerebellum is only 10 percent of the entire volume of the brain, it contains more than half of all of the neurons in the brain. The cerebellum is a spitfire and ounce for ounce packs a walloping punch. Measured by neurons rather than by volume, it is actually the larger brain. Whatever the cerebellum is doing, it is doing a lot of it. Never underestimate the power of the down brain, the cerebellum.

Cerebellar means relating to or located in the cerebellum. This is the sister word to *cerebral*, which means relating to or located in the cerebrum. I believe *cerebellar* should be a household word just like *cerebral*, because it is equally important. Being equally cerebellar and cerebral is the key to fluid athletic performance. I am on a crusade to make people aware of their cerebral and cerebellar thinking. I am a champion of the underdog, and the cerebellum has been one for too long. I want this book to get you thinking about your cerebellum and your human animal—to help you create athletic genius so that you can play like a champion.

> *Of this I am absolutely positive, becoming a neurosurgeon was the direct consequence of my eye for the ball.*
>
> RICHARD BERGLAND
> (MONTANA STATE TENNIS CHAMPION AND NEUROSURGEON)

That is not to say that the cerebrum, or up brain, is unimportant. On the contrary, the development of the prefrontal cortex, the advanced intelligence area just behind your forehead, gives humans the capacity for willpower, critical thinking, problem solving, and planning that other species do not have. The up brain is the key to sports psychology—strategy, scheduling, consistency, inner dialogue, and mental toughness. It also plays an essential role in the creativity that characterizes human beings. Further, the up brain or prefrontal cortex is essential for the proper functioning of our declarative working memory and conscious mind. The up brain allows you as an athlete to attach meaning and significance to the process. It is what makes you able to remember the rules of the game and allows you to be creative and inspired as an athlete.

Researchers have found that a state of fluid performance during rhythmic sport is achieved when the cerebellum and the prefrontal cortex are engaged and firing together in unison while the rest of the brain becomes very quiet. This is what you would call being in the zone or flow. Neurologically, this state of fluid performance is signaled by streamlined and finely synchronized firing patterns within synapses. During sport, the cerebellum should take center stage as the cerebrum quiets down and falls into step with cerebellar rhythms.

For an athlete, creating fluid performance is about being deeply rooted in your animal brain, the cerebellum. If you think too much as an athlete, YOU get in the way, because the cerebellum is a habit brain that learns through repetition. The key to sports will always be practice, practice, prac-

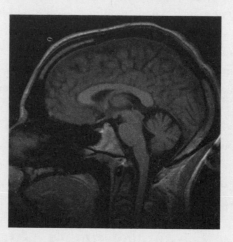

tice. You also need sleep for the memories to be stored. We will explore the importance of sleep more in chapter 11.

THE CEREBELLUM IS YOUR UNCONSCIOUS MIND THE ALL-KNOWING, NONTHINKING BRAIN

A little hidden door in the innermost and most secret recesses of the soul, opening into that cosmic night which was psyche long before there was any ego-consciousness, and which will remain psyche no matter how far our ego conscious may extend.

CARL JUNG

When I run, bike, swim, lift weights, or do yoga, I seat myself in my cerebellum. I see my brain as an iceberg, and I stay under the surface most of the time, hidden, tethered, and full of power. The tip of my consciousness is up in my frontal lobes like the tip of the iceberg. I peer out from there, too, but most of the time I am down below. In yoga, the word that describes the beginning of experience or the preparation for meditation is *prathyahara*, which means withdrawal of the mind from the senses. The analogy is to a turtle, which can pull its five appendages inside its shell and withdraw from the world. When the going gets really tough, the place I go is inside the reptilian brain. A withdrawal of the thinking mind from the senses involves going into a deep cerebellar state of trance.

Freud put the unconscious mind under the surface in an iceberg metaphor, but as far as I know, he never spoke of cerebellum. My original hypothesis is that our cerebellum is the seat of the unconscious mind and the cerebrum holds our conscious mind.

The iceberg metaphor works best for an athlete to visualize the cerebrum and cerebellum and realize that all the power is underneath in the cerebellum. This is my empirically discovered system of belief, and an educated guess as of now. Although my hypothesis that the cerebellum holds your personal and collective unconscious is original, whenever we refer to the unconscious mind we tend to say "deep, buried, primal, down, under, sub," but never put these memories into the cerebellum.

> I had a flashback to something that never existed.
>
> LOUISE BOURGEOIS

A female bird that is hatched and reared in isolation from other birds is still capable of building a perfect nest. Spiders can weave intricate spider webs, but this complex behavior is not learned, it is built-in neurological machinery. This is what Carl Jung referred to as the *collective unconscious*. These are ancient memories ("archetypes") passed on through our genes. Since the human brain is built like an archeological dig, when you break a sweat, you connect the deepest animal parts of your being. The highest form of humanness is stored in the prefrontal cortex, and it is the cerebellum that houses this primal knowledge.

REMEMBRANCE OF THINGS PAST
THE CEREBELLUM IS ALSO THE SMELL BRAIN

> Wide sea, that one continuous murmur breeds along the pebbled shore of memory.
>
> JOHN KEATS

Long-term olfactory memories linking smell to a time, place, or mood are housed in your animal, reptilian brain, the cerebellum. As an athlete, you can use the smell brain to trigger a state of peak performance. From an evolutionary standpoint, olfaction is our most primitive sense, and often the first warning sign of danger or safety, of friend or foe.

Smell is also often our first primal signal to take flight or fight or to tend-and-befriend. One reason you never want to let them see you sweat on a job interview is that humans can smell fear in the pheromones—even though we are not aware of it. This is leftover from our troglodyte days and is part of the cerebellum's sixth sense.

In *Remembrance of Things Past* Marcel Proust illustrates the neurobiological truth that smell is linked to early experiences that are deeply stored in our primal brain. Proust captures the power of forgotten childhood memories brought back to consciousness in their original intensity when the protagonist dips a madeleine into a cup of tea and has vivid flashbacks to his youth.

Recall the smells of your childhood. Don't the smells of Silly Putty and Play-Doh bring back huge waves of memory? I surround myself with scents that evoke positive psychology and ideal athletic mind-set. I have a collection of different scents that I've had since college: essential oils from Morocco and discontinued expensive perfumes in ninety-nine cent bins on Fourteenth Street. I have a cardboard box containing all these smells that are like time capsules. Each one can remind me of a specific race. I usually encode a scent for the months leading up to a big event, visualizing it day in and day out. When I arrive in New Zealand, Brazil, or Australia I whip out the smell and I feel like I'm at home. I bring these scents with me to races to help create a sense of familiarity and safety. I recommend that you pay attention to how smell is integrated into your athletic process and how olfaction affects your mind-set and mood. Make positive associations even to bad smells, like the locker room.

> *You never know when you are making a memory.*
> ABRAHAM LINCOLN

Coaches never seem to talk about using smell to create mind-set. People only comment on the smell of sweat in sport as if it is an unfortunate side effect. *The Athlete's Way* embraces smell as a powerful part of your athletic cognitive biology. For example, the smell of eucalyptus from the steam room reminds me of being relaxed, at a spa. I reward myself after a workout by sitting there. The smell of chlorine reminds me of the high school swim-team shirts that read "chlorine: the breakfast of champions" and makes me want to be Mark Spitz on a Wheaties box. The stink inside my bike helmet reminds me of my dad's squash rackets and my cousin Zander's hockey sticks. Olfaction is the human animal's most poignant sense. As an athlete don't underestimate its impact. Use it to trigger your athletic mind-set. Natascha Badmann, who has won six Hawaii Ironman races, agrees with me that the smell of plumeria in Kona is a prime motivating fuel and a deeply embedded memory.

SPLIT-LEVEL ARCHITECTURE
ENTER FROM UPSTAIRS OR DOWN

There comes a time in every rightly constructed boy's life when he has a regained desire to go somewhere and dig for hidden treasure.

MARK TWAIN

The split-brain model gives you a point of entry to start taking inventory. If what you are perceiving about the exercise process is coming from a gut level, it is coming from your down brain. You approach it objectively using behaviorism. If what you are struggling with involves issues of scheduling, motivation, planning, goal setting, or mental toughness, you know that it is an up brain activity, and you approach it with a psychology mind-set. As you familiarize yourself with identifying your motivations and inspirations, it will begin to become clear in most situations which approach you need to take.

Someone who is thinking too much on the field is being too up brain. You have to let it go or get out of the way, which means playing the game more from the down brain. If you let your brain psyche you out, it will cause you to choke or become overexcited. On the flip side, with practice you can change the script and dictate the cross talk sent down from your cerebrum. You can use its power to your advantage, but don't think too much.

There is a syndrome in sports called "paralysis by analysis."

ARTHUR ASHE

I watched Serena Williams lose in an early round at Wimbledon. As she shook her head in disbelief at her unforced errors, I realized she was thinking too much and her cerebellum was not doing what it needed to do. I noticed the more she tried to hold in her grunts, the more frustrated she became. The referees at Wimbledon had asked her to quiet down on the grunting, which may have stifled her cerebellum.

As the sets slipped through her fingers, she started grunting again, loudly, which made me hopeful that she might save the match. She had obviously said, screw it. The same thing happened in 2006 with Andy Roddick against Roger Federer at the U.S. Open. Grunting is part of the way the primitive cerebellum communicates, and it works well in sports. When you are performing from the cerebellum, you need only one or two trigger words, and you need phonemes, the smallest phonetic unit, also known as grunts. When people are hypnotized, they process bottom up from the primitive brain up to the cerebrum.

> *Good instincts usually tell you what to do long before your head has figured it out.*
>
> MICHAEL BURKE

The ideal state of performance, being in the zone, happens during sport when you are functioning primarily from the cerebellum with a direct link to the prefrontal cortex. The rest of the brain is quiet. This state of fluid performance can be seen on brain-imaging technology as being very efficient, without any wasted mental energy or clutter. Only the areas that need to be used light up. The brain is right and exact in its firing. Practice and repetition are what allows for this efficiency between neurons. When you feel a state of fluid performance, the synapses between your cerebellum and prefrontal cortex are firing at the same rate. They harmonize at a frequency above the din of the rest of the neuronal choir in your brain.

CHILDREN LIVE TO PLAY
RECESS!

> *If A equals success, then the formula is: $A = X + Y + Z$, X is work. Y is play. Z is keep your mouth shut.*
>
> ALBERT EINSTEIN

Try to remember that sport is play. As children we thought of running around and moving as play, and we loved to do it. As adults we call it exercise. The fun is often sucked out of it and the effort is perceived as drudgery. Bring the fun and playfulness back into the activity. Make it social. Join a club. Find a partner. Make it a game. How far can I go today? How fast? Take pride in the daily accomplishments and the power of transformation. Through sport you can get back in touch with your youthful, innocent, true self, get to know yourself better, and connect on that same level with other people.

This feeling is something that you share when you swim side by side, stroke for stroke with someone, when you run stride for stride or dance in synchronicity with another person, or rally a tennis ball. The cerebellum connects. Some neuro-philosophers think that the cerebellum may be the seat of the soul, which is why these connections feel so visceral.

In every real man a child is hidden that wants to play.
FRIEDRICH NIETZSCHE

CEREBELLUM AND SPORTS

THE FOUR PRIMARY ATHLETIC FUNCTIONS OF THE CEREBELLUM

1. *Maintains equilibrium and synchronizes head and eye movements*

2. *Coordinates and times appropriate muscular activity*

3. *Keeps track of your body's position in space (proprioception)*

4. *Knows without knowing; sees without seeing (intuition)*

The cerebellum is the physical genius in your brain. Peak athletic performance comes from letting the cerebellum do what it knows how to do instinctively. The concept of practice is to allow you to let go of your conscious mind and let your cerebellum take over.

Anytime you practice a skill or reinforce a behavior or mind-set, you are sending nutrients and blood flow to an area in your brain associated with that particular activity, behavior, or mind-set. With time, this current strengthens the neural networks involved in that activity. This engagement allows people to become masters of the things they practice—whether it's hitting a topspin forehand, running patterns on the football field, or distinguishing subtle differences between vintage bottles of wine. Our brain becomes better with practice, and these strengthened connections are not only pliable, but they are also tangible and can be seen on brain-imaging technology.

Cerebellum Keeps Rhythm and Time
It Snaps Your Fingers and Taps Your Toes

Where there is rhythm, there is grace.
Where there is grace, there is efficiency.

CHRISTOPHER BERGLAND

Your cerebellum is in charge of all timing and rhythm in your body. The cerebellum has long been known to play a critical role in the coordination of movement, especially skilled actions. New research shows that the cerebellum operates as an internal timing system, representing the precise temporal relationships between significant events that constitute an action, from reaching for a glass to hitting a baseball. The timing extends beyond motor control; the cerebellar timing system appears to be engaged in a variety of perceptual learning tasks that require a form of computation. For example, patients with cerebellar lesions are impaired in judging the duration of a sound.

The cerebellum is the rhythm keeper. From pouring a glass of milk to typing on the computer, precise timing, down to the thousandth of a second, is key to the brain's control of movement. By studying how monkeys track a visual target, Javier Medina and his colleagues at the University of Texas Medical School at Houston have gained new insights into the strategies the brain uses to measure time. Their findings indicate that the brain assesses the duration of a process using the equivalent of a neural stopwatch and computes the distance an object being tracked has moved. The cerebellum is responsible for this internal timekeeping and allows you to predict within a thousandth of a second the velocity of an incoming hockey puck or to return a 140-mph tennis serve.

The cerebellum is not only a timekeeper but is also a metronome that uses sight, sound, and proprioception to produce rhythm, tempo/cadence in aerobic sport, dance, and even coitus. I call the rhythm-making capacity of the cerebellum in sport the *loco-motor*. When you do any aerobic sport, try to feel the rhythm going through your joints and feeding back into the cerebellum. Sound it out like a tick-tick-tick in your head, and practice speeding it up or slowing it down. Saying the rosary over and over and over again has a similar effect as physical repetition—repeating a mantra pulls the mind into the cerebellum and quiets the cerebrum. In Sanskrit it is called *Japa*, which means the "repetition of the holy name." It blocks out other interests and allows you to concentrate on one thing.

The rhythm and tics and bobs associated with the repetitive motion of aerobic sports makes this function clear. I can spot a runner's idiosyncratic tics a mile a way. It's in the bob of the head, the flick of a wrist. Every runner has quirks that help him create a state of flow. When you run, your wrist becomes an adjustable metronome. Every limb and joint in your body is connected to this metronome, the rhythm keeper of the cerebellum. To go faster, speed up your wrist movements exactly with your leg turnover. The more experienced a runner is, the more fine-tuned the use of the inner metronome becomes. I can always tell veteran runners, not by how they move their legs, but by how definitively they snap and pop the wrist to keep cadence. Analyze the wrist movements of runners around you the next time you are jogging. Running, it turns out, is all in the arms.

> *America does not concern itself now with Impressionism. We own no involved philosophy. The psyche of the land is to be found in its movement. It is to be felt as a dramatic force of energy and vitality. We move; we do not stand still.*
>
> MARTHA GRAHAM

THE DAYTIME DREAM MAKER
REPETITIVE MOTION PUTS YOU IN A TRANCE

> *And if you gaze for long into an abyss, the abyss gazes also into you.*
>
> FRIEDRICH NIETZSCHE

Researchers have long wondered why repetitive motion tends to relax people and put them into what scientists call the trancelike default state. I read Herbert Benson's book *The Relaxation Response* in the early 1980s as I was beginning to run and have always been fascinated with his statement that repetitive muscle movement also slows brain waves. Now computer programmers, struggling to make robots that don't move with jerks, are realizing that the key to rhythm lies in the fluidity of the cerebellum.

USC neuroscientists studying discrete (one-time) and rhythmic movements recently discovered that the two types of movement are very different, including their points of origin in the brain. Their insights are aimed at producing more precise motion in robots and new methods of rehabilitation for the injured. The functional magnetic resonance imaging (fMRI) showed that the rhythmic motion of one hand tapping created activity only in the motor areas of the opposite brain hemisphere and the cerebellum. Remember, the left side of your cerebrum moves the right side of your body, but the right side of the cerebellum moves the right side of the body. The right cerebellum moves the right hand; the right cerebrum moves the left hand. One-time movements required much more extensive involvement on both sides of the brain and planning areas not directly connected with motor execution.

Stefan Schaal, associate professor of computer science in the USC Viterbi School of Engineering, led the international team that used fMRI scans to test a longstanding question regarding rhythmic versus one-time movement. "What our results indicate is that we really deal with two very separate systems in movement," Schaal said. "There is an automatic [rhythmic] system that, literally, functions without any thought; and a separate cognitive system that orchestrates more complex [one-time] movement." When people do the robot dance, these jerky movements illustrate the difficulty robotics experts have in trying to replicate the physical genius of the cerebellum. Diseases like Parkinson's and multiple sclerosis ultimately affect the cerebellum. Fluid, rhythmic athletic movements result from a well-developed cerebellum in action.

DASHBOARD GENIUS
UPSIDE DOWN AND ROUND-N-ROUND

Our physical body possesses a wisdom which we who inhabit it lack. We give it orders which make no sense.

                                                                HENRY MILLER

The unconscious perception of movement and spatial orientation is performed by the cerebellum. Proprioception is the ability to sense the position, location, orientation, and movement of the body and its parts, and the cerebellum is responsible for this. I view the cerebellum as a compass on the dashboard of a car that always knows north and stays level. It is like a gyroscope that keeps your balance. Drop a cat and it will land on its feet due to its cerebellum; trip on a tree root and your arms will fly out automatically to balance you.

Everything we do athletically is based on knowing the position of our body in space without having to think about it. The cerebellum does so by constantly monitoring hearing, sight, smell, taste, touch, heart rate, breathing, temperature, acceleration, equilibrium, gravity, and velocity. Your cerebellum knows your exact position in space even when you don't and works at quantum speeds to make appropriate adjustments.

Proprioception is instinctive, but it improves with practice. This is particularly evident in gliding and balancing sports like skating, skiing, and surfing. These athletes automatically shift their weight forward, lift the right arm to hold their balance, and fine-tune their position by moving the wrist a few centimeters. In this way the cerebellum is like the ballast in the bottom of a ship; it keeps your equilibrium. When you ride a bike, the cerebellum is telling you how to shift your weight to hold your balance. By conditioning the cerebellum, you learn to make fast and accurate adjustments without conscious thought. The ability of the cerebellum to control the coordination of muscles and tendons in milliseconds is the key to physical genius and athletic prowess.

Researchers have found that regions of the brain activated during sensory processing or self-reflective introspection are quite distinct and segregated. Specifically, the researchers have found that activity in the "self-related" prefrontal cortex is silenced during intense sensory processing, similar to what occurs in sports.

According to Ilan Goldburg of the Weizmann Institute of Science in Rehovoth, Israel, "During intense perceptual engagement, all neuronal resources are focused on sensory motor activity, and the distracting self-related cortex is inactive." Thus, the term *losing yourself* receives a clear neuronal correlate. This theme has a tantalizing echo in such Eastern philosophies as Zen teachings, which emphasize the need to enter into a mindless, selfless mental state to achieve a true sense of reality. When the cerebellum is engaged it appears that the ability to be introspective is lessened.

THE CEREBELLUM IS A KNOW-IT-ALL
OUR "NONTHINKING" OMNISCIENT BRAIN

A good hockey player plays where the puck is. A great hockey player plays where the puck is going to be.

WAYNE GRETZKY

The decision to make a movement starts in your cerebrum. Once we've decided to make a movement, the motor cortex in the brain sends out a command to the appropriate muscles to make them move. It doesn't stop there. Within one-sixtieth of a second, a message is sent back from the body's sensors into the cerebellum to report on how the movement went. Was it accurate? Too fast or too slow? Did it succeed? Based on this information, the brain responds by sending an updated command to improve the movement, which generates yet more feedback. This feedback loop system between the cerebellum and cerebrum is constant. We smooth out movements with practice and learn to fine-tune them. The precise and graceful movements of a black belt in karate, a ballerina, or a concert pianist come from the plasticity or muscle memory in the cerebellum.

Our reptilian brain automatically knows without knowing. For example, the primitive brain will be able to navigate your way home without knowing the names of any streets; the up brain would only be able to give MapQuest-like directions. When you give directions, you rely on the down brain to replay the sequence of moves from your memory and then translate them into declarative statements. The down brain is also the habit-learning brain and performs automatically, which frees up your cerebrum for executive function.

Some movements for humans are part of a primitive reflex passed on to us from the primal collective unconscious held in the cerebellum. Other movements do not come naturally. For example, riding a bike, driving a car, hitting a tennis ball, and playing the piano must be learned and practiced. Only with repetition can these skills become second nature. A system of conditioning based on repetition is key to the mastery of down brain skills

Have you ever gotten off the subway at an unfamiliar stop, and as you come up to street level find yourself unsure what corner of the intersection you're on? For a second, you are completely disoriented. You recognize landmarks, but you can't put them in proper context; you can't tell which way is north or south. The down brain is struggling to establish your position in space while your up brain is lost. You read the street signs but they are meaningless, because you don't know your orientation. When you suddenly figure out where you are, there is an "aha, now I get it. How could I have been so disoriented?" moment. Your down brain reestablishes orientation, and you begin to move. This is an example of bottom-up processing, and how we go through much of life. The memory box in the cerebellum is running the show.

Trust thyself: every heart vibrates to that iron string.
RALPH WALDO EMERSON

Cerebellum and Specific Sport Types

REPETITIVE MOTION (RUNNING, BIKING, SWIMMING): The cerebellum is your inner metronome and serves as the rhythm keeper, using its timing mechanisms to keep cadence. Remember: the elbows are the pistons on the train and the wrists are the locomotive. Your down brain supplies power to keep balance and coordinate movement. As with all sports, the muscle memory of each activity is held in the Purkinje cells of the cerebellum.

GLIDING SPORTS (SKATING, SKATEBOARDING, SKIING): The cerebellum works with equilibrium and balance to shift your center of gravity automatically. In gliding sports the cerebellum is the inner gyroscope and the ballast that keeps you balanced. The arms and hands will fine-tune the position by using the eight carpal bones in the wrist as a kind of GPS (Global Positioning System) for the cerebellum that keeps the horizon straight.

HAND-EYE COORDINATION (TENNIS, GOLF, BASEBALL, LACROSSE): The cerebellum focuses on timing by comparing the speed of an incoming object to the position of your body, limbs, racket, stick, or club. The blindsight capacity of the cerebellum is leftover from reptilian days. It lets you see without seeing, as a lizard catches a fly. This is how you hit a speeding ball in the sweet spot. The vestibulo-ocular reflex (VOR) is the automatic reflex of the cerebellum that produces an eye movement in the direction opposite to head movement. The VOR in the cerebellum is what allows you to focus and track an object. Without it we couldn't play hand-eye coordination sports .

ACROBATIC SPORTS (GYMNASTICS, TRAPEZE, PARKOUR): The cerebellum keeps track of where your body is in space so you can land on your feet. The sequential movements of a routine are also stored in the procedural memory of the cerebellum. As with all sports, the proprioception of where your limbs are in relation to the environment is crucial. Muscle memory is stored in the cerebellum.

THE NERVOUS SYSTEM
Invasion of the Body Snatchers
What a Tangled Web We Weave

It is as if the Milky Way entered upon some cosmic dance. Swiftly the brain becomes an enchanted loom, where millions of flashing shuttles weave a dissolving pattern, always a meaningful pattern though never an abiding one; a shifting harmony of subpatterns.

SIR CHARLES SCOTT SHERRINGTON (COINED THE WORD *SYNAPSE*)

More than 100 billion neurons are stretched throughout your entire body. When this chrysalis-like web of neurons twists with the three million feet of myelin-covered axons throughout your entire body, you can imagine the nervous system. As these cells connect, they are linked into neural networks or nets. Each neuron can be connected to thousands of other neurons, each simultaneously sending and receiving impulses to and from thousands of other neurons. One neuron can alter millions of other neurons in its network. Each axon, or nerve fiber, is one long hose. Some, like the sciatic nerve, stretch up to four feet long. An axon sometimes branches at the end into as many as a thousand separate nozzles into the synaptic gaps. Neurons never touch. Instead, neurotransmitters link them in networks.

(The neuron is) the aristocrat among the structures of the body, with its giant arms stretched out like the tentacles of an octopus to the provinces of the frontier of the outside world, to watch for the constant ambushes of physical and chemical forces.

SANTIAGO RAMON Y CAJAL (CREDITED WITH FIRST DISCOVERING THE NEURON)

THE NERVOUS SYSTEM: The nervous system is a network of neurons that tells the structures of the body what to do and when. It could be called a neuron system. Nerves are bundles of neurons encased in a myelin sheath. Myelin, the fatty, insulating material, wraps around some nerve fibers, making the brain more efficient and allowing messages to travel faster. Without myelin, the human brain would have to be ten times bigger and we would have to eat ten times more to maintain it.

Your central nervous system consists of the spinal cord and brain, plus a peripheral nervous system that branches out from the spine and down to your fingers and toes. The nervous system constantly monitors the internal and external environment and makes appropriate changes to create a stable internal environment called *homeostasis* (Greek for staying power).

NEURON STRUCTURE: There are generally three parts to all neurons: the cell body, the dendrites, and the axon. The cell body, containing the nucleus, carries out metabolic processes and houses neurotransmitters. Branched dendrites surround the cell and receive impulses from other neurons, bringing them into the cell body. Each cell generally has one axon that sends messages out of a cell. The axon of a motor neuron can be ten thousand times as long as the cell body is wide.

NEURONS: The nervous system is made up of neurons that communicate electrochemical signals throughout your body. There are three types of neurons. Sensory neurons receive messages from the body and carry that information to the brain. Interneurons, located in the brain and spinal cord, act as a bridge connecting sensory and motor neurons. The motor neurons carry instructions to your body to move.

SYNAPSES: Neural networks hook up by linking axons and dendrites in a chain using an electrochemical process across a tiny space called a synapse or synaptic gap. Dendrites and axons never touch. An electrical charge is sent down an axon in the form of positively charged ions. This releases a neurotransmitter into the synaptic gap that links together neural networks. All neurons saying yes to the charge link up and begin to pulse at the same firing rate. This chanting in unison creates a very specific neural ensemble that harmonizes like a choir and rises above the din of other neurons fighting for your attention. The neural assemblies at any time represent your state of consciousness at any given moment.

Anxiety Kills Brain Cells
Stress Is a Neuron Assassin

The key to winning is poise under stress.
PAUL BROWN

According to Ronald Duman, Ph.D. at Yale University, chronic stress, anxiety, and depression have been linked to atrophy or loss of neurons, and exercise has been linked to the growth of new neurons. The primary hormone triggering the degeneration of neurons seems to be cortisol, which appears to shrink the hippocampus, our memory hub. Under the rules of fight or flight, you need to burn off cortisol any time you have an alarm response. If you are wound up or stressed out, exercise is the best way to get rid of the cortisol.

Exercise has been proven to promote neurogenesis by increasing BDNF (Brain Derived Neurotrophic Factor) and lowering cortisol. BDNF is responsible for making your neurons stronger. Duman has observed the same level of neurogenesis in people who exercise as triggered by antidepressants. He hypothesizes that it may be the new cell growth that is actually lifting people's spirits, which would explain why it usually takes about two to four weeks for antidepressants to work.

Exercise Makes You Smarter
Running Boosts Brain Cells

You're smart too late and old too soon.
MIKE TYSON

By increasing BDNF, exercise boosts your memory, making you smarter and happier. BDNF is regulated by levels of serotonin and is known to be a prime candidate for causing serotonin delivering axon growth. Antidepressants work like exercise in that they increase BDNF, which may ultimately be why they are effective at elevating mood.

Justin Rhodes, Ph.D., a neuroscientist at Oregon Health and Science University in Portland, reports that "BDNF helps support and strengthen synapses in the brain. We find exercise greatly activates the hippocampus and grows more neurons there. In fact, the BDNF concentration in active mice increased as much as 171 percent after seven nights of wheel running. The more running, the more BDNF." But it can max out and backfire. Rhodes found that the ultra mice who run day and night perform terribly when attempting to navigate a maze. This is one of the things that convinced me to cut back on my running. If left to their own devices, the best-performing mice tend to run two to three miles a night, which I think is a great distance for humans, too.

When in doubt, punt!
JOHN HEISMAN

Scientists at the Salk Institute have shown that cardiovascular exercise can boost brain cell survival in animals. According to Carrolee Barlow, "Running appears to rescue many of these cells that would otherwise die. It suggests that staying active may help delay progression of neurodegenerative conditions."

The current study headed by Barlow builds on work directed by Salk professor Fred Gage. Barlow found that running leads to increased brain cell numbers in normal adult mice, elderly mice, and a genetically slow-learning strain of mice. Gage's studies showing that new cell growth occurs also in human brains suggests the boosting effects of running may occur in people as well. Miles logged correlate directly with the numbers of increased cells. In the study, the Salk team monitored the number of revolutions each mouse lapped on a running wheel placed in its cage.

"It's almost as if they were wearing pedometers," said Barlow. "And those that ran more grew more cells." She added that the current study demonstrated running's brain-boosting effects in the hippocampus, a region of the brain linked to learning and memory, known to be affected by Alzheimer's disease.

Research at MIT's Picower Institute for Learning and Memory showed that structural remodeling of neurons occurs in adult brains. Elly Nedivi, a professor of neurobiology at MIT, says, "Knowing that neurons are able to grow in the adult brain gives us a chance to enhance the process and explore under what conditions—genetic, sensory or other—we can make that happen. What's more, this growth is tied to use, so even as adults, the more we use our minds, the more robust they can become." In addition to exercise, you should flex your neurons every day by doing puzzles, brain teasers, problem solving, and just thinking.

Exercise stimulates the growth of new neurons in the hippocampus (memory hub) and prefrontal cortex (pleasure/free will). Exercise has also been proven to make the Purkinje cells of the cerebellum bigger and more efficient. Autopsies of patients confined to bed rest in the later stages of life show significant atrophy of Purkinje neurons and shrunken cerebellums. Cats forced to live in confinement lose 25 percent of Purkinje volume within six weeks of inactivity. New methods of moving bedridden patients on vibrating beds are utilized to keep the cerebellum strong by stimulating it. By sending blood flow and nutrients to specific parts of your brain, you fortify the neurons there.

Mirror Neurons
Monkey See, Monkey Do

*Any monkey can reach for a peanut. But only a human can reach for
the stars or even understand what that means.*

DR. RAMACHANDRAN (NEUROSCIENTIST)

Mirror neurons are specialized brain cells that allow you to learn by observing the actions of another person or imagining that you are doing those
actions. As I was running at the gym, old football footage was running on
ESPN, and I felt my body running in sync with the players on the screen. I
was also running stride for stride with the runner next to me. On another
screen a horse race appeared, and strangely enough, I felt myself begin to
run and bob my head with the horses. This happens in Central Park, too,
when I find myself jogging next to a horse-drawn carriage. This phenomenon is mirror neurons in action. During my run, my mirror cells locked in to
all three actions and my own reflection in the glass in front of me.

Mirror neurons are receptors placed in the frontal lobes of the brain.
They were discovered in monkeys in the late 1990s. Mirror cells allow you to
trigger the appropriate neurons associated with that movement to fire, the
fire-and-wire principle. Once these neurons fire, they become twisted together like vines of a hedge, and you can later reactivate the same pathway
that has been linked up when you actually perform the task.

The lead scientist on the discovery of mirror neurons was Professor
Giacomo Rizzolatti and colleagues at the university in Parma, Italy. During
their study of motor neurons, they placed electrodes in particular brain cells
of a monkey. Then they tried to measure the reactions of neurons to certain
movements by giving the monkey food. As with many other great discoveries, this one was made by accident. During the experiment, one of the researchers was standing next to a bowl of fruit. As the monkey observed the
researcher reach for a banana, the same neurons reacted in the monkey. Rizzolatti explains. "How could this happen, when the monkey did not move?
At first we thought it to be a flaw in our measuring, or maybe equipment
failure, but everything checked out okay and the reactions were repeated as
we repeated the movement."

These receptors are active when the monkeys perform certain tasks, but
they also fire when the monkeys watch someone else perform the same specific task. Mirror neurons are believed to be the basis of all imitations that
enable a child to learn to walk, talk, and behave like their parents or any

other adult. Scientists have found evidence of a similar system of matching observations with actions in the human brain. The mirror system is the first link between observing others performing a task and thereafter imitating or duplicating that very movement. Scientists studying human behavior and language learning all over the world agree that mirror neurons play a major role in the understanding of how we learn and empathize.

The mirror system is thought to play a key role in helping us to understand other people's actions and may also help in learning how to imitate them. To test mirror cells in the laboratory, a group of neuroscientists had one person observe another doing a tea ceremony and watched the pattern of neurons that fired as the person observed the systematic routine. Later, when the person actually performed the ceremony himself, the same set of neurons fired.

Neural action in the brain during observation matches that of the action itself. This is why athletes can improve their game by visualizing it. Visualization works in sports, because it triggers mirror neurons to mimic the neural pathway of an actual behavior without having to do it. When you are visualizing, you plan your actions before you do them. As a collective, mirror neurons are referred to as the mirror system. From an evolutionary standpoint, mirror neurons protect a species from repeating fatal errors observed in another, without having to die in the process. This ability to learn from other people's mistakes and triumphs without necessarily having to experience them firsthand is a function of the mirror neuron system.

There is a theory that part of the cause of autism might lie in a malfunctioning mirror system. The symptoms of autism include difficulties with social interaction, including verbal and nonverbal communication, imitation, and empathy. Autopsies of autistic children reveal shrunken cerebellums, enlarged cerebrums, and atrophied Purkinje cells. Neuroscientists believe the observation-execution matching system provided by mirror cells is a neural mechanism that allows others' actions, intentions, and emotions to be understood automatically.

Men acquire a particular quality by constantly acting a particular way . . . you become just by performing just actions, temperate by performing temperate actions, brave by performing brave actions.

ARISTOTLE

As an athlete, I have always watched my mentors closely and dissected their actions. I try to run with my chest and chin up like Steve Prefontaine;

hit a tennis serve with hip rotation and snap like Andy Roddick; hit a two-handed backhand like Chris Evert; swim with big arms and my legs kicking like the platypus Ian Thorpe; cup my hands, move my arms, and shuffle my feet like Heather Fuhr in an Ironman; get my shoulders at a right angle above my elbows on the aero bars, slide forward in the saddle, tilt my head, and shift my eyes like Paula Newby-Fraser; pedal up hills out of the saddle, light as a feather like Lance Armstrong. I begin to move like them. I begin to think like them. I have role models and mentors on whom I shape my mirror system in every sport. You should, too. Although I do none of these things as well as my role models, I feel them in my bones and every cell of my bone when I activate the mirror neurons.

As you observe your role models, put yourself into their bodies, go behind their eyes, and then transfer that feeling and perception into your own nervous system. Put it into your spine. I call mirroring the movements of role models a spinal transplant. My advice is to look for the small thing in a mentor's movements: the way they shift their eyes, move their wrists, tilt their head, hold their hands, distribute their body weight. Absorb their overall aura, how they sit on the sidelines, how they take off their helmet. Consciously hone in on one small thing while you soak up the big picture simultaneously. The mirror cells will take over and fill in the rest of the pieces in the puzzle. Think of it as a character study an actor would do. Sometimes you use external props, body language, a certain stance. Other times it is the mind-set, attitude, and aura that you emulate.

You have to defeat a great player's aura more than his game.

PAT RILEY

What We Do Ourselves,
We Understand in Others

Emulating mentors is about being able to identify and interpret the mind-set of your role models. Imagining what a role model is thinking or what his intentions are can be traced back to a simulation of the mirror neurons of the brain as soon as we observe a person in action. The actions of the observed person are imitated by these cells. We put ourselves in that person's shoes. We can best understand the actions of another on the basis of our own action inventory. This is why athletes of particular sports are simpatico. Our minds and bodies give us the foundation to understand what other athletes are doing, thinking, or feeling.

I was running in the rain one day and had a sympathetic exchange with another solo runner who was out there soaking wet, too. We both knew just what the other was going through. "The same area of the brain responsible for understanding behavior (the mirror neurons) can predict behavior as well," says Ahmanson Lovelace of UCLA. "Our findings show for the first time that intentions behind actions of others can be recognized by the motor system using mirror cells. They are an incredible tool. You become what you pretend to be."

Research findings suggest that once the brain has learned a skill, it may simulate the skill without even moving, through simple observation. An injured dancer might be able to maintain her skill despite being temporarily unable to move, simply by watching others dance. This concept could be used during sports training and in maintaining and restoring movement ability in people who are injured.

PART TWO: NEUROCHEMICALS

The Exercise Antidote
Time for Your Medication!

I see great things in baseball. It's our game—the American game. It will take our people out-of-doors, fill them with oxygen, give them a larger physical stoicism. Tend to relieve us from being a nervous, dyspeptic set. Repair these losses, and be a blessing to us.

WALT WHITMAN

The neurochemicals released during exercise are so strong that you could consider yourself a psychopharmacologist, self-medicating through exercise. There is a strong correlation between the quantity of certain neurotransmitters in your brain and your mood. Doctors like to alter brain chemicals by using drugs, which offer valuable treatment for many clinically depressed people. Recent studies have shown that the efficacy of these drugs is improved by incorporating exercise into a mental health regimen. Exercise has been shown across the board to improve the chemical environment of your brain in the long and short term. For people who are not clinically depressed, recent studies have shown exercise to be one of the most reliable long-term mood boosters on the planet.

It is widely accepted in the scientific and mental health community that there is a runner's high or general mood elevation immediately after exercise. The lasting ability of these mood-elevating effects is important to depression treatment as well as an overall healthy, happy lifestyle. The lasting effects are probably due to changes in microtubule delivery, neuron density, and neurogenesis—not just the influx of chemicals or reuptake inhibition.

Donna Kritz-Silverstein from the University of California at San Diego found that exercise must be done on a regular basis to maintain the positive benefits. She found that those who exercised had a lower Beck Depression Inventory (BDI), meaning they were generally in a better mood. Those who had stopped exercising eventually had BDIs similar to those who had never exercised, while those who continued to exercise were able to maintain a low BDI. The point is you need to keep exercising to sustain the benefits. Exercise needs to be part of your daily practice, like brushing your teeth.

The research on the chemical processes on the long-term effects of consistent exercise on mental health, learning, and memory is still being done. The study of these antidepressant chemicals helps to reveal the chemical properties of depression and mood. The psychopharmacologic power of exercise should not be underestimated, but it is not a panacea for all mental illness.

Estimated amount of glucose used by an adult human brain each day, expressed in M&Ms: 250. The brain is 2 percent of your body weight but uses 20 percent of its oxygen.

HARPER'S INDEX, 1989

Endogenous and Exogenous
Self-Produced vs. Externally Ingested

The magic moment is when "yes" or "no" may change the whole of your existence.

PAOLO COELHO

I give Nancy Reagan a run for her money in my "Just Say No" crusade. I am adamantly opposed to drugs. Any drug that works in your body does so because you already have the receptors to produce it yourself. Any exogenous (outside) drug that we ingest works because it docks with receptors for the endogenous (inside) version. Both endorphin and endocannabinoids get their name from endo (self-made), morphine, and cannabis respectively.

The problem with taking drugs is that if a receptor is bombarded enough times it gets smaller, and your body's ability to produce it decreases. This is a double whammy. Drugs create a vicious cycle. The more you take a concentrated exogenous drug, the higher your tolerance becomes and you need more of the drug to get high, which shrinks the receptors and produces less of the internal happy juice. The way to reverse this trend is to rely on the self-produced molecules your body makes to feel great. Exercise expands the receptors and increases your body's ability to produce even more receptors.

Remember, if you hijack any endogenous system with outside drugs, the natural function is crippled and eventually paralyzed. Life in the human body was designed to be an ecstatic process. Don't mess with with prescription or illicit drugs unless you have to for clinical reasons.

Runner's High
Beyond Endorphins

Most people never run far enough on their first wind to find out they've got a second.

WILLIAM JAMES

One of the groundbreaking revelations this book brings to the mainstream is that endorphin is not the primary cause of runner's high. As with every process in our body, the reaction results from myriad chemicals, but the spotlight of neuroscience is pointing toward the endocannabinoid system, and in particular anandamide, the bliss molecule. I recommend using the knowledge of anandamide flooding your brain when you exercise as a prime motivating force to lace up your sneakers and break a sweat. It is my number one motivator. Remember, your brain is a sponge for endocannabinoids, containing ten times more receptors than for endorphin. The harder you work out, the more cannabinoids you produce.

The runner's high has been described subjectively as pure happiness or elation, a feeling of unity with one's self and/or nature, peacefulness, inner harmony, boundless energy, and a reduction in pain sensation. These subjective descriptions are similar to the claims of distorted perception, atypical thought patterns, diminished awareness of one's surroundings, and intensified introspective emotional status made by people who describe drug or trance states. I call this state *athletic bliss*.

Rule Number 1 is, don't sweat the small stuff. Rule Number 2 is, it's all small stuff. And if you can't fight and you can't flee, flow.

ROBERT S. ELIOT

There are hundreds of neurochemicals in your brain; researchers have been able to give names to only about thirty. I have isolated a top five list of neurochemical molecules that affect your mood positively during exercise to produce bliss, and a top three that will help with anxiety. Depending on your personality type, certain neurotransmitters are going to be more important to your individual exercise prescriptive.

Take inventory daily and be your own brain chemist by deciding which ones you want to focus on releasing on any given day. An exercise-induced altered state of consciousness has long been appreciated by endurance athletes. The runner's high is a private experience, and the evidence for its existence rests mostly on anecdotal reports. Scientific research into the phenomenon has been restricted by its ephemeral nature.

The key is small. And small is key. Be a detective. Look for the pinhole—the swivel joint—and slip through.

CHRISTOPHER BERGLAND

THE TOP 5 NEUROCHEMICALS RELEASED DURING EXERCISE

1. *ENDOCANNABINOID:* The bliss molecule. *Euphoric, content, mellow.*

2. *DOPAMINE:* The reward molecule. "Score!" The "jackpot" feeling. Fluid moves.

3. *EPINEPHRINE (ADRENALINE):* The energy molecule. Eager, excited, psyched up.

4. *SEROTONIN:* The confidence molecule. Optimistic, confident, purposeful, secure.

5. *ENDORPHIN:* The painkiller molecule. Your body's natural morphine.

Endocannabinoids
Anandamide: "The Bliss Molecule"

Happiness is the meaning and the purpose of life, the whole aim and end of human existence.

ARISTOTLE

Endocannabinoids are the most potent neurochemical for creating the biology of bliss when you exercise. Endocannabinoids are not a household word yet, but I guarantee that by the end of the decade they will be as commonly known as serotonin, dopamine, and cortisol.

Cannabinoids are directly linked to feelings of pleasure and have analgesic and anti-inflammatory properties. Cannabinoids are released when you break a sweat; they linger in your system during and after the process. They are linked to neurogenesis, improved mood, bone density, and fine motor-control improvement in endogenous doses. The receptors in the brain for cannabinoids are called CB-1 and are everywhere, but are especially dense in the frontal lobes and cerebellum.

The feelings of contentment and well-being you experience after a workout occur because your brain is soaking in a cannabinoid cocoon. For reasons not completely understood, endocannabinoids have also been linked to bone growth and density by targeting the other cannabinoid receptor CB-2 in the immune system. Raphael Mechoulam of the Hebrew University School of Pharmacy, who was the first to isolate anandamide in 1992, discovered in 2006 that endocannabinoids also help to preserve bone density. Based on this finding, a prototype for a new drug to prevent osteoporosis (loss of bone density) without any psychoactive side effects has been developed and is in clinical trials. This is a breakthrough for people suffering from osteoporosis and offers a new area of drug therapy—and an additional reason to be motivated to exercise and release endocannabinoids through sweating.

DOPAMINE: THE "REWARD" MOLECULE

All moral learning is ultimately based on the pain and pleasure circuitry in your brain and your internal reward punishment system.

ROBERT HEATH (NEUROSCIENTIST)

Dopamine is a neurotransmitter that facilitates achievement, goal-oriented behavior, motivation, mood, and movement. It is the cause for the feeling that floods your body when you accomplish a goal. Dopamine is released during exercise naturally; it is also the culprit for creating drug addiction. Cocaine and other drugs hijack and fry dopamine receptors along the pleasure pathways from the mid-brain to the prefrontal cortex. By creating clear-cut goals as you move through the day, you can release a continuous stream of dopamine. Avoid reward deficiency syndrome by consciously identifying goals and achieving them.

There is a growing consensus that the dopamine network influences everyday behaviors. Pursuing certain behaviors, single-mindedly focusing on a project, for instance, increases the dopamine release. Richard Depue, Ph.D., professor of human development at Cornell University, points out that goal-directed behavior, or the lack of it, tends to present itself as a personality trait. There is a consensus that goal-oriented behavior is a key athletic trait. Depue believes that dopamine traveling along the reward pathways is what motivates people.

"When our dopamine system is active, we are more positive, excited, and eager to go after goals and rewards, whether it's food, sex, money, education, or professional achievement," he says. Depue also suggests that people who are goal-oriented not only tend to be more motivated but are also generally happier. "We have strong evidence that feelings of elation [that occur] because you are moving toward achieving an important goal are biochemically based, though they can be modified by experience."

Dopamine is what drives most athletes to set goals and achieve them. If I am working hard to qualify for the Hawaii Ironman—and pouring every ounce of energy into that and achieving mini goals day in and day out—it is incredibly rewarding; the actual race becomes the icing on the cake.

Eighty percent of dopamine is produced in a small region of the brain called the subsantia nigra (black stuff). Its axons thread like fire hoses through the brain, pumping dopamine to pleasure centers, where they cause a neural chain reaction that gives you a hit of ecstasy or reward. Dopamine also facilitates motor learning. Since autopsies of people with Parkinson's disease showed that the black stuff of the substantia nigra appeared lighter in color, researchers made the connection between dopamine and fluid movement.

Dopamine is key to fluid movement and reward. It is important to the athletic process and is in a close race with anandamide for top prize. Bottom line: set goals and achieve them. Finish what you start, and you'll release dopamine.

Too much dopamine makes a person schizophrenic; too little results in the shaky physical movements of Parkinson's. I have had delusions and hallucinations that are produced by an overload of dopamine after about twenty-four hours of nonstop exercise. I have experienced the illusion of snakes jumping out of rocks and blankets of shooting stars atop Father Crowley Point, which is the second five-thousand-foot climb that finally gets you out of Death Valley. During Badwater, these hallucinations are a form of exercise-induced schizophrenia triggered by too much dopamine. Regular, daily, goal-oriented movement will produce the perfect amount of dopamine.

EPINEPHRINE (ADRENALINE): THE ENERGY MOLECULE

God, do I love to hit that little round sum-bitch out of the park and make 'em say "Wow!"

REGGIE JACKSON

Adrenaline allows people to perform superhuman feats, improves mood, and gives you energy. Adrenaline is called epinephrine in the United States, because the word *adrenal* was a trademarked name by Parke, Davis and Co. Adrenaline and epinephrine are the same thing. Adrenaline is made in the adrenal glands just above the kidneys. In moments of sudden fear, excitement, or a near miss, the rush you get is from adrenaline. As an athlete, creating a sense of adventure and excitement will cause a surge of adrenaline.

Low adrenaline is directly linked to depression. Higher adrenaline levels are linked to happiness, but too much could make you anxious or jittery. There are two kinds of stress. Good stress (excitement) is called eustress and bad stress (anxiety) is called distress. Both release adrenaline. As an athlete, you want to channel good-stress adrenaline into motivation and inspiration. Adrenaline makes you eager and excited. This molecule is passion; use it to fuel your workouts and stay psyched up before and during athletic activity. Create eagerness and anticipation to release epinephrine.

SEROTONIN: THE CONFIDENCE MOLECULE

You gain strength, courage, and confidence by every experience in which you really stop to look fear in the face. You are able to say to yourself, "I have lived through this horror. I can take the next thing that comes along." You must do the thing you think you cannot do.

ELEANOR ROOSEVELT

Serotonin is the most talked about but one of the least understood neurotransmitters. It has many roles and is hugely important. For the purpose of practicality, I will focus on the role of serotonin in terms of confidence and a feeling of well being. The tonic amount of serotonin released during exercise is good for your mental health and literally builds a stronger, happier brain.

Low serotonin is directly linked to learned helplessness and rejection sensitivity. High serotonin is linked to learned optimism and chutzpah. Exercise will increase your serotonin levels, thicken the microtubules that deliver serotonin to the synapse, and make the neurons denser. Remember the feedback loop of higher serotonin and more confidence. You need to break the cycle of learned helplessness and rejection sensitivity. The more you work out, the more momentum you will have to create this upward spiral.

ENDORPHIN: THE PAINKILLER MOLECULE

The man who can drive himself further once the effort gets painful is the man who will win.

ROGER BANNISTER

Endorphin stands for endogenous (endo = self-made) morphine. Gram for gram, endorphin is three times more powerful than morphine. The more intensely you work out, the more this natural painkiller is released into your bloodstream. Endorphin makes you feel good physically, but it doesn't cross the blood/brain barrier. By pushing against your limits and breaking a sweat, you are triggering your body to release endorphin. The harder you work, the more endorphin you release. Endorphins have a huge impact on making your body feel great when you exercise.

I'm going to work so that it's a pure guts race at the end, and if it is, I am the only one who can win it.

STEVE PREFONTAINE

Stress Kills
Sweat Calms

Stressed is just desserts spelled backwards.

ANDRÉA TASHA (PASTRY CHEF)

Stress is the worst thing you can do to your body. It's better to drink a glass of wine than be wired, but it's better yet to go to the gym and blow it out on the treadmill, bang out some barbell curls, and then have the wine. Take it from someone who can get wound up really tight—stress is bad news. One problem with wanting to achieve and become the best that you can be is the constant pressure of it. This is why I combine two polar opposites to beat stress—extreme calm, as in stretching, and extreme exertion, as in anaerobic work and weights. This is how I do it. I stretch and breathe religiously, every day, because if I don't, my nervous system will short-circuit. The molecules listed below are directly linked to athletic calm. Think of these when you are thinking of the self-fulfilling prophecy of exercise, especially when stretching and doing anaerobic work. All cardio is a cortisol furnace. You have to burn up cortisol by exercising every day or getting into fistfights. The best thing is always to let it go.

Sometimes you've got to let everything go—purge yourself. . . . If you are unhappy with anything . . . whatever brings you down, get rid of it. Because you'll find that when you're free, your creativity, your true self comes out.

TINA TURNER

Exercise Squelches the Anxiety Triad

Not everything that is faced can be changed, but nothing can be changed until it is faced.

JAMES A. BALDWIN

THE TOP THREE NEUROCHEMICALS LINKED TO STRESS AND ANXIETY

1. *CORTISOL: The "stress" molecule.(⇊ Low level is good.) Too much makes you feel anxious.*

2. *MAOS (MONOAMINE OXIDASE): The happy-juice-eating enzyme. (⇓ Low level is good.) Too much of this eats away at your serotonin and dopamine levels.*

3. *GABA (GAMMA-AMINO-BUTYRIC ACID): The "anti-anxiety" tranquilizer. (⇑ High level is good.) Makes you feel calm.*

The three culprits behind high anxiety and high stress are cortisol, GABA, and MAOs.

CORTISOL: THE STRESS MOLECULE

Cortisol is public enemy number one. It interferes with your memory, increases weight around your midsection, lowers testosterone and estrogen, and increases blood pressure and cholesterol. The list goes on and on. Cortisol, like adrenaline, is used during exercise. You burn it off and get it out of your blood stream. Cortisol is released as part of our fight-or-flight response system. If it isn't burned up, cortisol festers and wreaks havoc in your body. Cortisol has staying power. A single anxiety-induced surge can remain in your body for twenty-four hours. You need to work it out of your system with physical labor in order to decompress and destress your endocrine system. Over time, cortisol builds up in the blood. Exercise brings these levels back to a healthy set point. The harder and longer you work out, the lower your cortisol level. Make this a prime motivation.

The fight-or-flight mechanism that releases cortisol is part of the general adaptation syndrome defined in 1936 by Canadian biochemist Hans Selye of McGill University in Montreal. He published his revolutionary findings in a simple seventy-four-line article in the journal *Nature*, in which he talked about eustress (good stress) and distress (bad stress) as well as the three stages of general adaptation syndrome. Once the bugle has sounded, the troops are mobilized, and there has to be a release.

Too much cortisol causes your hippocampus to atrophy, which will increase memory loss as you age. Psychiatric professor Sonia Lupien is a leader in the field of the cortisol/memory connection. Lupien, a researcher at McGill who collaborates with neuroscientists to chart the impact of high cortisol levels on memory and learning, emphasizes that stress is not the villain here. "We need [good] stress in our lives; without it, we couldn't even wake up in the morning." What we need is to harness the two types of stress in our daily lives.

MAO (MONOAMINE OXIDASE): THE HAPPY-JUICE-CANNIBALIZING ENZYME

MAOs live on a diet of dopamine and serotonin, what I call happy juice. MAOs eat serotonin molecules in the synaptic gap. This cannibalism is necessary, because we would all be manically delusional if we had too much serotonin. High MAOs are going to make you less happy. Exercise decreases MAOs, which is a good thing, because it allows more serotonin and dopamine to stay in the gaps that link up the neural nets of bliss. The antidepressant family of MAO inhibitors has the same effect. Strength training that completely exhausts muscles and stretching, deep breathing, and anaerobic work lowers MAOs extremely well.

MAO inhibitors (MAOI) were discovered by doctors in the 1950s when they realized that a drug called iproniazid, used to treat tuberculosis, made people feel happy and cheerful. That drug has since been removed from the market because it was found to cause health problems. People still take MAOIs in the form of drugs like Nardil and Parmate, although they are tricky to take because of interactions with certain foods containing tyramine, found in many pickled or cured foods.

Nicotine also lowers MAOs, which makes cigarettes doubly addictive, because smokers are often elevating mood by lowering MAOs with nicotine. In the absence of nicotine, mood goes below its natural set point. If you smoke, quit! Substitute sweat for cigarettes, and you will slay the tobacco dragon.

GABA (GAMMA-AMINO-BUTYRIC ACID): THE ANTI-ANXIETY MOLECULE

GABA is an inhibitory molecule that slows the firing of synapses and puts your brain into a calmer electrochemical state, like throwing water on a fire. Almost all antianxiety medications work by increasing levels of GABA. By means of aerobic, anaerobic, strength training, and deep stretching/breathing, you can also release this natural tranquilizer. You could liken GABA to foam from a fire extinguisher, spraying your neurons and into the synaptic gaps, slowing everything down. When doing relaxation work, visualize the actual rate of neurons slowing, and you will increase your GABA production. If too much adrenaline or dopamine are circulating in the body, GABA is released to control the flow rate of nerve impulses that manifest themselves as anxiety or even paranoia. When you breathe deeply and do relaxation techniques, you elevate your levels of this self-produced antianxiety molecule, which makes you feel calm. Anaerobic exercise in particular raises levels of GABA, which is why it is such a great stress buster.

PART THREE: ELECTRICITY

Mode Locking
Neurons Marching in Lockstep

He who joyfully marches in rank and file has already earned my contempt. He has been given a large brain by mistake, since for him the spinal cord would suffice.

ALBERT EINSTEIN

Different brain waves exist as a way of focusing and shifting states of consciousness. Each mood and thought has a specific frequency that connects a neural network. Brain waves reflect the firing rate of your neurons. Higher firing rates denote a very active, busy brain; lower rates, a calmer brain. Neurons tune themselves to a specific frequency of firing, and there is power in numbers. Every brain cell is vying for your attention. Your state of mind is democratic. The number of neurons that get together or the louder the signal is what gets your brain's attention. You have free will and ultimately you can decide in almost every situation what you want to think about, then turn up the volume of that neural ensemble.

Biofeedback and the Zone
Fluid Performance Is a Brain Wavelength

Reverse every natural instinct and do the opposite of what you are inclined to do, and you will probably come very close to having a perfect golf swing.

BEN HOGAN

The principle of biofeedback is to watch your firing rates and learn how to slow them down through trial and error. When you learn to slow or speed up the firing rate of neurons to create a specific state of consciousness, they change the frequency to a different channel, a lower gear. Like any feedback loop, you can focus on slowing the firing rate down and feel a shift in consciousness, or you can change the state of your body by deep breathing to slow the firing rate. Remember that GABA is going to be the tranquilizing molecule, slowing the firing rate of synapses like throwing water on a fire.

Wes Sime, professor of health and human performance at the University of Nebraska at Lincoln, focuses on creating peak performance in many golfers by using the EEG Spectrum and biofeedback methods. Sime is an avid golfer. He uses his handheld EEG on and off the golf course. By watching electrical waves on a handheld device, golfers are able to see when they are tense and can then practice relaxation and focusing methods.

Sime and his colleagues found a clear correlation between certain wave states and unsuccessful putts. Armed with the data of what created the most successful putts, Sime began to hone in on a brain wavelength of peak performance. Once the players knew what the ideal mind-set felt like, they were able to encourage that particular state. According to Sime, the most effective setting for golfers across the board is to inhibit all settings that encourage activity at all the major frequencies. It's the EEG equivalent of being in the zone, getting your mind out of the game and letting your muscle memory do its work unimpeded. From my perspective, what Sime describes is classic down mind activity. The up mind of the neocortex becomes very quiet, almost in hibernation, when you are in a state of peak performance.

They say golf is like life, but don't believe them. Golf is more complicated than that.

GARDNER DICKINSON

In his book *Mind Wide Open*, Steven Johnson, on seeing Tiger Woods at the fourth round of a PGA championship at Medinah Country Club in Illinois, remembers, "I was standing among the throngs lining the path between the sixth green and the seventh tee, reveling in the noise and the rhythmic chanting ("Tiger! Tiger!"), when the man himself walked down the narrow aisle carved through the crowd. For a second or two I saw him up close as he made his way to the seventh tee. I have never in my life seen a wider chasm between the look in someone's eyes and the surrounding environment. He had five hundred boisterous fans chanting his name from two feet away, and he looked as though he were halfway through a transcendental meditation session."

Johnson's story reminds me of watching Steffi Graf entering the court at the U.S. Open, setting up her towels and rackets, and beginning her warm-

up with the most incredible sense of poise and precision. She was very methodical and moved with the calm alpha waves of a cat about to pounce. Between games, she would sit for a few minutes and remain in a complete
state of composure and stillness—and then explode onto the court like a
panther.

The Volition Switch
The Spark Plug of Free Will

My candle burns at both ends;
It will not last the night;
But ah, my foes, and oh, my friends—
It gives a lovely light!

                    EDNA ST. VINCENT MILLAY ("FIRST FIG")

The idea that there is a localized region of the brain that is the seat of
free will began in the 1960s. A recent study using new brain-imaging technology offers the strongest evidence yet that what sets humans apart from
other primates may be found in a small cluster of neurons in the brain's
frontal lobes. This small area just behind your eyes in your prefrontal cortex
is the seat of free will and decision making. I call it the *volition switch* and
imagine a traditional on/off light switch.

In 1963 John Eccles won the Nobel Prize in medicine for finding specific
signal transmissions among neurons in the brain. In the 1970s his research
focused on the cerebral cortex, the brain's highly developed outer layer,
which is the seat of higher reasoning and oversees movement of the body. A
few milliseconds before a person decides to carry out a willful action, specific neurons in the cortex discharge an electrical readiness surge signal that
cues the appropriate motor neurons to fire. But what was the flint that
sparked the intent? That is the divine spark of human intent.

Eccles believed that the signal of the mind to tell the cerebrum to fire
the motor neurons that would make the body move came from the mysterious source of human volition or the self-willed mind. Eccles claimed that
the volition neurons are continuously ready to fire. Just triggering a single
one of these specialized nerve cells creates a domino effect, a chain reaction
that spreads like wildfire from a few thousand neurons to engaging billions
of synapses.

Let's Make a Deal
Bartering with Volition

If you can't fly, then run. If you can't run, then walk. If you can't walk, then crawl. But whatever you do, keep moving.

MARTIN LUTHER KING, JR.

When I do Ironman races, I let myself walk about ten yards at every aid station, once every mile during the toughest portion of the marathon, which for me always tends to be around mile fourteen to mile twenty-two. This is a deal I make with myself to break the run into doable doses. As I shift from a jog to a walk at the aid station to refuel on Gatorade, Coke, or Gu, I can feel my volition switch go off. Then a millisecond before I take my first jogging step, I feel it go on again. When I'm walking in a race, I always use physical landmarks like a tree, a lamppost, or a line in the road as the point that I *have to* (no ifs, ands, or buts) start jogging again.

I visualize the volition switch to be a huge light switch just behind my forehead with on and off, go/stop on it. Practice keeping it in the up and locked position. This is one of the easiest tricks for kick-starting a workout and getting through it. Once that trigger switch is turned off, the synapses along that network will stop firing. This is quitting, or giving up. Don't reinforce that habit; always fight to the finish. Keep the volition switch in the up and locked position.

The key to flicking the volition switch lies in previsualizing the movement and sending your inner dialogue down from your frontal lobes. Researchers have found that the thicker and denser the neurons get with exercise, the easier it is to guide positive cross talk and to trigger the volition switch.

Researchers can literally see the spark of volition in an fMRI, just as you can feel it. Anytime you decide to go, remember you have flicked the volition switch. Anytime you decide to quit, you have turned it off. The next time you decide to do something like get up from the couch or break from a walk to a jog, pay attention to the millisecond of volition that precedes the muscle movement.

MICROTUBULES
TRANSPORT TUBES OF BLISS MOLECULES

When nothing seems to help, I go and look at the stonecutter hammering away at his rock, perhaps one hundred times without as much as a crack showing in it. Yet at the hundred and first blow it will split in two, and I know it was not that one blow that did it—but all that had gone on before.

JACOB RIIS

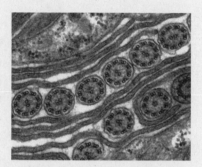

This is an image of cilia microtubules, which are slightly different from the microtubules in a nerve axon, but easier to photograph. This image is included because it clearly illustrates the "intracellular pipelines" that current brain-imaging technology has trouble photographing as clearly in a nerve axon.

Over time, with continuous daily practice, exercise strengthens—pumps up—the microtubules to transport more effectively the neurochemicals associated with bliss. The improved delivery system can result in more amplified feelings of bliss because the pipes run faster and cleaner.

These waterproof pipelines can transport a substance from the body of a cell to its synapse end-terminal up to three feet away. Inside each axon are about a hundred microtubules that lie flaccid like a flat fire hose. With a neurotransmitter cargo inside, they become rigid and stiff. These pipelines will swell within 1/10,000 of a second when a neuron springs to life and begins to communicate using the chemicals pumped through millions of neurons like wildfire, each linking at the tips of these microscopic channels to create an engram, a neural net. Within each axon, there are actually a hundred separate delivery systems squirting messages into the synaptic gap in milliseconds. This is how all the neurotransmitters transport chemical messages and deliver cargo to pleasure and pain centers.

When you exercise, microtubules pump serotonin into the frontal lobes—this makes you happier and smarter. Researchers at Johns Hopkins have recently discovered that the strengthening of axons in the frontal cortex because of more serotonin is probably what makes SSRIs (Selective Serotonin Reuptake Inhibitors) like Prozac work. Although it is too early to say, the real power in antidepressants may actually lie in the microtubules becoming a better delivery system because of serotonin, which also occurs with exercise.

Breaking a sweat makes your microtubules bigger, stronger, and more efficient. My dad used to say, "People like you and Lance Armstrong who do a lot of exercise have bigger microtubules than the rest of us." You need microtubules to be able to deliver large quantities of cargo quickly. They get stronger and bigger when you overload them. This cutting-edge concept is just beginning to be studied by other neuroscientists.

PURKINJE CELLS
THE KEY TO MUSCLE MEMORY

Learn by practice.
MARTHA GRAHAM

Number of Purkinje cells = 15 to 25 million (relatively small number)
Number of synapses made on a Purkinje cell = up to 200,000 (relatively huge number)

Muscle memory is stored in the Purkinje cells of the cerebellum. Purkinje cells are named after Johannes Purkinje, who first identified these neurons in 1837. Dr. Purkinje was also the first person to identify the individuality of the human fingerprint. He had a gift for discovering relatively obvious things everyone else had overlooked. Purkinje cells are the most distinctive neurons in the brain; their dendrites fan out into Chinese fans. Dendrites are arranged at right angles to the parallel fibers of the molecular layers, forming tens of millions of synapses. But they never touch.

You could think of one thousand purkinje cell dendrites as a "receiving dish" from many wide and varied places in you body. The single purkinje cell axon could be seen as one outgoing wire sending signals from all over the place through a consolidated pipeline. The dendrites of Purkinje cells are parallel but never touch. They oscillate like fishtails and push signals up the axon, out of the cerebellum, and up into the cerebrum. The power of these "fishtails" oscillating in unison could also be seen as a car engine with thousands of cylinders (the dendrites) channeling information into a single drive shaft (the axon.)

The synaptic plasticity of Purkinje cells is in your hands. They are re-shaped daily through practice and repetition. The Purkinje cells work at a quantum speed. The amplification of more than two hundred thousand incoming signals through one axon offers parallel processing capability from the cerebellum up into the cerebrum.

This lightning-fast processing in a goalie's cerebellum allows him to leap for a soccer ball while reaching out his hands, keeping his eyes locked on the target. His cerebellum monitors postural control, muscle tensions, velocity, and gravity before he grabs the ball and rolls as he hits the grass. The final output of any given Purkinje cell is via a single axon, but all the Purkinje cells are working autonomously, but simultaneously. They oscillate together and march in lockstep. These cells take sensory information from all parts of the body and send it to the cerebrum.

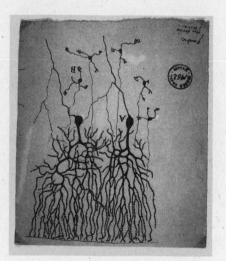

The Purkinje cells are beautiful to look at. They look like one tree trunk (the axon) with hundreds of roots. The long extended branches (dendrites) of the Purkinje cell are what allow it to collect input from two hundred thousand other cells. This incredible power of amplification directly connects all the information from your body to your mind, by sending all the signals from hundreds of dendrites up a single axon.

CHAPTER FOUR

POSITIVE PSYCHOLOGY

You're not going to make me have a bad day. If there's oxygen on earth and I'm breathing, it's going to be a good day.
COTTON FITZSIMMONS (FORMER HEAD COACH OF THE PHOENIX SUNS)

LEARNING OPTIMISM THROUGH SPORT
GETTING HAPPIFIED THE ATHLETE'S WAY

Experiencing pleasure in a smiley-face way isn't really a big part of happiness. As William James said, "If merely feeling good could decide, drunkenness would be the supremely valid human experience." In the long haul, you need to strengthen other virtues besides just seeking pleasure in order to feel fulfilled. Chasing bliss has a place, but it always needs to be rooted in a bigger picture. You don't want to end up alone in a rapturous athletic vacuum; I've made that mistake, as have many of my athletic peers. It is a sublime place to be, as we will explore in chapter 12, but you need to stay connected to other people.

Both individual ideals and interpersonal needs should coexist as a part of your athletic mind-set and behavior as part of *The Athlete's Way*. The bonding molecules oxytocin and vasopressin are as important as the bliss molecules dopamine, endocannabinoids, adrenaline, and serotonin. We will explore ways to make you genuinely happy and fulfilled.

Positive psychology, which has its roots in humanism, is based on building human strengths and fostering the conditions that make humans flourish. Martin E. P. Seligman of the University of Pennsylvania, a champion for this movement and the head of the American Psychological Association, says the goal of traditional psychology is to get people "from a minus five to a zero." The goal of positive psychology is to get people "north of zero." Similarly, *The Athlete's Way* is a way to get north of zero.

The Athlete's Way has its roots in ancient values of the Greek Spartans as well as the humanist movement founded by Abraham Maslow in the 1950s. There are two definitions to humanism—one is believing in the "values, characteristics, and behavior that bring out the best in human beings," and the other is an innate "concern for the needs and well-being and interests of people." These two definitions of humanism come together in *The Athlete's Way* and are at the core of the philosophy of the program.

The year was 2081, and everyone was finally equal.

KURT VONNEGUT

The Three Musketeers' maxim "One for all, and all for one" sums up the collectivism of *The Athlete's Way* philosophy. Since as adults only 3 percent of us play team sports, all too often athletes isolate and withdraw. The ideal is to bring both sides of the humanist coin to your athletic process, individual strength, and a sense of purpose in belonging to a community. The win-win of *The Athlete's Way* is that you can use sport as a vehicle to learn about yourself, experience the joy of being alive, and bond with other people. In this chapter, we look at the key components of human fulfillment as a combination of personal resilience combined with a sense of purpose and belonging to a community.

Joining an athletic culture is a way for you to feel fulfilled, engaged, and meaningfully happy by having a sense of purpose and feeling part of a group. You can do this as a fan of a home team, a member of a team, or as a role model for someone. Ultimately, you need to be connected to the daily process of lacing up your sneakers and getting through a workout. Exercise in and of itself creates a synaptic state of positive psychology. *The Athlete's Way* is a program for creating solid spokes on the wheels of your life, enabling you to accelerate and cushion your ride over the speed bumps.

Everyone knows that on any given day there are energies slumbering in him which the incitements of that day do not call forth. Compared with what we ought to be, we are only half awake. The human individual usually lives far within his limits.

WILLIAM JAMES

As Abraham Maslow said, "Man is a wanting animal—what humans can be, we must be." It is human nature to reach for the stars. Athletics is a way to become self-actualized and have peak experiences because it taps the human spirit and human will. It is also a way for you to bond with other humans and collaborate as you strive for your peak performance. *The Athlete's Way* is about dreaming big, pulling your own weight, and working together. This is how we build skyscrapers and jumbo jets or send men to the moon. It is also why we invented athletics—no other animal has a need to play sports.

Throughout this chapter I will look at lessons of resilience and talk about fear conditioning and avoidance learning, coping with rejection sensitivity (intimidation), and overcoming low self-esteem. We will look at the neurobiology of intimidation and the ability of serotonin to bulk up the neurons in your frontal lobes and help you to have a more optimistic outlook and inner dialogue.

> *Man is the only creature that strives to surpass himself, and yearns for the impossible.*
>
> ERIC OFFER (U.S. PHILOSOPHER)

The Athlete's Way is not a panacea for all life's woes. We all need to seek balance on the tightrope of life. Remember not to isolate yourself in your blissed-out vacuum. There is no fun to be had alone on your lotus leaf of nirvana. I've seen people sacrifice family, friends, and career for an exercise fix and I've been there myself. Don't do it.

True strength is being strong enough to admit when you are weak. Ideally as an athlete you want to be sensitive and magnanimous but also tough as nails, with a spine of steel. This state of coexisting opposites—wanting to win but playing fair, and being completely independent but working as part of a team is all part of the athletic paradox. There is an art to *The Athlete's Way* and it is often a high-wire balancing act. You get better at with practice.

> *In spite of illness, in spite even of the arch enemy sorrow, one can remain alive long past the usual date of disintegration if one is unafraid of change, insatiable in intellectual curiosity, interested in big things, and happy in small ways.*
>
> EDITH WHARTON

THE RELIGION OF SPORT
BINDING PEOPLE TOGETHER

Human beings are born into this little span of life of which the best thing
Is its friendship and intimacies, and soon their places will know them no
More, and yet they leave their friendships and intimacies with no cultivation,
to grow as they will by the roadside, expecting them to "keep" by force of inertia.

WILLIAM JAMES

The word *religion* is derived from the Latin *religio*, which means to bind together. To me sport is a religion, in a community-building way. I encourage you to look at sport as a way to bind together both as a participant and a fan. Rooting for your team or an individual athlete you admire or know and love is an important part of bonding through sports. The catch is, you don't want to be just a benchwarmer or couch potato. Find a balance between just observing the sporting life and participating.

VASOPRESSIN AND OXYTOCIN
(THE BONDING MOLECULES)
TEND AND BEFRIEND IS KEY TO SURVIVAL

There is always something to do. There are hungry people to feed, naked people to clothe, sick people to comfort and make well. And while I don't expect you to save the world; I do think it's not asking too much for you to love those with whom you sleep, share the happiness of those whom you call friend, engage those among you who are visionary and remove from your life those who offer depression, despair and disrespect.

NIKKI GIOVANNI (AMERICAN POET)

If there is a molecular explanation for tending and befriending it is probably found in vasopressin and oxytocin. Shelley Taylor of UCLA Westwood has done extensive research on the "tending instinct" and uses the term *tend and befriend* as a way to juxtapose our other key survival mechanism, fight or flight. Making friends is just as important to our survival as defeating or avoiding enemies. The general adaptation response, which allows us to spring to life to protect ourselves, or flee when we are in danger, has been well documented in many creatures. Recently brain researchers have begun looking at what neurochemicals make creatures bond together. To examine the neurobiology of attachment they have focused on the prairie vole, a small rodent from the midwestern United States, because it bonds for life with its first mate.

After mating, prairie voles remain monogamous, which is rare in the animal kingdom. In the male prairie vole, vasopressin serves to make the lifelong link stronger. In the female it is oxytocin (not to be confused with the barbituate oxycotin). Research has long shown that oxytocin is released in life situations that have emotional significance. It is probably also released when your team wins a championship, during a spin class, swimming with the masters team, doing a local race, or smiling and nodding to a fellow runner on a jogging path.

Living the sporting life and joining the physical culture creates community. The feeling of being part of a collective is one of the most beneficial aspects of becoming physically active. Your path crosses with like-minded individuals, even if the camaraderie is a nod and a wave exchanged between two solo runners or running stride for stride with the stranger on the treadmill next to you without speaking a word. Understand the power of unspoken communion through sport but foster the solidarity by making it tangible whenever you can. There is a lot of positive energy generated between athletes and sports fans. Harness it and soak it in. The combination will create a positive psychological, spiritual, and biological bond.

> *The best index of a person's character is (a) how he treats people who can't do him any good, and (b) how he treats people who can't fight back.*
>
> ABIGAIL VAN BUREN ("DEAR ABBY")

The Spartans were a collective society that has deeply influenced my mind-set as an athlete. As I coach, I take many lessons from the Spartans that are reflected throughout this program. Kinship was a key part of Spartan society, and what most likely led to their longevity. Both young boys and girls were trained to be athletic. Spartan men and women remained active in the community and civil duties well into their sixties. You should look for kinship through sports as the Spartans did.

Sometimes the bonds are obvious, like being part of the same team, but sometimes they are discreet. Be proactive about forming bonds with other athletes, including animals. Being with pets is very good for your health, too. In the early 1970s I had a horse named Commander, who taught me how to run. If you don't have a person with whom you can work out, think about doing exercise with a dog or a horse, and you'll both stay healthy a lot longer. My mom structures her fitness regimen around morning and evening walks with our black lab, Solo. The companionship of exercising with the family pet with the purpose of keeping both fit keeps Mom motivated and on schedule. As Hippocrates said, "Walking is the best medicine."

> I started early—
> Took my dog—
> And visited the sea—
> The Mermaids in the basement
> Came out to look at me.
> EMILY DICKINSON

THE UNIFIED FIELD
UNIVERSAL ATHLETIC WAVELENGTHS

> I, not events, have the power to make me happy or unhappy today. I can choose which it shall be. Yesterday is dead, tomorrow hasn't arrived yet. I have just one day, today, and I'm going to be happy in it.
> GROUCHO MARX

This morning, I got up early and was running in East River Park at sunrise. Since I don't usually run that early, it was a new experience on very familiar turf. I enjoyed the new angle of light and seeing pockets of people from Chinatown doing Tai Chi along the esplanade, saluting the sun as it came up over Brooklyn and Schaefer Landing. It was beautiful to see the juxtaposition of these ancient movements under the industrial bridges and highway overpasses amid the stench of the fish market and random joggers, bikers, and inline skaters.

They were perspiring on this hot and humid morning as they went through the motions. Our actions were very different, but I realized that their routine was invigorating their nervous systems in different but similar ways to my jog. We were out there for the same reason: mental and physical harmony. I felt connected to them and drew strength from that.

To absorb is better.
JOHN BURROUGHS

I see the human spirit bursting out of athletes out of the corner of my eye every day. To me, people working out are on a neurochemical and electrical unified field. Watching them and seeing the glisten of sweat on the nape of someone's neck makes me feel like an athlete vicariously. I sink myself into their spine and feel as if I ride the cascade of their athletic bliss for a few seconds. I see the essence of *The Athlete's Way* everywhere in full-body movements, small gestures, rhythmic tics, the tilt of a head, or slant of the eyes. I can't help thinking of lines from the Walt Whitman poem "I Sing the Body Electric" when the athletes I see engirth me, and I engirth them. The poem sums up *The Athlete's Way*.

I SING THE BODY ELECTRIC

But the expression of a well-made man appears not only in his face;
It is in his limbs and joints also, it is curiously in the joints of his hips
  and wrists;

It is in his walk, the carriage of his neck, the flex of his waist and
  knees—dress does not hide him;
The strong, sweet, supple quality he has, strikes through the cotton and
  flannel;
To see him pass conveys as much as the best poem, perhaps more;
You linger to see his back, and the back of his neck and shoulder-side.

The sprawl and fulness of babes, the bosoms and heads of women, the
  folds of their dress, their style as we pass in the street, the contour of
  their shape downwards,
The swimmer naked in the swimming-bath, seen as he swims through
  the transparent green-shine, or lies with his face up, and rolls silently
  to and fro in the heave of the water,
The bending forward and backward of rowers in row-boats—the
  horseman in his saddle,

Girls, mothers, house-keepers, in all their performances,
The group of laborers seated at noon-time with their open dinner-
  kettles, and their wives waiting,
The female soothing a child—the farmer's daughter in the garden
  or cow-yard,
The young fellow hoeing corn—the sleigh-driver guiding his six
  horses through the crowd,

The natural, perfect, varied attitudes—the bent head, the curv'd
  neck, and the counting;
Such-like I love—I loosen myself, pass freely, am at the mother's
  breast with the little child,
Swim with the swimmers, wrestle with wrestlers, march in line with
  the firemen, and pause, listen, and count.

                                                    WALT WHITMAN

Remember, sweat is your passport to sing the body electric. It doesn't matter how fast or slow you are, or what activity you are doing. If you are out there moving you are tapping the nervous system—the body electric—and you are doing it *The Athlete's Way.* You are part of the athletic culture. Kinship, physical activity, and energy balance are the three pillars of longevity, and they are all part of a modern Spartan life lived *The Athlete's Way.*

With life and nature, purifying thus the elements of feeling and of thought, and sanctifying, by such discipline both pain and fear, until we recognize a grandeur in the beatings of the heart.

                                               WILLIAM WORDSWORTH

POSITIVE PSYCHOLOGY
EIGHT WAYS TO MOMENTOUS HAPPINESS

To me, there are three things that we should do every day of our lives. Number one is laugh. You should laugh every day. Number two is think. You should spend some time in thought. And number three is, you should have your emotions moved to tears, could be happiness or joy. But think about it. If you laugh, you think and you cry, that's a full day. That's a heck of a day. You do that seven days a week, you're going to have something special.

JIM VALVANO (AMERICAN BASKETBALL COACH, NORTH CAROLINA STATE
UNIVERSITY)

The essentials to human fulfillment are always going to be: family, friendship, love, and respect—a sense of purpose and belonging to a community. Nothing sums up these traits in sport as well as the starting line of any local race. For me, the starting line of the weekend races in Central Park embody individualism blended with collectivism, which are the heart of *The Athlete's Way*.

Sport is about people coming together to push against their own limits, to cheer one another on, to feel part of a group, and to earn respect while family and peers either run by them side by side or cheer from the sidelines. Central Park on any given weekend morning is a very cosmopolitan pagan ritual of villagers communing to move together, laugh together, gasp for air, grunt, burst open with delight, cheer, and sweat together.

Happiness is an attitude. We either make ourselves miserable, or happy and strong. The amount of work is the same.

UNKNOWN

Through my work as an athlete and as a coach I have come up with eight points that are the source of positive psychology. Put up your antennae and think of ways to incorporate this list into your life. If you live by these rules your life will be in good shape. Be creative and think of ways that you can include these into your daily athletic routine.

1. *TAKE CARE OF YOUR BODY: Get seven to eight hours of sleep, exercise for at least twenty to thirty minutes most days of the week, maintain energy balance, drink plenty of water, don't do drugs or smoke. Practice safe sex. Respect yourself. Don't be self-destructive.*

2. *FAMILY AND FRIENDS: Strong personal relationships mean more than money, status, or your job title. Family, friends, and community are essential to happiness and longevity. Fortify your sense of community as an athlete and nonathlete. Join a club or a class at a local gym or community center. Be open and friendly;*

make new friends every day. Spread good cheer in every human encounter you have.

3. *LAUGHTER AND LEVITY: People laugh thirty times more when they are in the company of others than when they're alone. Laughter heals, stress kills. Lighten up. Make it a conscious effort to smile and laugh a lot. You'll live longer. Have fun working out with people. Exercise puts people in a good mood. Trigger neurobiological joy by smiling when you work out. Smiling and laughing sends a signal to your nervous system that all is well and you're having fun. Put the cart before the horse. This is called the facial feedback loop. Use it. Smile and the world smiles with you—it's true.*

4. *LOOK FORWARD TO SOMETHING: A sense of anticipation makes people healthy and happy. Put things on the horizon that you can look forward to. A sense of curiosity and eagerness gives you a sense of purpose and a reason to seize the day. Pick a race or have a group exercise event on your weekly or monthly calendar. Play it forward in your mind—and get yourself psyched up.*

5. *GRATITUDE AND SIMPLE JOYS: Take time to count your blessings from little things like a good meal to big things like watching your children grow up. Music and pets are also a key to improving your mood and lowering blood pressure. Take pleasure in every breath and the celebration of being alive—the joy of movement and sweat. Watch the world news and realize that of the 6.5 billion people on Earth, odds are that most are probably worse off than you.*

6. *DO SOMETHING WELL: You want to hone a skill and become really good at something. Find your calling in life and become the absolute best at it that you can. Work hard and pour your heart into it. Mastery is the key to fulfillment. Mastering an athletic skill is an easy place to start, even if it is just becoming the best spinner in spin class or the best stepper in step class. Master it.*

7. *DEVELOP COPING MECHANISMS FOR HARDSHIPS: The mechanism for getting through hard times is threefold: a belief that you are a survivor, an understanding that it is temporary, and a willingness*

to reach out for your support network. Face the dragon head-on and do not hide under the covers, and you'll weather any storm. Sport gives you tenacity and resilience, just by getting from point A to point B and finishing what you start. Remember, these changes happen at a neural level.

8. *GIVE SOMETHING BACK: Try to practice selfless acts of kindness toward family, friends, and strangers every day. This can be altruistic—and should be—but it also creates a positive feedback loop of feeling generous and appreciated and will bring you reciprocated kindness. Create more systematic ways of philanthropy by finding a regular activity like being a mentor or volunteering that you can use to make a contribution to the world. Once you start doing it The Athlete's Way, recruit other people, show them why you love sport, and how to make it a part of their lives.*

THE HUMANIST ATHLETE
INDIVIDUALISM AND COLLECTIVISM

Seven sins: wealth without work, pleasure without conscience, knowledge without character, commerce without morality, science without humanity, worship without sacrifice, politics without principle.

                                                          MAHATMA GANDHI

The Lance Armstrong "LIVEstrong" phenomenon exemplifies the perfect blend of individualism and collectivism in sport . By spending one dollar to buy a yellow rubber bracelet, any individual can donate to the Lance Armstrong Foundation for cancer research and become part of a group with an ethos and credo that could be identified across the room. The small bright yellow band of rubber serves as a daily reminder of the code of conduct the wearer has committed to and an ever-present memento to stay on course.

A soul without a high aim is like a ship without a rudder.

                                                          EILEEN CADDY

Individualism is a philosophy in life that stresses the priority of personal goals over those of a group. There is a desire to remain autonomous from others' influence and to form loosely knit social networks. Collectivism stresses the priority of group needs over individual needs and requires a willingness to sacrifice individual wants for what is in the best interest of the group and the formation of tight-knit social networks. Currently 70 percent of the world's population lives in societies with a collective orientation. The ideal of *The Athlete's Way* is to blend individualism and collectivism in an even fifty-fifty split.

The human species evolved because of our ability to form tight social groups and work together. Over time there has been a struggle to balance individual needs for survival and a selfless desire to ensure that your gene pool thrives and to recognize that you need your neighbors' help to protect your well-being and that of your community. As René Dubos said in 1972 when he was an adviser to the United Nations: "Think globally, act locally." Protecting your group protects you, too. But individuals need to shine.

> *At bottom every man knows well enough that he is a unique being, only once on this earth; and by no extraordinary chance will such a marvelously picturesque piece of diversity in unity as he is, ever be put together a second time.*
>
> FRIEDRICH NIETZSCHE

Individualism becomes megalomania when people forget the needs of the group. Each of us is a dynamic and original force of nature, but we are also a part of the collective. Over time a delicate balance has evolved that automatically keeps these conflicting tendencies in check. The ideal is to be a maverick and not a lemming, but also to be a team player. Any team sport is a perfect metaphor for practicing and exploring this equilibrium between the individual and the collective. Don't fall into the "every man for himself" mentality of me, me, me individualism.

> *If we could read the secret history of our enemies, we should find in each man's life sorrow and suffering to disarm all hostility.*
>
> HENRY WADSWORTH LONGFELLOW

LEARNED OPTIMISM VERSUS
LEARNED HELPLESSNESS

Between the optimist and the pessimist, the difference is droll. The optimist sees the doughnut, the pessimist the hole.

OSCAR WILDE

You can learn to be optimistic by choosing to take that perspective. You have the choice to decide what your perspective is going to be. Whenever you are angry or negative, you can be assured that it is not only a present state of mind, but also that you have encouraged a habit. Your brain will architecturally be more likely to think that way in the future. Thoughts move along the neural pathways most frequently traveled. By making a decision to see the glass as half-full, you can rewire your brain to be inclined toward that explanatory style. Learned helplessness or learned optimisms become habits the same way. Through repetition, the grooves are carved into your synapses and welded together. You have to break the chains that bind you to negative thinking or passivity.

Learned helplessness is the giving-up reaction, the quitting response that follows from the belief that what you do doesn't matter.

ARNOLD SCHWARZENEGGER

With learned optimism you can reshape your mind-set by changing your explanatory style from pessimistic to optimistic. Simply see the glass as half-full, find silver linings, make lemonade from lemons, look on the bright side; you know the clichés. They work. Optimists and athletes believe that they are the rulers of their destinies, rather pessimists, who take the deterministic view that what they do doesn't matter because they are backseat passengers in life.

There is always a lot to be thankful for, if you take the time to look. For example, I'm sitting here now thinking how nice it is that wrinkles don't hurt.

UNKNOWN

Optimists tend to believe that bad events are temporary, specific, and generally caused by external factors. Pessimistic people tend to see bad events as being permanent, universal, and caused by internal flaws and good events as lucky, caused by temporary, specific, and external factors. As Seligman describes: "It comes down to this: people who make *universal* explanations for their failures give up on everything when a failure strikes in one area. People who make *specific* explanations may become (temporarily) helpless in that one part of their lives, yet march stalwartly on in the other."

OF MICE AND MEN:
MICE RUN FOR LEARNED OPTIMISM
. . . HUMANS DO, TOO

If you don't like where you are, change it! You're not a tree.
JIM ROHN (MOTIVATIONAL COACH)

Learned helplessness has been linked to lack of exercise in studies on mice. In one experiment, mice who ran on a treadmill would repeatedly attempt to escape from a puzzle box that gave a shock, even if their attempts were futile. Mice that were deprived of access to a running wheel would give up and passively accept the shock. Running made mice resilient and determined, optimistic that they could escape even when it was futile.

makes me

A positive attitude may not solve all your problems, but it will annoy enough people to make it worth the effort.
HERM ALBRIGHT (SATURDAY EVENING POST WRITER)

Learned optimism is within your conscious control. You have the ability to create the perspective of reality that you want. Breaking a pattern of thinking is about breaking apart the neurons associated with that neural network. You lose about eighty-five thousand neurons a day, every day. Why not send the ones associated with the pessimistic explanatory style to the neural Darwinism termination center and make them extinct?

PRAGMATISM
REALISTIC OPTIMISM

If you keep a cool head in these times perhaps you don't understand the situation.

PRISON WARDEN'S DESK SIGN

The optimistic perspective of *The Athlete's Way* is not just about being an unrealistically optimistic Pollyanna. The potency of sports as a way of building a solid positive psychology is that the athletic process creates a sense of realistic optimism.

As an athlete you learn to tactfully walk the high-wire between optimism being productive and being counterproductive as a method of denial to overlook failure or flaws. Keeping it real by learning how to avoid self-deceptions while maintaining a sense of realistic optimism is the main goal of *The Athlete's Way*. In sports, the outcome and results speak for themselves.

THE ATHLETE'S WAY *EXPLANATORY STYLES*
PUT THESE IN YOUR TOOLBOX

What's shaking, chiefy baby?
THURGOOD MARSHALL (CUSTOMARY GREETING
TO CHIEF JUSTICE WARREN E. BURGER)

Below is a sampling of explanatory styles I created for *The Athlete's Way* based on the ideas of positive psychology, neuroscience, and ideal athletic mind-set. Use this list as a quick review and decide what angle would best suit you for achieving your objectives on a given day. Your perspective changes from day to day, week to week, and even during a workout. Keep taking inventory and try different perspectives to keep you motivated. Create more perspectives of your own in your workbook. Say, "This is the perspective I need to take" and define it. Give it a name and make it tangible.

I will elaborate on these perspectives throughout the book. You can use these as a reference, but please expand on this list with your own ideas. Remember that for all these positive explanatory styles there are negative ones, too. If you find yourself taking a negative perspective, consciously switch your point of view using these:

- THE ATHLETE'S WAY *PERSPECTIVE: I promise to work hard, play fair, and love the game.*

- THE "BIOLOGY OF BLISS" *PERSPECTIVE: Sweat=Bliss. Endocannabinoids are sublime.*

- THE NEURO-PLASTICITY *PERSPECTIVE: My thoughts/actions shape my brain and who I am.*

- THE OPTIMISTIC *PERSPECTIVE: Silver linings, the bright side . . . the glass is half-full*

- THE WOE-IS-ME *PERSPECTIVE: No more pity parties. No more violins. Snap out of it!*

- THE COLLECTIVISM *PERSPECTIVE: United we stand, divided we fall. One for all, all for one.*

- THE SPARTAN *PERSPECTIVE: Discipline, austerity, loyalty. I am tough as nails.*

- THE BRING-IT-ON *PERSPECTIVE: This hurts, but pain releases analgesics, so crank it up!*

- THE HUMANIST *PERSPECTIVE: Maximize my potential and foster the best in all humans.*

- THE GREEN *PERSPECTIVE: I use my own energy to transport myself whenever possible.*

- THE BARTERING *PERSPECTIVE: Let's make a deal: Run for three minutes, walk for two.*

- THE QUID-PRO-QUO *PERSPECTIVE: Balance calories in, calories out. Create energy balance.*

- THE EXCELSIOR *PERSPECTIVE: Higher, harder, faster. You can always do more.*

- THE FUN-LOVING *PERSPECTIVE: Sport is play; this is a game. I'm having fun.*

- THE ROMANTIC *PERSPECTIVE: The essence of yearning and struggling is joyful but bittersweet.*

- THE SUPERFLUID *PERSPECTIVE: No friction/viscosity. Trance and transcendence. Piercing through.*

These perspectives are simple and concise. Take the perspective you need to balance out where you are going. Sometimes your perspective supports where you are and makes it more tangible. Sometimes it changes your course. Remember to be intuitive but also intellectual. It is a dance between your cerebrum and your cerebellum.

RAINDROPS KEEP FALLIN' ON MY HEAD
ACCEPTING THE WEATHER

I can't change the direction of the wind, but I can adjust my sails to always reach my destination.

JIMMY DEAN

Being resilient and sticking with it by having a variety of coping mechanisms is key when you are faced with obstacles or intimidation. I have an endless array of coping mechanisms and defense strategies for dealing with any type of fear or struggle. Below is the systematic checklist I go through when I face a heavy headwind or crosswind on a bicycle. Wind is every biker's number one nemesis and source of resistance. I am pragmatic about wind. Sometimes the wind seems to be personally attacking me when I'm on the bike. I have four things that I say systematically when facing a headwind and feel myself slipping into pity party, woe-is-me mode:

1. *"THAT WHICH DOES NOT DESTROY ME MAKES ME STRONGER."*

2. *"IT MUST BE A GREAT DAY FOR SAILING." "If I was in my Sunfish sailing, I'd be psyched about the wind." This is my way of looking at it from a different point of view. I remind myself that the electrical wind turbines would be storing up tons of power, and that the wind is good.*

3. *"I FELT LIKE A BIRD." (Noting what Natascha Badmann— six-time Hawaii Ironman winner—said to me when I asked, "How did you deal with the wind today?" "I just pretended that I was a bird and that it allowed me to soar," was what she replied. With those words in my head, I pretend it's just the wind beneath my wings.*

4. *IF I PUT MY HEAD DOWN AND KEEP DOING WHAT I'M DOING, I WILL GET THERE EVENTUALLY. I just keep pedaling, plow along, and*

hang in there. The time and miles will roll away until I reach the end. This struggle is finite—I will reach my destination and rest again.

Consider a man riding a bicycle. Whoever he is, we can say three things about him. We know he got on the bicycle and started to move. We know that at some point he will stop and get off. Most important of all, we know that if at any point between the beginning and the end of his journey he stops moving and does not get off the bicycle he will fall off it. This is a metaphor for the journey through life of any living thing and I think of any society of living things.

WILLIAM GOLDING

VALOR
ONE FOR ALL, ALL FOR ONE

Mental toughness is many things. It is humility because it behooves all of us to remember that simplicity is the sign of greatness and meekness is the sign of true strength. Mental toughness is spartanism with qualities of sacrifice, self-denial, dedication. It is fearlessness, and it is love.

VINCE LOMBARDI

The goal of *The Athlete's Way* is that through the valor of our individual pursuits we improve the collective. As athletes we look at our own self-improvement as a way to make the world a better place.

In President Teddy Roosevelt's speech "The Strenuous Life" he said, "Pray not for lighter burdens but for stronger backs," and this idea of toughness summed up his credo. Roosevelt's words reiterate the ideals of the athletic mind-set and behavior—the choices that you make about your health affect us all. How we treat our bodies is a political statement. Take responsibility for the cost your health choices have on those around you. The obesity epidemic is a national crisis that we all pay for. Take responsibility for your energy balance and girth. If you eat more than you burn, eat less. If you smoke, quit. If you do drugs, stop. These three things alone cost our nation hundreds of billions a year—and we all pay. So on days when you don't feel like exercising for your own mental health and physical well-being, do it for the collective —a loved one, a family member, a fellow citizen. As Roosevelt put it:

A life of ignoble ease, a life of that peace which springs merely from lack either of desire or of power to strive after great things, is as little worthy of a nation as of an individual. We do not admire the man of timid peace.

We admire the man who embodies victorious effort; the man who never wrongs his neighbors; who is prompt to help a friend; but who has those virile qualities necessary to win in the stern strife of actual life.

It is hard to fail; but it is worse never to have tried to succeed. In this life we get nothing save by effort.

I love this quote for its humanism, high aspirations, and collective ideals, but I'm also aware of its over-the-top machismo. I get a kick out of Roosevelt's unabashed bravado, but it's not just about virility. We need to be sensitive and humble, too. You need to coexist from a point of fearless grit and determination, but also be sensitive, nurturing, and tender to yourself and others.

He that respects himself is safe from others.
He wears a coat of mail that none can pierce.

HENRY WADSWORTH LONGFELLOW

To be meaningfully happy as an athlete, you need to blend the ideals of striving to achieve your maximum individual potential with interpersonal ideals that include kindness, laughter, and a capacity for bonding to family and friends. The principle of *The Athlete's Way* is to combine the ambitious mind-set of individual performance with the universal, biological need to bond with other humans.

Darkness Within Darkness
An Athlete Dying Young

And salted was my food, and my repose, Salted and sobered too, by the bird's voice. Speaking for all who lay under the stars, Soldiers and poor, unable to rejoice.

EDWARD THOMAS

When I was in college my cousin Sam committed suicide. Sam was a terrific athlete, a wonderful human being, and a role model for me. Sam suffered from paranoid schizophrenia. Real clinical depression or mental illness creates a completely different neurobiological landscape beyond learned optimism and positive psychology.

The thing that constantly tears me apart about Sam is the pain and the suffering he endured because of his brain's chemical, architectural, and electrical imbalances. No amount of exercise or sweat was going to readjust the environment of his brain or his perceptions of reality. I think the worst feelings a human being can have are those of insecurity and inadequacy, or of being threatened and unable to cope when everybody else seems to be coping beautifully. That was my cousin Sam all the time. Although he did his best to look perfect to all of us on the outside, and succeeded well at that, internally he was tortured. So he drove himself maniacally as a student and as an athlete. Sam got straight A's and would do things like run up and down the steps of the Penn football stadium for three hours at a time to strengthen his legs and release some of his demons. Or just to feel something.

> This is the hour of Lead—Remembered, if outlived,
> As Freezing persons, recollect the Snow—
> First—Chill—then Stupor—then letting go—
> EMILY DICKINSON ("AFTER GREAT PAIN, A FORMAL FEELING COMES—")

Sam said that leg muscles were the most important body part to a rower, even more important than muscles in the arms and back. He also needed to be very light. So he worked himself to the bone, and had the leanest, strongest legs and chiseled features I'd ever seen. He poured himself into sport, and they made him captain of the lightweight crew at Penn. It was probably the happiest period of his life.

Sam was a hero to me. He was who I wanted to be when I got to college. I had been the family ne'er-do-well all through high school, but Sam always seemed like he had it so together. I emulated him after my athletic conversion. I think about him a lot when I push myself too hard, or beat myself up by trying to overcompensate, or strive to be perfect and feel completely inadequate. Anytime I think sweat may be the answer to all my problems, a way to numb all my pain or help me to achieve all my dreams, I remember Sam, and how alone he was, and I remember it's not.

> "Dust thou art, to dust returnest," was not spoken of the soul.
> HENRY WADSWORTH LONGFELLOW

Many people, especially obligatory exercisers, treat mental health problems with exercise. Be on the lookout for the warning signs of compulsive behavior, and if you think there's a problem get help to sort it out. Please understand that a lot of what I accomplished as an athlete was my way of dealing with life, a coping mechanism for me. In many ways it was a substitute for not being able to really let people into my life. Instead of connecting intimately to other humans, I had an ongoing love affair with "the other."

If you are clinically depressed and looking for a cure-all to mental health issues, you are not necessarily going to find it in this book or in exercise. This program can be a part of your strategy but is by no means a panacea. When life throws me a curveball, I have learned from experience to be proactive and reach out to friends and mental health professionals to help me through.

Darkness cannot drive out darkness; only light can do that. Hate cannot drive out hate; only love can do that.

MARTIN LUTHER KING, JR.

When you are in the blackest of blackness the light seems like it will never enter your brain again. But it will. The light will flicker again. That is the human spirit; it always, always comes back. I've been there myself. If you are depressed or suicidal do whatever you have to do to stay vital and get yourself back on track. You were born to be alive. Don't isolate. Reach out. Ask for help. There will be sunbeams in your soul again. Ride out the storm—but don't do it alone. People will take care of you. Let them. And make a vow, when you're back on top, to give something back.

My winter world, that scarcely breathes that bliss. Now yields you, with some sighs, our explanation.

GERARD MANLEY HOPKINS

CHAPTER FIVE

THE TRAINING
PROGRAM:
AN OVERVIEW

*You have to stay in shape. My grandmother, she started walking five
miles a day when she was sixty. She's ninety-seven today and we
don't know where the hell she is.*

ELLEN DEGENERES

D uring the past twenty years of training, coaching, and competing, I
have learned a lot about the athletic process. In the following chapters, I will share with you all the basics you need to tackle your cardio, strength, and fitness regimen. To get started, you will need the right
equipment and need to be familiar with the fundamental principles of *The
Athlete's Way*. This chapter presents an overview of the program and the
building blocks of *The Athlete's Way* in a ten-point prescriptive. The principles of this prescriptive can be applied to any level of workout. Later, we
will look individually at cardio, strength, flexibility, and nutrition, and I will
show you ways to apply these core tenets to each of those pursuits. This program has been road tested and can be plugged directly into your athletic
process. I have isolated the core tenets of the athletic success.

*Always keep fit! Study your sport deeply, and only pay attention to
the advice of those who do things. Leave those who theorize se-
verely alone. Practice and compete with your superiors at your
sport and emulate them. Observe your inferiors and learn from their
mistakes.*

MAXICK (*HOW TO BECOME A GREAT ATHLETE*
BY EARLY-TWENTIETH-CENTURY PHYSICAL CULTURE GURU)

EQUIPMENT
KEEP IT SIMPLE, BUT RIGHT AND EXACT

A place for everything, everything in its place.

BENJAMIN FRANKLIN

In this section we will go over all the things you need in terms of equipment to be on *The Athlete's Way* program. Remember, as always: Use common sense, be a wise consumer, and keep it simple. A core philosophy of *The Athlete's Way* is spartanism and simplicity. This should be reflected in your gear. Don't believe the hype and waste tons of money on lots of gear that you won't use. Buy high-quality, low-status gear that is functional and durable. Get the most out of it. I learned this lesson the hard way. For years I was a total gearhead and spent tons of money collecting more and more stuff, thinking it would make me a better athlete. It didn't, of course. Invest your time and energy in the actual work, not in gadgets, supplements, or clothing. All you need is a few key pieces.

I have a philosophy which is "play the melody." It means don't over-arrange, don't make life difficult. Just play the melody, I play it the simplest way possible.

JACKIE GLEASON

Keep your athletic gear separate from the regular clothes. One of the first things to do is to clear a drawer or shelf for your athletic equipment. Get a gym bag to transport gear. Packing this bag each day will serve as a prime reinforcer in terms of ritual and habituation. Remember the five stages of the daily athletic process—anticipation, preparation, action, perspiration, and completion. The equipment plays a key role in all phases.

You want to have the right fabrics and garments that are appropriate for specific workout environments and conditions. Having the right clothes for every condition is one fewer excuse to avoid working out. Get a good pair of sneakers; buy them at a store that either lets you try them out on a treadmill or that has a return policy that allows you bring them back if they do not fit properly.

It pays to invest in specific technical gear for different conditions: indoor training during which you sweat a lot, cold weather when you'll need layers, or if aerodynamic gear if you're racing. I encourage you to make your workout gear a uniform and an extension of your athletic persona.

> *I don't like my hockey sticks touching other sticks, and I don't like them crossing one another, and I kind of have them hidden in the corner. I put baby powder on the ends. I think it's essentially a matter of taking care of what takes care of you.*
>
> WAYNE GRETZKY

LOCKER STUFF

THE ATHLETE'S WAY SPORTING GOODS CHECKLIST

1. *SNEAKERS: Always try on athletic shoes. Find a pair that fits well; take your time choosing them. Go to a local running shop with knowledgeable staff.*

2. *MUSIC: Choose anthems; make a soundtrack for your workouts. Mix it up.*

3. *COMFORTABLE, CLIMATE-APPROPRIATE CLOTHING: Wicking fabrics work to transfer moisture away from the skin, which keeps you dry and comfortable.*

4. *SPORTS WATCH: Work out by time and intensity more than distance. Always use a stopwatch.*

5. *HEART-RATE MONITOR (OPTIONAL): Get to know your perceived exertion levels as they correspond to your heart rate (beats per minute)*

6. *SUNSCREEN: Apply thirty minutes before exposure—reapply after more than forty-five minutes of outdoor swimming or perspiration.*

7. *SUNGLASSES: Protect eyes from UVA-UVB, even on cloudy days.*

8. *WEIGHT-TRAINING GLOVES: Most underrated weight-lifting tool— use them.*

9. *TRAINING LOG: Keep tabs on your progress, personalize your log.*

10. *SAFETY GEAR: Wear a helmet (for biking and skiing) and light yourself up like a Christmas tree with reflective materials and battery-operated lights anytime after dusk.*

Find the Right Shoes

Never underestimate the benefits of a good pair of running shoes. Follow these tips:

- *WEAR MEDIUM-WEIGHT SHOES: Look for shoes that weigh ten to twelve ounces. While some shoe experts recommend that the heavier you are, the heavier the shoe you should wear, for most people a pair of fourteen-ounce shoes will feel like you're carrying a potato on your foot and will disrupt your gait. When it comes to shoes, less is often more.*

- *AVOID ORTHOTICS IF POSSIBLE: Even if you overpronate as many runners do, I think that orthotics make feet weak and lazy, as will motion-control shoes. Pronation is a natural shock absorber and too much motion control interferes with this. Most people need a little stability, and some people really need motion-control shoes, but you want to get as close to a neutral shoe as possible. Think of keeping your feet strong without too much support and you can help keep them injury-free.*

- *FIND A SHOE BALANCED BETWEEN CUSHIONING AND DURABILITY: Shoes with a firm heel strike combined with good cushioning on the forefoot but firm, durable EVA outsoles are great for running. I personally don't like mushy heel strikes but prefer a beefy midsole with a firm poplike feel while running on the hard sand near the surf line at the beach. This is opposed to the sinking feeling in soft sand, which requires more effort to spring out of and is actually harder on your joints.*

YOUR WORKOUT UNIFORM
USE IT. OWN IT.

Opportunity is missed by most people because it is dressed in overalls and looks like work.

THOMAS EDISON

Use your workout clothes like a surgeon in his scrubs, a soldier in his fatigues, an actor in her costume, or a police officer in his blue to transfer your mindset when on athletic duty. Putting on exercise clothing is the strongest reinforcer to signal your nervous system that you are in athlete mode and about to work out. With consistent ritualization, putting on these clothes will trigger a physiological shift that releases neurochemicals to energize your body to move. Trigger your volition switch to go! Attach a psychological significance to your athletic gear. You want to be able to say, "That's my uniform." But remember to keep it subtle, and keep it simple. No one else needs to know that a gray cotton tank top or a faded cap is part of a uniform, even if it is.

- *SHIRTS: Cotton is fine if you're not sweating a lot. Wear a Coolmax wicking fabric or knits that have a piqué texture knit weave if you are running indoors or will be sweating a lot. Sheer fabrics will cling to your skin like Saran Wrap.*

- *SHORTS: Look for fabrics that are not going to chafe. And if you are going to sweat a lot, wear lightweight shorts that don't absorb too much water.*

- *COMPRESSION SHORTS: Wear compression fabrics with Lycra or Supplex to reduce muscle fatigue on long workouts and to prevent chafing.*

- *SOCKS: Cotton socks are fine if you're not sweating a lot—if you are, try a lightweight crew made out of a wicking fabric like Coolmax.*

- *RUNNING CAP: Running caps are great for blocking the sun, keeping your head cool, and keeping sweat out of your eyes. They also serve to block out peripheral distractions (I call it "blinder's down" mode) and make it easier to stay focused.*

- *A LIGHTWEIGHT, WATERPROOF SLICKER/ANORAK: Buy it big so that you can wear it over cold-weather gear.*

- *SWEATPANTS: Great for lifting weights or running outside in weather under seventy degrees.*

- *HAT AND GLOVES: Mandatory for outdoor training in temperatures under forty degrees.*

- *WEIGHT-LIFTING GLOVES: Most important accessory for effective strength training.*

- *LAYERING: In cold or inclement weather: Always start with a base layer of a wicking fabric; use a second layer for insulation, and a third layer for protection from the elements.*

- *VEST: Great for keeping your core temperature up while allowing mobility of your arms.*

NO SUCH THING AS BAD WEATHER
. . . JUST BAD GEAR OR A BAD ATTITUDE

Gray skies are just clouds passing over.

FRANK GIFFORD

A favorite Norwegian saying of mine is, "There is no such thing as bad weather, just bad gear," which is heard often in Scandinavia in response to complaints about the cold, wind, and snow. With the advances that have been made in synthetic fabrics, there is no excuse not to dress in a way that makes working out in any climate possible. If the weather outside looks ominous and your dread factor is high, just bundle up or waterproof. You'll feel great once you're out there if you have the right gear. I repeat my Norwegian saying every time I bundle up to bike crosstown in frigid temperatures, and it always puts the weather in perspective, and makes me feel in control of it, not a victim of it.

The sea was wet as wet could be, the sands were dry as dry. You could not see a cloud because no cloud was in the sky.

LEWIS CARROLL ("THE WALRUS AND THE CARPENTER")

USE A SPORTS WATCH METHODICALLY
MAXIMIZE EVERY SECOND

We are going to get in two good hours of practice even if it takes six hours.

LOU HOLTZ

Time is one of the most valuable commodities in everyone's lives, and you don't want to waste it. Use the stopwatch as a way to keep yourself on schedule and to break a workout down into doable doses. The physical act of clearing and starting your stopwatch will directly trigger your volition switch. Starting the watch will trigger the small clusters of neurons that fire like a gun going off at a starting line. Ready, set . . . go!

SAFETY
HELMETS, REFLECTIVE GEAR, BLINKING LIGHTS

Safety should always be a top priority when you are working out. Wear a helmet any time you are biking. Buy other appropriate gear to keep yourself injury-free: wrist guards, reflective clothing, and blinking lights. You are invisible to drivers at night if you are out walking, biking, or jogging. Light yourself up like a Christmas tree, which is the term used by Chris Kostman, race director of Badwater races. In ultra-racing, you learn to be covered in reflective materials and blinking lights at night. Do the same on your nighttime workouts.

- *The Centers for Disease Control (CDC) states that there are three hundred thousand sports-related brain concussions in the United States each year.*

- *Wearing a helmet reduces the risk of brain injury by as much as 88 percent.*

- *Never dive into water in which you can't see the bottom.*

- *Follow the traffic rules when you cycle; ride on the right-hand side. When you walk, jog, or run, stay on the left side and move against traffic, so you can see the cars coming toward you and move out of the way if you have to.*

Below are the core tenets of *The Athlete's Way* prescriptive—this is the philosophy in a nutshell. You can apply these principles to your cardio, strength, and stretching routines that I will go into detailed description of in chapters 6, 7, and 8.

"THE ATHLETE'S WAY" *PRESCRIPTIVE*

1. *SET GOALS/ACHIEVE THEM: Long-, short-, and present-term goals; micro and macro wins*

2. *ANTICIPATION/EXPECTATION: Create eagerness; expect success*

3. *MENTOR/MASTERY: Role models. Practice, patience, persistence*

4. *DAILY PRACTICE/SACRALIZE: Ritual and routine. Consistent behavior*

5. COMPETITION/CAMARADERIE: *Do your best. Build kinship*

6. CREATING FLOW/STAYING PRESENT: *Lose yourself in the present tense. Concentrate*

7. CROSS-TALK/EXECUTIVE FUNCTION: *Guide inner dialogue. Learned optimism*

8. REWARD CIRCUITRY/TOKEN ECONOMY: *The carrot vs. the stick. Reward*

9. TRIGGERS AND CUES: *Create a spark and chain reaction*

10. MENTAL TOUGHNESS/RESILIENCE: *Fight to the finish; bounce back*

1. Set Goals/Achieve Them
Long-, Short-, and Present-term Goals. Create Micro-macro Wins

Find something that you're really interested in doing in your life. Pursue it, set goals, and commit yourself to excellence. Do the best you can.

                                                CHRIS EVERT

Setting goals and achieving them is the foundation of any successful athletic process. It guarantees a constant supply of dopamine, which is released during goal-oriented behavior and upon achieving a goal. Reward deficiency syndrome is marked by low dopamine and a feeling of malaise when someone is not cognizant of the need to achieve goals. Making your bed in the morning can be a dopamine releaser if you acknowledge it as such. Set up the playing field every day to release dopamine by setting lots of mini goals and achieving them.

Set up three tiers of goals: long term, short term, and present term. Consider the accomplishment of each a macro or micro win. The long-term goal hovers as the prime motivating force that is played out day by day. This would be a race for which you're preparing or your commitment to working out most days of the week for a month. The daily process itself becomes the short-term goal every morning when you wake up and renew your commitment to follow through with the daily practice. Once you are actually working out and inside the athletic process, you need to compartmentalize the entire workout into doable doses—or mini molehills—chunks of time or distance that represent the present-term micro goal and micro wins. Each goal will release a hit of dopamine. This could be finishing one set of three when you are lifting weights.

Nothing is so fatiguing as the eternal hanging on of an uncompleted task.

WILLIAM JAMES

The playing field should be set up so that you are constantly nudging gently against your own limits, which will engage you by being challenging but not overwhelming. To create positive reinforcement, you want to finish what you start and achieve what you set out to do. Don't sabotage yourself by setting unrealistically high goals. One of the key principles of tailoring *The Athlete's Way* program is for you to create goals that are challenging but achievable. Only through this success are the cascade of neuropeptides released. Lifelong changes are just a series of daily recommitments strung together. Regroup from failure and keep moving forward. Reassess and rebound; modify the goal if you have to.

2. Anticipation/Expectations
Create Eagerness. Expect Success

I couldn't wait for the sun to come up the next morning so that I could get out on the course again.

BEN HOGAN

Anticipation creates excitement, eagerness, and arousal, which gives you the epinephrine (adrenaline) to get you psyched up and the momentum to start working out. Creating anticipation starts by flashing forward in your mind's eye and composing mental snapshots of each stage of the athletic experience, imagining how it will feel, and seeing yourself succeeding. See yourself starting the workout, going through the motions, breaking a sweat, getting through it, and feeling great when it's done. Bring the workout to life and always picture yourself finishing.

It is fatal to enter any war without the will to win it.
GENERAL DOUGLAS MACARTHUR

Make success your only option. To do this, you must see yourself completing the action. Success becomes hardwired. Once the ball is in motion, you move with the volition that you will succeed, *and* keep self-doubt at bay throughout the process. Anticipation, eagerness, and expectations give you the velocity to create a self-fulfilling prophecy.

3. Role Model—Mentor/Mastery
Character Work. Practice, Patience, Perseverance

The best and fastest way to learn a sport is to watch and imitate a champion.

JEAN-CLAUDE KILLY

Use mentors and role models to mold yourself into who you want to be. This is done primarily by stimulating the mirror neurons. Identify the specific character traits you admire in your athletic heroes and integrate these qualities into your own belief system and daily behavior.

Mastery is the process of the protégé becoming experienced and trained. To do this, you need to adopt the athletic credo and renew a commitment to stick with it every day. Mastery requires that you be patient. Only through consistent daily practice will the neural grooves be carved deeper and deeper and make thinking like an athlete innate.

Mastery is about having the dedication to practice a lot and stick with it even through the plateaus; to push against your own limits and constantly strive for excellence. Through mastery you will evolve and improve, and your efforts will make you a role model for someone else. Remember, as Paul Coffey said, "Nobody's a natural. You work hard to get good and then work to get better." Be patient. Practice every day.

If people knew how hard I have had to work to gain my mastery, it wouldn't seem wonderful at all.

MICHELANGELO

4. Sacralize Daily Practice
Ritual and Routine. Consistent Behavior

*Do every day or two something for no other reason than you would
rather not do it, so that when the hour of dire need draws nigh, it
may find you not unnerved and untrained to stand the test.*

WILLIAM JAMES

The key to creating good habits is to develop personal rituals and routines that become almost sacred to you. Make your routines ceremonial.
These routines create synaptic changes in your brain that will make you
hardwired. The process of creating good habits leads to consistent behavior.
We are all creatures of habit, and the associations connected to behavior are
strong reinforcers of a positive routine. It is important to commit every
morning to daily practice, because for neuroplastic changes to stay hard-
ened, they must be reinforced.

The goal of having a ritual and routine is to create a Pavlovian response
or a chain reaction of synapses firing in a particular sequence that causes the
mind to click over into an automatic athletic state. Packing the gym bag, setting up the iPod, putting on sunscreen, smelling the eucalyptus in the locker
room, lacing up your sneakers . . . are small and seemingly insignificant, but
taken together are a big part of helping your brain click into athletic mode.

*Excellence is not a singular act, but a habit. You are what you re-
peatedly do.*

SHAQUILLE O'NEAL

Rituals and routine wire your brain in what is called contiguity. The
neurons get used to firing in a certain sequence. If you stop and buy a
Gatorade or an espresso every day before your workout, this action cocks
the trigger. Your nervous system begins preparing for the gym by pumping
adrenaline. Equally important to the process of creating good habits is
breaking bad ones by disengaging from them and causing their neural
pathways to atrophy and disconnect.

As part of your sacralizing, try building a shrine on a dresser or put pictures of things that inspire or motivate you on your refrigerator door. Attach
significance to these images and objects. On my fridge I have pictures of
Lance Armstrong, the Hawaii Ironman swim start, family and friends, a
Norwegian flag, funny postcards people have sent me, a Superman magnet.

These things remind me every morning of my mission to aspire and give back. On my dresser, I have souvenirs from races and mementos I've collected my entire life. Begin to surround yourself with things that remind you of why you do it. *The Athlete's Way* is about having fun, being happy, and achieving goals. I urge you to use anything and everything that inspires you.

5. Competition/Camaraderie
Always Do the Best You Can. Build Kinship

Call it a clan, call it a network, call it a tribe, call it a family: Whatever you call it, whoever you are, you need one.

JANE HOWARD

Bonding with other human beings through sport is a cornerstone of *The Athlete's Way*. It releases feel-good Oxytocin and Vasopressin. Camaraderie, loyalty, and magnanimity are characteristics that you should strive for as you go through your daily athletic process. Be generous about spreading around the joy of life you get from sport with everyone you come in contact with. That said, *The Athlete's Way* is also about maximizing your own potential and the best way to do that is to be competitive with yourself and with your comrades.

Competition is a good thing. Although athletic rivals are the enemy on the playing field, they are usually teammates, friends, comrades, and a part of your social network. Athletics is a great way of making friends and becoming part of a social network. Friendship and belonging to a community are at the top of the list for creating happiness and longevity. Find camaraderie in competition.

People work out together but they are often competing, too, which is a perfect dynamic. The sweaty bodies in the spin class room represent the individual and the collective to me; there is something tribal about sweating together. For times when you are training alone, under the fluorescent lights of a gym, out on the road, in your house, you are obviously just competing against yourself. This intrinsic desire to achieve your personal best is key to *The Athlete's Way*.

I'm trying as hard as I can, and sometimes things don't go your way, and that's the way things go.

TIGER WOODS

When training indoors, the level of resistance or the blinking light of a pacer is going to be your competition. Remember always to push your limits. I've raced the digital, red, blinking lights on the dashboard of a cardio machine around the globe a couple times at this point. They keep you challenged and rewarded. Set the pace so that you have to focus and fight to the finish. When you do lose to a person or a pacer, don't feel defeated. Instead, feel inspired to work harder to avoid it happening again.

6. Creating Flow/Staying Focused
Lose Yourself in the Present Tense

We must not just be in the world and above the world, but also of the world. To love it for what it is . . . is the only task. Avoid and you are lost. Lose yourself in it, and you are free.

HENRY MILLER

Flow can happen in anything you do, but especially in sport when you create a tonic level of exertion in which the skill level and challenge are perfectly balanced. When you are in a state of flow, you are engaged and focused. Anytime you feel listless, you need to increase the level of challenge, which will force you to concentrate and lose yourself. Flow is a paradox of being totally present, but also far gone. In a state of flow, you are always moving forward. When you are in the zone of your flow channel, you get things accomplished.

Concentration, confidence, competitive urge, capacity for enjoyment are the key. What do I mean by concentration? I mean focusing totally on the business at hand and commanding your body to do exactly what you want it to do.

ARNOLD PALMER

Creating flow will calm the electrical firing rates in your brain and release endocannabinoids to create a state of bliss. I call it *fluid performance*. Flow occurs when a person's skill level is perfectly balanced to the challenge level of a task that has clear goals and provides immediate feedback.

You'll want to make the state of flow a daily goal; it is one of the most sublime and therapeutic aspects of the athletic process. People enter a flow state when they are fully absorbed in an activity, during which they lose their sense of time and to a certain degree become what they are doing.

Make the state of flow an objective—when you get there take note, and tag everything surrounding the time, place, and circumstance that created it so you can re-create it. Use a trigger word like *yes* as a marker that you are in a state of flow.

Pass into nothingness.
JOHN KEATS

Being in a state of flow when you exercise is the key to making exercise a pleasurable experience because it allows you to lose yourself in the moment. You are totally engaged; time flies. If you ever get bored working out, the cure is simple—increase the level of difficulty. On the flip side, if you're overwhelmed, decrease the level of challenge. These perimeters are your flow channel. Flow is a state of mind and a feeling that you tune almost like a radio frequency by guiding thoughts and either increasing or decreasing the level of challenge. This process is very simple. Don't complicate it; you either want to go faster or slower (easier or harder) to create flow.

HOW TO CREATE FLOW

- Find the physical exertion level between boredom and feeling overwhelmed.

- Surf the cusp between your skill and the level of challenge.

- Gently nudge up against your comfort zone.

- Note the corresponding heart rate and perceived exertion that feels like tonic level.

- Allow the rhythm and repetition of cardio to put you into a trance.

- Learn to stay focused and engaged in the moment.

- If you are bored, increase the level of challenge.

- If you are overwhelmed, decrease the level of challenge.

- Let go, and lose yourself.

I have broken flow into two tiers. With fluid performance there is the regular state of flow, which is a launching pad to superfluidity, which feels ecstatic. Superfluidity is a point marked by the loss of all friction and viscosity and is a feeling that comes in waves. Superfluidity is an episodic ecstatic wave akin to an orgasm that you should strive for daily within the flow experience. To me it is the goal of flow, just as orgasm is the goal of intercourse. You build to superfluidity; you keep going and it comes around again. We will talk more about this elevated state of flow called superfluidity in the final chapter and compare it to what others have called peak experience and epiphanies in chapter 12.

7. Cross Talk/Inner Dialogue
Learn to Guide Self-Talk

As a kid I always idolized the winning athletes. It is one thing to idolize heroes. It is quite another to visualize yourself in their place. When I saw great people I said to myself, "I can be there."

ARNOLD SCHWARZENEGGER

In every workout there is going to be cross talk between the two main parts of your brain, the cerebrum and the cerebellum. The dialogue will go from the top down or from the bottom up. Your job as the athlete is to learn to hear your inner dialogue, and then guide it in a way that achieves your target mind-set or behavior. The cerebrum (up brain) is your center for volition and says what you should do. This is your autobiographical self talking, and it has ideals, ethics, and willpower. The cerebellum (down brain) is impulsive and intuitive and could be viewed as your primal self. This cross talk can be played out in a dialogue from down below saying, "I don't want to run up that hill." Your up brain sends the message: "You have to run up the hill, but you can walk when you get to the top."

Talk low, talk slow, and don't talk too much.

JOHN WAYNE

The higher serotonin levels in the frontal lobes have been linked to giving people the upper hand to guide inner dialogue constructively, because these levels make the tough neurons there stronger and more optimistic. This makes it easier to take an optimistic stance from the up brain to the down brain (called top-down processing). In any given workout an athlete encounters an array of situations, moods, peaks/valleys, and low points that need to be addressed. You can learn how to be creative about it.

You will learn to use many different voices to steer your inner dialogue but most important, you need to hone a master-and-commander voice that rules with an iron fist and says, "I'm the boss around here." Cross talk is a skill based on negotiating and making deals. Once you have gotten a signal that something needs to be addressed, use your executive decision making to correct the problem. More than anything else, this requires the use of your imagination.

A man's character may be learned from the adjectives which he habitually uses in conversation.

MARK TWAIN

Self-talk is different from cross talk. Self-talk is when the voices in your head are not in a dialogue. This can take the form of trigger words, or talking to yourself in the third person and actually using your name as a coach would. Self-talk usually consists of phrases that are generally no longer than three words and sound sophomoric outside the athletic process. When used inside the game, their power is profound—and sometimes profane. Also, talk to yourself in the third person like a coach would. I often add "Chris" to the end of most of these triggers or use my full name, including my middle name, Karr. I speak to myself in the tone a parent might use when reprimanding a child in a "go to your room" kind of way.

SOME OF MY FAVORITE TRIGGER WORDS I SAY TO MYSELF

Yes.

You can do it.

That's right.

Go.

Move swift.

Come on.

Move it.

Hang on in there, baby.

Feet, fail me not.

Keep it together.

Keep doing what you're doing.

Don't give up now.

You can make it.

You suck.

Don't fuck with me.

Don't fuck up.

Under certain circumstances, profanity provides a relief denied even to prayer.

MARK TWAIN

Sometimes the tough love of a drill sergeant is the best approach. I am not a believer in always talking positive. Now and then you need to be hard on yourself and kick your own ass. Find your own trigger words and phrases inside the athletic process. Remember these are very personal. Keep a list of phrases that work. These phrases are state dependent. You have to see what bubbles up for you inside the athletic process and use those.

8. Reward Circuitry/Token Economy
The Carrot vs. the Stick

The most difficult thing is the decision to act, the rest is merely tenacity. The fears are paper tigers. You can do anything you decide to do. You can act to change and control your life; and the procedure, the process is its own reward.

AMELIA EARHART

In terms of triggering your reward circuitry, you are always going to use positive reinforcement (the carrot) to create an incentive to exercise. When you activate your reward circuitry, you get a hit of dopamine. Once the goal is set, the trigger is cocked for reward mechanism and the surge of adrenaline to move kick-starts the cycle of urge-action-reward-relief. The relief will be the hit when you achieve your goal. Flash-forward to a reward or a token that you'll receive after the workout to create the urge to take action. With practice, you'll figure out how to create a token economy in which you are rewarded for specific behavior and learn to associate that with pleasure psychologically but also neurochemically.

The dopamine pathway is activated when you anticipate working out and sparks the cascade of neurochemicals that will lead you into a state of bliss. Not only should there be a prize at the end of the workout, like a cold glass of water, a hot shower, a meal, downtime on the couch, but there should also be mental molehills and bartering for micro wins or eager anticipation of the reward as you move toward the goal. Play game-show host by breaking a bigger workout into mini wins. Okay, two miles down, I'm at the turnaround. Two more to go. I'm heading home. This would be a micro goal within a bigger workout. You should practice chunking the run into much smaller doses. Each stage has a much different psychological angle. Maximize your approach to each.

9. Triggers and Cues
Create the Spark and Chain Reaction

The inner fire is the most important thing that mankind possesses.

EDITH SODERGRAN

You need to find external and internal triggers or cues to get you motivated. These could be anything from a thought, a song, a piece of jewelry, a rubber band, a smell, or even a cup of coffee before a workout (caffeine works, in moderation). If used effectively, all these serve as reinforcers to help maintain an attitude and behavior that lead to peak performance and achieving your goals. Begin to move with intent and find props that can be trigger your psyche to click into athletic mind-set.

People with rejection sensitivity who feel intimidated tend to slouch, reinforcing a state of insecurity and low serotonin. My advice is stand tall— shoulders back and chin up. This sends signals from your nervous system that you are in control and releases neurochemicals associated with a state that will make you calm and relaxed. Lifting your head high and opening up your shoulder width will not only give you great posture, but that posture will also create a feedback loop and signal your nervous system to create that motivated mood. Imagine a triangle from the top of your head connecting to your shoulders; then make the sides of the triangle each as long as possible. Plant your feet firmly and imagine another triangle from shoulders to toes so you are stretched like a kite.

Success is not the result of spontaneous combustion. You must set yourself on fire.

REGGIE LEACH

Since every person is lifted or motivated by his own unique combination of triggers, you have to find what works for you through experience. The goal is to begin creating an arsenal or toolbox of internal (psychological), external (tactile), and physical (bodily) triggers and cues that will help you stay upbeat and strong through every workout. Keep track of these mentally and in your workbook. The lesson work here will be done mostly on note cards; it is crucial to document which triggers and cues work for you while they're still fresh, ideally from inside the athletic process itself. When you have access to state-dependent memory, have pen and pad handy to jot down insights ASAP after a workout.

10. Mental Toughness/Resilience
Fight to the Finish

Suffering becomes beautiful when anyone bears great calamities with cheerfulness, not through insensibility but through greatness of mind.

ARISTOTLE

Mental toughness and resilience is often just about sheer force of will, but it is also about the ability to choose your point of view by rearranging and selecting perceptions of reality. Mental toughness is cerebral; it originates in your cerebrum and is sent top down.

Ask yourself the ultimate quitter barometer question: "Is quitting now a matter of can't or won't?" If you can't do it, you can't do it. But if it's a matter not wanting to, then try to do it. Rate on a scale of one to ten how bad it really is. Usually you realize it's not that bad. Part of mental toughness and resilience is based on an ability to adapt or to learn how to dwell on the positive and accept the negative things that can't be changed. The weather is a perfect example. Since the weather is something that is out of your control, the athlete has two choices: to associate/attach (dwell on it) or dissociate/detach (let it go). Letting it go and choosing to think about something else is obviously the best thing to do.

You must guide and sift your thoughts based on a cognitive executive decision that you have no control and the visceral understanding that attaching to positive thoughts gives you energy and that negative thinking is draining. If you begin to think with an optimistic perspective, the neurons associated with that frame of mind will get fortified.

> *You become what you think about.*
> **EARL NIGHTINGALE**

SPORTSMANLIKE CONDUCT
THE GOLDEN RULE

> *Live so that you wouldn't be ashamed to sell the family parrot to the town gossip.*
>
> **WILL ROGERS**

In closing, I bring up the importance of always being a good sport as part of *The Athlete's Way* code of conduct. Play fair and be a gracious winner and an equally gracious loser. Live by the Golden Rule: "Do unto others as you would have them do unto you."

Athletics is a perfect venue for anyone to foster the core values of fairness and respect, especially if the emphasis is on loving the process and taking pride in good sportsmanship, not just whether you win or lose. "Once upon a time, parenting was largely about training children to take their proper place in their community, which, in large measure, meant learning to play by the rules and cooperate," said Alvin Rosenfeld, a child psychiatrist. "There was a time when there was a certain code of conduct by which you viewed the character of a person," he said, "and you needed that code of conduct to have your place in the community." Being a good sport is hands-down one of the key traits of the athletic mind-set. *The Athlete's Way* represents a code of conduct based on integrity, good manners, fairness, and respect.

> *Sometimes when we are generous in small, barely detectable ways it can change someone else's life forever.*
>
> **MARGARET CHO**

CHAPTER SIX

THE CARDIO PROGRAM

Whenever I get the urge to exercise, I lie down until it goes away.
ROBERT MAYNARD HUTCHINS (FORMER PRESIDENT, UNIVERSITY OF CHICAGO)

THE CARDIO PRESCIPTIVE
EXERCISE IS A BRAIN TONIC

FREQUENCY: *Three to five days per week.*

TIME: *Twenty to sixty minutes of movement daily. Done continuously or broken into chunks.*

INTENSITY: *Tonic level, which is around 60 to 80 percent of your maximum possible heart rate (maximum heart rate [MHR] is generally considered to be 220 minus your age).*

TYPE: *Continuous, aerobic, rhythmic movement using large muscle groups with a few anaerobic bursts every week. Aerobic means in the presence of oxygen. The bulk of your cardio workouts should be at this tonic exertion level, where your muscles are using oxygen as fuel. Anaerobic exercise takes place in the absence of oxygen. At intense levels of exertion your body doesn't use oxygen in the muscles to produce movement. Anaerobic exercise is intense, but in small doses extremely beneficial.*

Cardiovascular exercise should be the keystone of your health and fitness program. In this chapter, we will cover all the specifics of a cardio program. I will give you detailed advice on structuring and getting through workouts. Regularly moving your body by doing aerobic-rhythmic movement using large muscle groups is crucial for staying healthy. This chapter teaches you the nuts and bolts of structuring workouts and gives you the know-how to put together a training calendar. The most useful tool for gauging your exertion level and structuring workouts is heart rate.

The most valuable feedback to gauge how hard you are working is beats per minute (BPM). There are many formulas for calculating your maximum heart rate and then finding a level of exertion based on a percentage of that rate. None of these is perfectly accurate.

Just do something! Do! Something!
JOHN PASSERO, HAWTHORNE PREMIERSHIP-WINNING
COACH

The ballpark formula for calculating your maximum heart rate is 220 minus your age. The numbers can be misleading, so use them as a starting point. There are so many factors involved in calculating your heart zones that you need to be tested using lactate in blood levels to get accurate readings on your maximum heart rate potential. On the flip side of maximum heart rate, resting heart rate (taken in the morning before you sit up in bed) is the best benchmark of improved fitness. Keep tabs on this. If a downward trend reverses, this is the first warning sign that you are overtraining, or not training enough, depending on your modus operandi

I encourage you to purchase a simple heart-rate monitor and pay attention to the specific BPMs you see at various levels of exertion. The most basic Polar model is my favorite. Get to know your heart rates related to perceived exertion and power output (calories/watts). Remember, you are your own universe when it comes to heart rate. Don't compare yourself with charts or athletes around you. I tend to have a very low heart rate; however, athletes running at the same speed as I am but with a higher heart rate could have a lower perceived rate of exertion based on their physiology. It's all relative to your unique physiology. Once you know your own baselines you can use this information to monitor your progress and keep tabs on your target zones.

Being strapped into a heart-rate monitor for every workout can become tiresome because you feel constricted. The key to associating sweat with bliss is learning to find your tonic level of exertion intuitively. Interpreting feedback from heart rate, energy output, and perceived exertion is good for getting started and to use for peak performance and honing in on your flow channel. Once you know what your target heart rate feels like, and what level opens the door to superfluidity, you should be able to tune into that frequency without the use of any gadgets. Remember to make your desired mental state your pilot. Make a fluid and superfluid performance, and the state of mind that goes with it, the destination of every workout.

> *Success or failure depends more upon attitude than upon capacity. Successful men act as though they have accomplished or are enjoying something. Soon it becomes a reality. Act, look, feel successful, conduct yourself accordingly, and you will be amazed at the positive results.*
>
> WILLIAM JAMES

The most important factor in your success will be creating a program that fits your personality. You have to find physical activities you enjoy doing in a comfortable environment. If you are extroverted, work out with other people. If you enjoy exercise as a time away from the world to sift your thoughts, do something solitary. Remember to mix it up. Variety is going to keep you engaged and interested, not to mention injury-free. If you have different options, you can vary your routine to fit your state of mind and will be much more likely to stick with it.

MINIMUM GUIDELINES FOR CARDIO BENEFIT

> *You've got to stick at a thing, a particular thing, until you succeed. I feel that's the only way to succeed—by concentrating on something in particular. Once you know what you've got to do you will succeed, you will succeed.*
>
> BETTY CUTHBERT

The minimum weekly time commitment you need to make is 120 minutes of cardio, broken up in any way that fits your schedule. Aim for at least twenty minutes most days of the week, but also keep tabs of your weekly time totals. The cumulative time spent moving each week is the most important gauge to keep track of over the long haul. Jot down the total minutes per week spent on cardio in a special column of your workbook. This way you can look for trends in your behavior and chart your averages like a stock market analyst. If you don't like to write things down, keep mental tabs. If you are a fastidious log keeper, you can also jot down your overall time and then have a subcategory of time spent working out anaerobically above 80 percent of your maximum heart rate. Aim for a minimum of twelve minutes per week spent exercising at an anerobic level, or "red lining it" as I like to say. To make the high level of exertion easier to cope with, break it down into smaller units, or intervals, of one to six minutes over the course of three to four workouts. Again—the harder you work in the shortest amount of time, the more bang you'll get for your buck. Make anaerobic exercise part of your weekly routine and you'll get faster, stronger, leaner, and happier.

Just remember, 100 percent of the shots you don't take, don't go in.
WAYNE GRETZKY

THREE TIERS OF CARDIO TRAINING

THREE OPTIONS BASED ON TIME AVAILABILITY AND YOUR OBJECTIVES

1. *BEGINNER/MAINTENANCE (2 to 3 hours weekly) 2 to 3 percent of week*

2. *INTERMEDIATE/MASTERY (3 to 5 hours weekly) 3 to 5 percent of week*

3. *ADVANCED/COMPETITIVE (5 hours weekly) 5 percent of week*

*Based on 8 hours of sleep a night and a 112-hour-awake week.

The three tiers of *The Athlete's Way* cardio program are based on your time availability and your personal goals. Choose the level of time commitment that fits your lifestyle, then make a schedule based on these weekly commitments. As your life changes from week to week, month to month, or year to year, you can adapt the amount of time you spend working out. Remember, you want to aim for a minimum of 120 minutes of cardio per week. Look at your calendar and see where you have windows of time available to meet the requirements of the level that you choose.

STRUCTURING WORKOUTS
INTENSITY, DURATION, FREQUENCY

The Three Pillars to Structuring a Weekly Program

1. DURATION: *How long you work out.*

2. FREQUENCY: *How often you work out.*

3. INTENSITY: *How hard you work out.*

DURATION: You should aim to do cardio for between twenty and forty-five minutes a session for a total of 120 to 240 minutes (two to four hours) per week. The thirty-minute workout four to five times a week is ideal for most people. The forty-five-minute workout to me is the gold standard if you have time, because it allows for a proper warm-up, thirty minutes of flow, and a cooldown.

FREQUENCY: How many times you work out will most likely depend on your schedule. You should aim for thirty minutes of cardio most days of the week. Look at your calendar and see what days you can work out. Remember to sneak in a six-minute anaerobic burst any day you are short on time. These are highly beneficial to your heart and stress level.

INTENSITY: Establishing the intensity at which you are working out requires feedback. When you are exercising indoors, the display panel in front of you offers direct external feedback to the level of intensity of your workout. The mechanisms for monitoring intensity indoors on a machine are going to be heart rate, perceived exertion, watts (energy expended), speed, cadence, level, and calories burned (expanded on below). If you exercise outdoors, your intensity will generally be monitored only by heart rate, speed, and rate of perceived exertion.

Monitoring Feedback

There is a vitality, a life force, an energy, a quickening, that is trans-
lated through you into action, and because there is only one of you
in all time, this expression is unique.

MARTHA GRAHAM

In structuring a workout program, you need to monitor feedback and establish your baselines. Remember that you are unique. Get to know yourself
without comparing yourself too much to others. You can start by simply establishing three basic zones: easy, medium, and hard, with a plus or minus
on either side. Most people have three basic gears that have a heart-rate zone
and a level of perceived exertion attached to each. To fine-tune your training
zones, you must get to know the feedback associated with each zone. Try to
spend most of your time in the medium zone, your flow channel.

If you are training inside, the gym's equipment gives you the best instant feedback and makes it easy to stay in your flow channel, which is between 60 and 80 percent maximum exertion. This level of intensity is where
exercise is going to feel just right. This is the level between boredom and
anxiety where you are engaged and challenged but not overwhelmed.

On the following page is information you can use on the machines at
your gym to give you the feedback you need. In general, I recommend ig-
noring the charts pasted on the machines. Establish your personal zones instead. Remember that you are your own universe when it comes to heart
rate and perceived exertion. Get to know your body. Don't think about fat-
burning zones or guide your workouts based on charts or formulas, which
tend to be inaccurate. Learn through trial and error what various heart rates
feel like to you.

Rating Perceived Exertion (RPE)

For fast acting relief try slowing down.

LILY TOMLIN

No one knows you better than you know yourself. Whether or not you
wear a heart-rate monitor, you should get in the habit of rating perceived exertion on a 1 to 5 (+/−) scale. The term RPE refers to exactly what it says;
you'll rate the level of exertion based on your own perceptions. It is designed
to be subjective. Some days, your regular workout is a breeze, some days, it's

a bitch. The good news is that many days when you go into a workout feeling like total crap, it turns out to be incredible. And on the flip side—you go into some workouts feeling elated and they end up being mediocre. The unpredictability of what is going to happen inside the athletic process should inspire you to work out, and hang in there, instead of aborting the mission prematurely. On days when it's feeling much harder, rate it with a harder RPE. In general, though, as your level of fitness improves, your RPE of the same level of exertion will result in a lower rating of perceived exertion because you are stronger and more efficient and it feels easier.

You can learn to rate your exertion by paying attention to the cues of lactic acid—muscles burn, breathing deepens, and you gasp for breath. Inner dialogue becomes scattered or overwhelmed, as does your overall explanatory style at that level of exertion. Generally, when you're working out at a tonic level you can be contemplative and have a wide-angle lens of thought and vision to the world around you. The harder your workout, the smaller the aperture becomes, and you begin to be more microscopic in your focus. At a high level of exertion you can't think about much other than the task at hand, and how much it hurts. If you are working out with a partner, or if you like talking to yourself like I do when working out, you can use the talk test described below:

THE 5-POINT RATING PERCEIVED EXERTION SCALE AND TALK TEST

1. *VERY EASY: You could sing a song (40 to 50 percent maximum heart rate).*

2. *EASY: You could carry on a regular conversation (50 to 60 percent).*

3. *MODERATE: You could speak four- to six-word sentences (60 to 80 percent). *Tonic Level**

4. *HARD: You could express short two- or three-word thoughts (80 to 85 percent)*

5. *VERY HARD: You could grunt and use sign language (85 to 100 percent)*

You want to spend most of your time working out at level 3 on the perceived exertion scale. This is going to be your tonic level. Anyone who exercises regularly nestles into this level of exertion intuitively. It is the point of balanced challenge. Constantly nudging up against the upper end of level 3 is going to be the key to creating flow. Work out just hard enough to get your juices going. As you improve, remember to increase the level of challenge to stay engaged.

External Feedback

All feedback on cardio machinery is going to be interconnected. If you keep your bike in the same gear and increase your cadence, your energy production (watts) goes up, as does your speed and your heart rate. Use all the feedback effectively to structure your workouts.

WATTS: The number of watts that you produce when exercising is a measurement that is directly linked to how much power you are producing. If there were a lightbulb attached to a generator on your stationary bike, the harder you pedal, the more watts you create, and the brighter the bulb will shine. Watts are directly linked to calories burned. Both are measurements of energy expenditure. Wattage is the best tool to gauge exertion, because it is a constant. Professional cyclists attach watt meters to their pedals so they can get a clear gauge of how much power they are pushing through the pedals at a given time. Even if he is biking into a headwind or uphill and the miles per hour looks slow, the biker knows that the rate of exertion is staying consistent if the wattage is consistent.

CADENCE-RPM: Revolutions per minute. This is how many times you do a repetitive motion in sixty seconds—it is also called cadence or turnover. In all cardio sports you have a rhythm that is set by turnover or cadence. In general, the faster the cadence, the faster you go. Bike cadence should be around 80 to 90 RPMs for biomechanical efficiency. Anything under 70 RPMs is called mashing and is bad for your joints and ineffective. Above 100 RPMs is too fast to be biomechanically efficient for most mortals. But you should aim for a high turnover. Move swiftly and keep it peppy to make the pedal stroke fluid and put less stress on your knees. Push as hard going down on the pedal as you do pulling up. In biking, you want to float on the pedals; to do this you need to exert equal pressure throughout the 360 degrees of the pedal stroke. The same cadence with a lower gear produces higher wattage and faster speed, so if you can keep it peppy in a high gear you will put out more energy and go faster.

MPH/LEVEL: Whether you're running, biking, or working on a stationary machine, look at miles per hour or level as part of your energy exertion equation. On a treadmill, the speed and grade are your level. I recommend running at .5 percent or 1 percent incline to emulate what it feels like to run outside. A 0 percent incline is almost like running downhill. The faster and steeper the grade, the higher the watts/calories being burned. On other equipment, the level is going to be the gear you are in. Increasing cadence, or turnover, at the same level is going to increase wattage/calories burned. They are all linked.

CALORIES PER HOUR: Most of the machines at the gym will give you a number for calories burned. This number is hypothetical but a good benchmark within the universe of that particular machine and your personal metabolism. If you use the same piece of home exercise equipment, seeing 200 calories burned at the end of a workout may not be accurate, but if you burn 250 the next day, you can be assured that you expended about 25 percent more calories. For keeping tabs on energy out I recommend writing down the numbers in a training log, not because they are accurate, but because you can keep tabs on your estimated calories out. Remember, one pound of fat equals 3,500 calories. Burning 350 calories a day—and keeping caloric intake the same—would result in losing a pound of fat in ten days.

CARDIORESPIRATORY FUNCTION
THE NUTS AND BOLTS OF PHYSIOLOGY

Few are those who see with their own eyes and feel with their own hearts.

ALBERT EINSTEIN

Many people don't realize that the heart is actually comprised of two pumps that work independently of each other. Aerobic and anaerobic exercise is called cardio-respiratory because the heart and lungs are directly linked as part of the circulation loop that delivers oxygen to every cell in your body. It takes about sixty seconds for one red blood cell to complete a loop inside your body. Here's how it works:

1. *The right-ventricle chamber of the heart receives deoxygenated blood from the body and pumps that blood down into the lungs*

for aeration, the removal of carbon dioxide, and addition of oxygen.

2. As you breathe out, the lungs exhale the carbon dioxide and with the inhalation, you take in oxygen, which is put into the hemoglobin of blood in the lungs. This oxygenated blood is then sent back up to the heart.

3. The left-ventricle chamber of the heart receives the oxygenated blood and pumps it out through the body. The substance that human blood resembles most closely in terms of chemical composition is sea water.

THE FORTY-EIGHT-HOUR "INERTIA TRAP"
TWO DAYS WITHOUT SWEAT = SLUGLIKE STATE

Luck is a dividend of sweat. The more you sweat, the luckier you get.
RAY KROC

Whenever I feel a bead of sweat come off my skin I have a habit of saying "Take that to the bank." To me each drop of sweat is an investment in feeling healthy and happy. You have a twenty-four to forty-eight-hour grace period after a workout to feel the benefits in your bloodstream and in your state of mind. After twenty-four hours, blood levels return to a sedentary, dyspeptic mode. Ideally, you should be working out within a thirty-six-hour window as you move through the week. If you work out on a Monday night, you can feel the benefits all day Tuesday, but by Wednesday morning they will be wearing off. Use this knowledge to motivate you not to let more than forty-eight hours pass without exercising.

THE SWITCH POINT
WHEN THE BLISS MOLECULES KICK IN

First comes the sweat. Then comes the beauty.
GEORGE BALANCHINE

The hormones and neurotransmitters associated with the biology of bliss tend to kick in systematically at around seven to eight minutes into a workout—I call this the switch point. The first five minutes of working out is kind of like chewing glass and walking on hot coals for everyone—it is a shock to the system. That is why you should always start really, really slowly. This is the warm-up. Always warm up and cool down for at least five minutes each! I use the exclamation point here for emphasis. People neglect to do either. Give your body time to ease in and ease out of every workout. After seven to eight minutes, the *exocrine* system releases the first beads of sweat. You will see your skin start to glimmer if you work out indoors. This external signal is a cue that the *endocrine* system is revving up the neuro-transmitter pumps. Sweat is the external symbol of internal harmony of bliss hormones. Use this as a motivator.

The switch point is when you click over into an aerobic mode, into a state of fluidity. Take note of the switch point in every workout. Sometimes it takes longer to click over. Be patient! When you do click over, have a trigger word or gesture that symbolizes the switch. When you slip through that pinhole, say something like "I'm in." Flick your wrist, or your snap your neck to let your nervous system know that the workaday world is light-years away. Condition yourself to crave this transition, and your cerebellum will seek it intuitively. All animals seek pleasure and avoid pain. By conditioning the pleasure associated with this bliss you will learn to crave it. Stay conscious of the shift from the workaday world to the feeling of being inside an athletic vortex from which the vantage point on your life seems different. Everything tends to seem more beautiful from there.

ESTABLISHING YOUR BASELINES
YOU ARE YOUR OWN UNIVERSE

From the beginning I was an overachiever. That is to say, if you flatter me, or if you look at me the right way—I will kill myself to please you. It's very painful to be an overachiever.

LOUISE BOURGEOIS

- *RESTING HEART RATE: Your resting heart rate is an excellent way to gauge your level of fitness. To establish true resting heart rate you want to take your pulse before you sit up in bed after a full night's sleep. Find your pulse on your wrist or jugular vein, count the beats for six seconds, and multiply by ten.*

- *PERCENTAGE BODY FAT: In general your percentage of body fat is more important than your weight. The average man has 15 to 17 percent body fat, while the average woman has between 18 and 22 percent. Typical scores for elite athletes are 6 to 12 percent for men and 12 to 20 percent for women. You can get measured using calipers at most health clubs. There are also home scales that can measure body fat.*

- *FLOW CHANNEL: This is the level where exercise is going to feel blissful based on the biological electrochemical environment of your brain. And psychological engagement.*

- *TONIC LEVEL: Establish the level of exertion that corresponds to feeling engaged but not overwhelmed by the athletic process. Think of it as a groove of cannabinoids, endorphins, dopamine, and serotonin. Electrical rate of synapses is firing steadily.*

- *THE SWITCH POINT: This is the point when you've slipped into a state of fluid performance.*

- *THE PIERCING POINT: This is the point in any workout at which you feel yourself having a superfluid episode—when there is no real time or space for a second. This is the moment of bliss. You have slipped through the pinhole into Narnia or Wonderland. Always take note of the exact circumstance, so that you can re-create it. This is the holy grail of every workout and going back to this place provides a lifetime of yearning, inspiration, and daily recommitment.*

- *BASAL METABOLIC RATE: The minimum level of energy required to sustain the body's vital functions in the waking state. In general the equation for basal metabolic rate is your weight times 15 (e.g., 150 pounds × 15 = 2,250 calories a day). Remember strength training and cardio combined boosts metabolism most.*

- *BODY MASS INDEX (BMI): This is a general ratio of your height to weight. These charts are very misleading, and I don't recommend using them. You want to create as much lean body mass as possible. A pound of fat burns two calories a day; a pound of muscle burns thirty to fifty calories a day. That is why lifting weights is so important.*

MIX IT UP: CROSS-TRAINING AND VARIETY

Anytime you see someone more successful than you are, they are doing something you aren't.

MALCOLM X

Every athlete should cross-train. You want to pursue varied physical activities regularly not only to keep your muscles in balance, but also to keep you from getting bored. Cross-training is the best way to stay injury-free, exercise different muscle groups, and keep yourself interested. Be sure to build cross-training into your program. Runners who cross-train have stronger muscles, fewer injuries, and healthier cardiovascular systems than runners who don't. Excellent cross-training exercises for runners include strength training at the gym, biking, elliptical machines, cross-country ski and rowing machines, and upper-body machines like the arm bicycle and the upper-body exerciser (UBE), a terrific machine. Try to do a few minutes of upper- body cardio every day. I finish most bike rides or indoor runs with five to fifteen minutes of rowing or UBE before I stretch. It's a good cooldown.

Working out at various intensities and durations is the way to improve your level of fitness. You need to mix it up. Your body is constantly striving to maintain homeostasis and will adapt to the workload that you regularly put on it. Keep your body guessing by shuffling things around, overloading your system from different angles. Remember that overload is how we improve; just remember to give your body time to recover and rebuild.

If you are just working out to feel good and stay healthy, you can mix up your routine whimsically—do whatever you are in the mood for or have time for on a given day. Sometimes being pressed for time is the best impetus for having a short, high-quality workout. If you are planning to compete in a race, you should consider mixing up your workouts every day to cover the five types of workouts for a competitive training program. Also, mixing up the intensity and volume will keep you vital and protect you from injuries.

Listed below are the terminology and symbols I use in my coaching training logs. You can put them symbols on your training calendar to remind you of what that day's workout is. The pattern of symbols on a calendar will help you to make sure you are mixing it up.

♥ ***Base*** *(medium intensity-medium duration) The bread and butter of cardio work done at tonic level.*

△ **Interval** *(cycle of hard bursts, or hill work, followed by recovery, repeat) A series of intense anaerobic bursts followed by period of recovery.*

⇑ **Tempo** *(short and fast) A workout done at race pace—consistently high output.*

∞ **Endurance** *(long and slow) A run done at the lower end of the base-level exertion, but for a longer time.*

⇓ **Recovery** *(short and easy) Almost like a day off—a very short and easy workout.*

Anyone training for multi-sport rotates these five basic workouts weekly. Mixing up your workload in terms of volume, intensity, and frequency keeps your body guessing and improving. Use common sense to rotate these workouts into your training program.

The bulk of all conditioning is done in the base zone, around sixty to seventy percent of maximum heart rate, but the key to getting faster and stronger is to mix it up. Endurance runs are followed by recovery runs, tempo runs at race pace are followed by a day at base level. Intervals are interspersed with base level aerobic training to raise your VO_2. VO_2 max is the maximum amount of oxygen in milliliters that one can use in one minute per kilogram of body weight. VO_2 max is important because it represents how much oxygen you can deliver to your muscles efficiently. With proper training your VO_2 rises and you can maintain a constant level of exertion with less effort because your delivery of oxygen to muscles becomes more efficient with consistent training, which makes harder work seem easier.

Remember that in a thirty-minute workout, if you do five three-minute intervals at an anaerobic level of, say, nine mph, your body records the total for that workout as fifteen minutes at nine mph. During the course of a month, you can put those intervals together for a fifteen-minute run straight at nine mph. This is how athletes improve. If you train at base or endurance level, you will feel great and be happy, but you won't ever get faster. Getting faster may not be your goal at all.

ANAEROBIC EXERCISE = STRESS-BUSTING EUPHORIA
CALCULATED BURSTS OF ANAEROBIC EXERCISE ARE SUPREME

Effort is only effort when it begins to hurt.
JOSE GASSET

Anaerobic means without oxygen. Going anaerobic feels intense. Sometimes it hurts, but it ultimately floods your system with blissful, pain-killing, and calming neurochemicals. When your body works above a certain level, it switches from using oxygen to using other sources of fuel. The surge of anaerobic exercise when you attack, increasing output, sends a flood of very powerful neurochemicals into your brain. I call it slam dunking because the floodgate literally opens up and saturates your brain first in adrenaline, then endocannabinoids and endorphin, and finally the anti-anxiety triad that gives you a sense of calm. Anaerobic cardio is the best stress buster on the planet.

The four factors that you are dealing with during cardio work are:

- *Oxygen debt*

- *Lactic acid buildup*

- *Stroke volume*

- *Tidal volume*

Oxygen debt occurs when your body cannot deliver oxygen to muscle quickly enough, and you get the burn of lactic acid. Stroke volume is how much blood your heart can pump into your body with every beat. Tidal volume is the amount of oxygen your lungs can take in. Over time, all of these systems will improve, benefitting your overall health. Your ability to perform at the anaerobic level will improve as well. All these signals should be embraced as a sign that physical exertion is under way, and you are going places.

During anaerobic work, the body is working so hard that the demands for oxygen and fuel exceed the rate of supply, and the muscles have to rely on the stored reserves of fuel. In this case, waste products accumulate, the chief one being lactic acid. The muscles, being starved of oxygen, take the body into a state known as oxygen debt. This point is often measured as by the onset of blood lactate accumulation (OBLA). When you walk up a set of stairs you are feeling the effects of oxygen debt and lactate buildup in the muscles. Oxygen debt also releases neurochemicals. The more oxygen debt, the harder your body works to maintain homeostasis, which makes it the best anti-anxiety fix on the planet. You should aim for a total of twelve minutes of anaerobic work a week in an anaerobic zone that is generally anywhere above 80 percent maximum heart rate.

Most experts agree that a moderate to low amount of regular aerobic exercise can ease personal tension and stress. A new study by researchers at the University of Missouri–Columbia shows that bursts of relatively high-intensity exercise are superior in reducing stress and anxiety that may lead to heart disease. The researchers found that high-intensity exercise especially benefits women. Make sure that you get checked out by your doctor before doing anaerobic, or any new exercise for that matter, if you have been inactive or might have heart disease or high blood pressure.

Let us not underestimate the privileges of the mediocre. As one climbs higher, life becomes ever harder; the coldness increases, responsibility increases.

FRIEDRICH NIETZSCHE

A very small amount of anaerobic work will make a huge difference to your health and the electrochemical environment of your brain. Intense exercise opens the floodgates of all the major neurochemicals and increases the firing rate of synapses. Short bursts of intensity can be physically and psychologically tough—but the payback is huge. Create a system of motivation based on this knowledge.

I call the six minutes of an aerobic work the "Take 6," meaning that you take a total of six minutes a week and pick up the pace at least three times a week. I find it helpful to tell clients, "Okay, today we are going to Take 6." It makes the goal tangible. Then you decide how you want break up the six minutes. Remember, anytime you break up a workout into intervals, the time goes much faster. You can break the six minutes into thirty seconds done throughout a workout, at two-minute intervals. Think of it as a "4 or 4+" on the perceived exertion on a one-to-five scale. You inner dialogue should be saying: "This is just about the hardest I can go right now."

SPORT-SPECIFIC ADVICE

Born to Run
Chimps Like Us

*One step by one hundred people is better than one hundred steps
by one person.*

LOICHI TSUKAMOTO

Of all the sports I do, running is my favorite. As an ultra-runner I have
conquered mountains, but still have some hills to climb. Watching other
people run is my favorite pastime.

I learn so much by seeing what it takes for others to reach their goals.
Researchers have found that our ancestors' ability to run long distances
across the African savanna influenced the shape of our bodies from head to
toe. Humans are born to run. We are, in fact, running machines. Interest-
ingly, women and men are equally matched as ultra-runners. This may be in
response to our need to travel long distances together on foot. Odds are we
evolved to be able to stick together over the long haul as we traveled in
bands.

Our bodies have evolved specifically to run as a form of locomotion.
The ability to spring through the air is what sets us apart from primate
cousins. It is this pogo-stick ability of each leg that allows us to travel long
distances and to hunt and gather a high-protein diet, using relatively little
fuel. We are very fuel-efficient machines. As our brains grew, so did our prefrontal cortex, the seat of human intelligence, and we became better hunters.
Endurance running is, in fact, unique to homo sapiens among not only primates but also all other mammals except for dogs, horses, and hyenas.

Drs. Lieberman and Bramble, paleontologists at Harvard, established
that our slender legs, shorter arms, narrower rib cage and pelvis, skulls with
overheating prevention features, and the nuchal joint that keeps our heads
steady when we run set us apart from chimpanzees. Our uniquely huge gluteus maximus (our butts), the biggest muscles in our body, make us able to
run. Dr. Lieberman explains, "Your gluteus maximus stabilizes your trunk
as you lean forward to run. A run is like a controlled fall, and the buttocks
help control it." Monkeys don't have butt muscles. The scientists compiled a
list during the thirteen-year-long study of twenty-six traits that made early
homo sapiens specifically connected to running.

I re-lived my ecstasy again and again . . . at the first pale light I got up; and ran, yes really ran, in sandals, far beyond Mustapha; a kind of lightness of the body and soul did not leave me all day.

ANDRÉ GIDE (SI LE GRAIN NE MEURT)

Scientists concluded that running improved our chances of survival and reproduction. Although we were not as swift as our four-legged competitors, we could (and still can) outrun and hunt over greater distances than other predators. Lieberman says, "Endurance running may have made possible a diet rich in fats and proteins thought to account for the unique human combination of large bodies, small guts, big brains, and small teeth." Running, it turns out, is another thing that makes us uniquely human.

RUN, BIKE, SWIM TIPS
TIME-TESTED TRICKS OF THE TRADE

You can work at something for twenty years and walk away with twenty years' worth of valuable experience, or you can walk away with one year's experience twenty times.

GWEN JACKSON

Below are some tips on running, biking, and swimming that I've gained doing triathlons:

Running

- *Don't think too much about running. Don't try too hard to correct your gait. Your biomechanics are often set. Try to be relaxed and graceful, and over time you will become an efficient runner and find your natural stride.*

- *Lean forward a bit and shift your center of gravity to catch your fall.*

- *Create torque! Power in most sports comes from torque. Think of a boxer throwing a punch when you run. The arms move more as a unit with your torso. They create an optical illusion of moving more than they are as they rotate with your torso on the axis of your spine.*

- *The wrist is the metronome. Set pace with the snap and pop of your wrist. Remember that your cerebellum maintains rhythm and timing.*

- *The elbows are the pistons on a train. Think about your elbows more than your knees.*

- *"Hands high, feet low . . . hands high, feet low"—Say this mantra as you shuffle along, falling forward. Unless you're a sprinter, shuffle your feet and keep hands near your chest.*

- *Don't flail your arms. They should have a nice wrist pop—but keep it tight and fluid. Or like locomotive pistons when sprinting.*

- *Move swiftly. Run like you're on hot coals. Keep your turnover high. Land on the midsection of your foot and feel more of a pop as you toe off—and less of a roll from heel to toe.*

- *Learn to feel the windlass mechanism when your foot becomes a lever and pushes you off the ground. Consciously keep the point from the ball of the foot to the heel actively engaged as you spring into the air on every stride.*

- *Imagine leaning and spinning like a dreidel. Don't lean forward directly but pivot your torso so you fall a few degrees left or right. Use that gravitational pull and torque to pull you forward.*

- *Think about reaching back with your feet as you take off—imagine an invisible wall behind you that you are extending your stride to tap. Bringing the left foot back this way pushes the right foot forward and vice versa.*

- *Imagine a tick/tick/tick/chop/chop/chop tempo in your head that sets the pace.*

- *Think "Float like a butterfly, sting like a bee." Stay airbound as much as possible. Imagine you are running but your feet are barely touching the ground.*

- *Mix up your gait. Don't always hit the ground exactly the same way.*

- *The hand harness: To practice keeping your hands up near your chest and rotating your spine: take a small hand towel, wrap it around your neck, and grab it at the corners just below your chest, like a harness. This is easy to do on the treadmill, where you can put the towel down.*

- *Watch your own reflection if you have a mirror or glass in front of the machine. Work on your form and strength by watching yourself run.*

- Cross talk: Keep it upbeat and third person often. Today's line for me: "Can you kick it? Yes! I can." Have an arsenal of words you use to keep yourself motivated.

- Lace shoes snugly but not too tightly. Think of a boxer taping up his hands. You want everything to stay in place on impact. Always double-knot your laces.

- Feel the physics of your body move against forces of gravity, velocity, pendulums, and momentum, but don't think too much about it. Feel the forces intuitively, and use them. Create dynamic tension of forces.

- Find your most fluid tonic speed. Slower running is often actually harder on your joints.

- Kinetic energy: Remember when running fast that you coil energy up and then let it spring out of you. Running power is held in the rotation of shoulders and hips on an axis. You rotate, coil, and snap. The energy is in your core; you rotate and flick it out like a bullwhip. This kinetic principle plays itself in most sports. It is like serving a tennis ball, hitting a golf ball, or pitching a baseball—coil, pause, release. Think of yourself as being spring-loaded like a jack-in-the-box.

- Think of your sternum as the center of gravity like a gyroscope. Everything rotates around the sternum, like the web of a spider rotates around its core.

- Your spine should float when you run. Remember the central nervous system is composed of your brain and spine. The cerebrum is the helmet of intellectuality. Be pragmatic always, but let the cerebellum and the tail slither down your spinal cord.

- Keep track of where you tend to hold tension (I hold it in my right shoulder/hip), and let it go. Constantly relax these points. Run a head-to-toe checklist periodically to find tension spots and let them go.

- Think like a horse when you run. Watch horses closely and emulate their behavior if you want to be a good runner. They are the best runners, and great teachers. Get on top of a horse and you will learn what it's all about at a cerebellar level.

- Keep a happy inner smile on your face, by relaxing all the muscles in your face, to trick your nervous system. Don't grimace or tighten your face. Stay relaxed.

• I like to run with rolled up towels in my hands when I run indoors, and always with ice-cold sponges from the aid stations in Ironman races. I learned this from Heather Fuhr, who has won more Ironman races than anyone on the planet, other than her good friend Paula Newby-Fraser. I call things I hold in my hands "the grips." They make me feel grounded. Other people like to run with sticks. See if running with things in your hands works for you. I hold things about half the time if I have some-place to put them down.

Biking

• Keep your cadence between 80 and 90 rpm. Not everyone is Lance. One hundred+ rpms is too fast for most people to have good form and efficiency.

• Make sure the seat position is right: high enough so your knees bend and your hips don't rock to reach the downstroke.

• Engage your core. Use your abs and triceps to support your weight. Don't use pedals to hold you up. This will block your fluid pedal stroke.

• Don't block the opposing pedal by delaying on the downstroke, trying to catch a fall. Use triceps, core, and the seat to support your body weight.

• Imagine pedaling with pistons attached between your heel and butt. Do not just push down with your quads into the pedal with the ball of your foot. Pull up by imaging a piston shortening between your heel and butt. Make this a fluid motion.

• Scrape the bowl—as you pull up and down with the pistons from be-hind, imagine equal pressure at every part of the 360-degree revolu-tion as if the pressure is pushing against the outside.

• If you're a guy, sit to one side of your perineum by twisting the saddle five degrees to one side and sitting perched on the nose of the saddle. Don't squash your perineum.

• Exert an equal amount of pressure on all your joints with each pedal stroke. Think of your hips, knees, and ankles (left and right). This sounds tricky but you'll get the knack. Visualize this with every stroke.

- Realize that the cerebellum is going to keep you balanced like a ballast.

- Think like a locomotive.

- Laundry tip: To save water and energy—and avoid workout clothes getting really skanky—walk directly into the shower wearing everything you worked out in. Stand under the water in your clothes rinsing off the sweat. Disrobe, soap up the clothes and socks and then wring them out. If your gym has a swimsuit spinner, spin them in the machine to get rid of most of the water. Otherwise just wring them out well, then put them in a plastic bag and hang them up the second you get home. They'll dry in a couple of hours and be ready for you to grab and go in the morning. There is no need to have a week's worth of stinky, wet, moldy clothes in your hamper. Hand wash your workout gear after every use like a Spartan would.

Swim (Freestyle Advice)

- Create very little turbulence. When you swim, you want to slither. Grab the water with your forearms and kick it back with triceps, but not with a lot of thrashing or splashing.

- Imagine swimming in a tube. Keep yourself contained. Point your toes like an arrow.

- Practice drills every swim. Technique is key. Unlike running or biking trying harder in the water doesn't mean you go faster. In fact, the opposite is true.

- During freestyle, keep one eye underwater when you turn to breathe. Don't lift your head; turn your neck.

- Think like a fish.

- Rotate at the spine around the spine like when you run. I think of my torso as rotisserie chicken on a skewer, which is my spine. The same torque of running or serving a tennis ball applies. Coil the energy and snap it out of your shoulders and into your hands.

- Imagine punching forward with your shoulders.

- Remember like with running and most sports—it's all in the wrist—stiff wrist underwater, delicate and limp above waterline.

- Learn how to feel the water. Use it like a wall you press against.

- Power is in the hips. Rotate torso on spine and churn hips back and forth like a turbine.

- Don't overkick—imagine an elastic band around your ankles and keep it tight. Keep your kick tight by kicking toe to toe and having big toes touch with each kick.

- Practice foot flexion by sitting on ankles—point your toes.

- Catch the water. Learn to feel when you hold it with your forearms.

- Keep your elbows high and thumbs up the side.

- Shoot off the wall like a torpedo. Tuck head, overlap hands, and point toes.

- Put your goggle straps under your cap. Buy goggles that create suction without the straps attached. No pair of goggles fits every face. Try lots of pairs.

- Start with bone-dry goggles and see if they stay fog-free. If not, just rinse and reseal by dunking underwater—or try saliva and a rinse.

- Ear plugs. If you are prone to ear infections (like me) I recommend the kind that are firm rubber. Find ones that create a tailored fit for your ear canal. Don't use the puffy ones. They suck.

- Transfer muscle memory from other sports. I did not swim well as a kid. When I learned as an adult, it was the motion of serving a tennis ball that taught me how to coil, pause, and snap the power rotation from my hips to my arms during freestyle. It's the same principle as running to a degree, but you have a wall of water to use like ladder rungs to climb and slip through simultaneously.

- Practice sighting by looking like an alligator over the top of your goggles at the waterline.

- Lose yourself in the sensory deprivation of it. Think altered states. Lose yourself. Return to base! Swimming is one of the purest cerebellar experiences because it is goes back to our amphibian roots.

- Beauty tip. Chlorine is great for your skin. Like a chemical peel—I'm not kidding. The trick is a warm shower and exfoliating with a soaped-up hand towel in small circles, then applying a moisturizer. I recommend using a moisturizer with Squalane, which is a highly refined olive oil similar in its chemical structure to your skin's own oils. It is good to exfoliate with a little soap on a towel after you break a good sweat; use small towels if your gym has them, or the corner of a big towel.

- Rinse your suit in the shower, then drop it in the swimsuit spinner to get rid of excess water.

SPORTS PSYCHOLOGY

Scheduling/Game Plan
This is the Day

Do not wait; the time will never be "just right." Start where you stand, and work with whatever tools you may have at your command, and better tools will be found as you go along.

NAPOLEON HILL

Finding the time to work out is going to be a constant struggle. Schedule the slots of time you have available each week. Have a game plan every day. Write down the windows you have available to work out at the beginning of each week for the first eight weeks in a calendar. Put the calendar someplace conspicuous and check off the completed workouts. Make a schedule to exercise and stick to it with no questions asked. Whether or not you are going to work out is not up for debate.

Some people like to record every appointment down in detail and know weeks in advance what they will be doing on the third Tuesday of the month. Others like to play it a bit looser. Either way is fine as long as you have worked out by the end of the day.

Idleness is the devil's workshop. Want to get the job done?
Give it to the busiest person.

RICHARD BERGLAND (NEUROSURGEON)

Just Do It!
No Discussion. No Debate

Action is character.

F. SCOTT FITZGERALD

Researchers at the University of Alberta in Canada have revealed that the Nike advice to "Just do it" is the wisest athletic maxim of all time. The study by Dr. Sandra Cousins, professor of physical education and recreation, discovered that people who are successful at exercising regularly don't stop to think about it; they just do it. Dr. Cousins explains, "We used to think that positive self-talk was important to promote individual exercise participation, but when it comes to the general public, you don't need a pep talk. You need a plan. If you plan to meet a friend every Tuesday at three P.M. for a walk, you will show up so you don't let them down." Make a weekly schedule that becomes a routine—"Mondays I meet Joe after work for a walk—Tuesdays I take Nadia's class."

According to Dr. Cousins, regular exercisers stick to a routine because when something doesn't go according to plan, like bad weather, a minor injury, not getting your favorite bike in a spin class, you improvise and adjust to it. Stay flexible and adaptable within your routine. Don't be a slave to it. You want to own it, not have it own you. Find ways to make cardio a part of your daily life—take the stairs, bike to work, walk instead of taking a cab. These small bursts of activity are cumulative and add up to a daily quotient of activity that can be substantial.

> *If you do what you've always done, you'll get what you've always gotten.*
>
> ANTHONY ROBBINS

Flow
Creating Fluid Performance

When you start working, everybody is in your studio—the past, your friends, enemies, the art world and above all your own ideas. But as you continue, they start leaving one by one and you are left completely alone. Then, if you are lucky, even you leave.

JOHN CAGE (AMERICAN COMPOSER)

People experience flow doing all types of things. Bakers, painters, surgeons, window washers, and athletes can all lose themselves in what they are doing and create what I call fluid performance, which is flow.

The Six Characteristics of Fluid Performance

Stung by the splendor of a sudden thought.

ROBERT BROWNING

The key with any state of mind is being able to give it a name when it happens so that you can take inventory on the ingredients in place and recreate it. Below are the six characteristics that are used to describe a state of flow. By Mihaly Czikszentmihlyi and others.

1. *ACTION AND AWARENESS MERGE: You become so engaged in what you are doing that the actions become spontaneous, almost automatic.*

2. *CLEAR GOALS AND POSITIVE FEEDBACK: You want to have well-defined goals and tangible feedback that they have been achieved.*

3. *LASERLIKE FOCUS ON THE TASK: You want to concentrate and be focused on the task at hand; you want to exist in the present tense.*

4. *THE PARADOX OF CONTROL: The paradox of being in control as an athlete is that the less you consciously worry about being in control, the more in control you will become. This is how the cerebellum works. If you try too hard to micromanage your movements cerebrally, you will choke. Let it go. Don't think too much. Stay cerebellar.*

5. *LOSS OF SELF-CONSCIOUSNESS: The elevated amount of serotonin in a flow state lowers self-consciousness. Impressions of your self seem to vanish when your attention is directed mostly on the task and you are in a fluid state. Anytime you feel a loss of self-consciousness, it is a good sign in sport. It means you have created flow and are being more cerebellar than cerebral.*

6. *DISTORTION OF TIME: As Roger Bannister noted during his sub-four-minute-mile run, perceptions of time disappear when you are in a state of flow. Since the tick tock of time when you're doing cardio can be torture, creating flow will allow you to create a time warp where minutes can seem like seconds. This may also be a function of anandamide creating a distortion of time.*

The Halfway Tipping Point
Go Fetch, Then Bring It Home

Whistle your way back home.
WALT DISNEY

Always take note of the halfway tipping point in a workout. When you turn around to come home, your perspective is always different from when you headed out. If you do an out-and-back run—pay attention to the go-fetch feeling of reaching the halfway point and turning around to bring it home. This is a key psychological shift; you always feel different with 50 percent of a workout or race under your belt. Remember that within each stage of working out you have a different inner dialogue and you need to have different cognitive strategies. I generally break each workout into four quarters to start—and then dissect it into smaller bite-sized pieces if need be. Pay attention to the clock indoors and out and notice the shifts in mind-set that go along with each stage of the process. Your perspective is much different in the last five minutes than it was in the first five. You also have the option to think about nothing at all, to cover the time display, or not even think about how far you have to go. A nonthinking state is the best option—use these methods when you need a new perspective.

SEVEN WAYS TO BEAT BOREDOM WHEN TRAINING INDOORS

Someone's boring me. I think it's me.
DYLAN THOMAS

1. *ACCEPT IT: Consider the time doing cardio indoors as a job. Look at it as if you are on the clock at work; you leave when the shift is over. Don't open it up to discussion. It ain't over till it's over. Don't stop till you're done. The good news is that no matter how much discomfort you're in, when you finish, it will end. Be patient and give yourself something to look forward to when it's done—even if it's just the fact that it's over. Always finish strong, cool down for five minutes, and do five to ten minutes of stretch and balance work.*

2. *DISTRACT YOURSELF: Use anything at your disposal to distract yourself—magazines, TV, music, people watching, chewing gum—*

whatever works for you. Cover the display some of the time or all of the time; play around with it. I like to watch sports on TV when I'm working out at the gym. Programs with a plot often make the time go slower. Music is the best way to stay entertained. Put on energizing songs near the end; pump up the volume and finish strong.

3. LOSE YOURSELF: By finding your flow channel and going into a trance with the rhythmic movements and breathing, you should lose sense of time. Remember to find your tonic level and patiently wait for a state of flow to kick in. Then hope for a piercing point to superfluid performance. That is the gold ring you reach for and stay on till the end. It is a great time to think about stuff and enjoy time alone to sift your thoughts. Pretend you're somewhere else or flash forward to when it's over. You'll be relaxercising on the couch or in bed again soon enough. Slow down, if you have to, but never quit.

4. INTERVALS: Break up your workout into doable doses by setting up a series of intervals. Be creative in how you break it down. I generally like three minutes hard, two minutes recovery—a thirty-minute workout becomes six single units and you check them off one by one. Mix it up. You will always be eager for the interval to end and you'll love the downtime. This is normal. Use interval mode on machines. This will create automatic fartleks (Swedish for speedplay), which will get you in good shape and make time fly.

5. PARTNER/BUDDY: Use conversation or working out side by side as a way to make the time go faster. Also try competing with a friend to bring out a higher effort. Take a class with an instructor and a group. Always mix it up.

6. CHUNKING: Always break the workout into smaller segments that you can wrap your mind around. The halfway point is the tipping point and crucial as a shift in perspective to bringing it home. The last fifteen minutes should be a piece of cake; think of how fast a fifteen-minute coffee break goes. Break the fifteen into three five-minute chunks. The key is to dissect and barter to keep an optimistic perspective. Typical dialogue for sixty minutes of cardio: "Okay, excellent, I'm three minutes to the halfway—and then I only have two fifteen-minute chunks left. That's three songs on my iPod. I can get through that."

7.   CROSS-TRAIN/MIX IT UP: Do two or three different machines. Try
     twenty minutes on two for a forty-minute workout, or three
     machines for fifteen minutes each.

Apply the rules above and time will fly!

You must first have a lot of patience to learn to have patience.

STANISLAW J. LEC

Stake Your Turf
Build a Fortress

*My center is giving way . . . my right is in retreat, my left yields—
situation excellent. I shall attack. "Attack! Attack!"*

FERDINAND FOCH (FRENCH MILITARY GENERAL)

You want to feel secure at the gym, and one way to do that is to set up
some boundaries around your personal space, almost like a fortress. To do
this, use your imagination more than anything. But you can also put down a
towel or a water bottle as a boundary that defines your personal turf. Make
it your domain. A few small things will symbolize to your cerebellum that
this is home, on familiar turf. It can settle into the clickity-clack of fluid performance right off the bat.

If you travel, these routines can create a familiarity that will put your
brain at ease so that you can lose yourself in a workout wherever you are.
With indoor training you can transplant yourself anywhere and feel like
you are at home in a completely foreign environment. The panel of an elliptical trainer or treadmill looks the same in Chicago as it does in Shanghai or
Tasmania.

*When I heard the learn'd astronomer, When the proofs, the figures
were ranged in columns before me, When I was shown the charts and
diagrams, to add, divide, and measure them, When I was sitting
heard the astronomer where he lectured with much applause in the
lecture-room. How soon unaccountable I became tired and sick, Till ris-
ing and gliding out I wander'd off by myself, In the mystical moist night-
air, and from time to time, Look'd up in perfect silence at the stars.*

WALT WHITMAN

CHAPTER SEVEN

THE STRENGTH PROGRAM

Every man is the builder of a temple, called his body, to the god he worships, after a style purely his own, nor can he get off by hammering marble instead. We are all sculptors and painters, and our material is our own flesh and blood and bones.

HENRY DAVID THOREAU

THE STRENGTH-TRAINING PRESCRIPTIVE

FREQUENCY: *Two to three times a week.*

INTENSITY: *One to three sets of eight to twelve repetitions. Exhaust each muscle to point of failure.*

TIME: *Twenty to sixty minutes.*

TYPE: *Ten to fifteen different exercises covering different muscle groups.*

In this chapter, we will go over all the basics of lifting weights. Strength training should be an integral part of your weekly exercise regimen. Many people who are religious about cardio will put weight training on the back burner and neglect to do it regularly. This is a big mistake. *The Athlete's Way* program is incomplete if you are not lifting weights at least twice a week. This isn't an option. In this chapter, I will give you reasons to want to lift weights and show you how to create effective and safe workouts. You will learn about the basics of form, technique, major muscle groups, your two types of muscle fibers, how to exhaust a muscle completely, and the simple gold standard full-body workout.

Lifting weights offers you a huge return on your time investment. As little as twenty minutes twice a week will give you significant life-changing benefits. Cardiovascular exercise requires time. You can go anaerobic and get more bang for your buck, but in general cardio is an hourglass situation. With lifting weights you get substantial results without a Herculean effort. Invest a minimum of forty minutes a week in strength training and bank high dividends in return. You can't afford not to be weight lifting. It's never too late to start. If you don't lift weights currently, start today.

A year from now you will wish you had started today.
KAREN LAMB

Resistance training with weights will tone and strengthen your muscles, but the most important benefits involve things you can't see—bone density, hormones, neurotransmitters, metabolism, improved self-esteem, and overall sense of well-being. Lifting weights is going to make you feel great. It floods your body with lots of blissful, energizing molecules and calming ones, too. This is a neurobiological phenomenon that you will experience firsthand as you float out of the gym after a good weightlifting workout. Strength training invigorates your nervous system.

The guidelines set forth in this prescriptive section are straightforward. The finish line is always where you set it. Set the bar high and achieve. There tends to be a lot of hype surrounding weight lifting; don't psyche yourself out. The bottom line is that anytime you overload a muscle, and then give it time to recuperate, it is going to get stronger. Keep it simple. Educate yourself on the muscle groups and exercises I share with you here, and then do the exercises at least twice a week with proper form and technique.

If you remember only two things about strength training these should be:

1. *The last three to four reps are the most important. You want to exhaust the muscle completely.*

2. *You want to lift weights at a steady, controlled speed between gravity and momentum. Never throw or drop the weights.*

That's weightlifting in a nutshell. Don't dog it or stop lifting when it starts to burn near the end of a set. Push through. Save time by doing fewer sets with proper form and get better results. If you exhaust each muscle completely on each set by lifting in a steady controlled manner, you can be out of the gym in less than thirty minutes for a full-body workout.

> *The last three or four reps is what makes the muscle grow. This area of pain divides the champion from someone else who is not a champion. That's what most people lack, having the guts to go on and just say they'll go through the pain no matter what happens.*
>
> ARNOLD SCHWARZENEGGER

There are shelves full of books in any bookstore or library dedicated solely to the subject of lifting weights. This chapter will cover the basics, but I recommend doing more research on specific exercise to broaden your knowledge base and give you more ideas of exercises to add to your regimen in addition to the building blocks covered here. Just remember, don't believe the hype of the latest, greatest discovery. Stick to the fundamentals. It never hurts to subscribe to twelve months of a fitness magazine to keep yourself updated on new exercises you could incorporate into your regimen.

Remember to slow down and think clearly about your joints and how muscles move. Lift your arm, extend your leg, and feel the muscles used. Then think of where you would put the resistance to strengthen that muscle. Use common sense and educate yourself. Study the body parts listed here and then familiarize yourself with how they work in your own body. Always focus mentally on the muscle you are working on when you're working it. Attack weight lifting with vigor—it is a very invigorating experience. It makes you soar. Stick with it.

It is a myth that lifting weights is automatically going to make you musclebound or bulky; lifting weights actually increases flexibility and can lengthen muscles. Don't lift weights that are too heavy because you'll end up getting injured and not isolating the muscles properly. You want to focus on form and completely exhausting both your slow-twitch (Type 1) and fast-twitch (Type 2) muscle fibers with every set, which you'll learn how to do in this chapter. We'll review the fundamentals of strength training in a straightforward, no-nonsense way.

BUILD SELF-ESTEEM
PUMPING IRON MAKES YOU LESS REJECTION-SENSITIVE

Rejection. Rejected. Reject. Rebound.
LOUISE BOURGEOIS

Pumping iron makes you feel more confident and less prone to rejection sensitivity, or intimidation, than anything I know. The neurochemical culprit behind rejection sensitivity is low serotonin. The vicious cycle of low serotonin coupled with rejection sensitivity makes you less confident, creating a vicious downward cycle because you avoid the gym. The daily athletic process, especially lifting weights, can reverse this trend chemically and psychologically. The less serotonin, the more rejection-sensitive you become.

Pumping iron sends more serotonin to your prefrontal cortex via plumped-up microtubules. The mini-pipelines that deliver serotonin get more efficient at their job when you break a sweat regularly. More serotonin thickens the density of neurons that guide the optimistic discussion and facilitates optimistic cross talk inside your head around the clock, giving you tenacity to take the bull by the horns. Regular exercise will strengthen your frontal lobes and make you less rejection-sensitive and intimidated in all life situations.

*My passions were all gathered together like fingers that made a fist.
Drive is considered aggression today; I knew it then as purpose.*
BETTE DAVIS

Stepping into a gym—or onto a weight floor—can be overwhelming and nerve-wracking if you've never done it before. Exercising in public is one of the most intimidating things we do as adults, because we are exposed and vulnerable. Don't be intimidated. If the fear of rejection or being judged is preventing you from joining a gym or the sporting life, it is time to get over it. While reading this section, consider areas in your life in which you feel insecure and personalize a strategy to cope with these situations. The worst thing you can do when feeling rejection sensitivity is to try to blend in and go under the radar. Don't do it.

I'm the fucking boss around here.
MADONNA (BLONDE AMBITION TOUR, 1990)

People who are rejection-sensitive try to make themselves invisible. Then even if they do something well, nobody notices. Not that you are necessarily doing things to impress other people, but you want people to be proud of you and you want to be a role model. Strive to be a maverick and a trailblazer, never a lemming. This is something I have consciously pounded into my head and reinforced through my daily behavior. The insecurity never goes away completely but you can handle it. The alternative would be living a life based in fear. Lead a life that makes you proud and that people would admire.

> *A life lived in fear is a life half lived.*
> **BAZ LUHRMANN**

I have struggled with paralyzing fear at many times throughout my life and I have bouts of insecurity every day. It has been helpful for me to have role models who substitute bravery and mental toughness for rejection sensitivity. My father, astronaut Chuck Yeager, and Madonna have been my mental-toughness, rejection-sensitivity role models for decades. When I feel emotionally hypersensitive, I think of the nerves of steel my dad had as a neurosurgeon, "the right stuff" of Chuck Yeager, or some of Madonna's "blonde ambition."

> *Nobody roots for Goliath.*
> **WILT CHAMBERLAIN**

For anyone who feels ostracized or intimidated for whatever reason, remember, it's OK to feel rejection sensitivity and experience the pain of it. There is power in feeling like an underdog. It makes you fight harder. Feeling like an underdog teaches you how to be tough and stay strong. Identify the feelings of rejection sensitivity as being just that; give it a name so you can conquer it. Think like a Spartan youth; train hard to become brave. Have courage and respect yourself. Don't let the judgment of other people or the fear of failure stop you.

TWELVE REASONS TO LIFT WEIGHTS
A LEAN, MEAN, FIGHTING MACHINE

When you're playing against a stacked deck, compete even harder. Show the world how much you'll fight for the winner's circle. If you

*do, someday the cellophane will crackle off a fresh pack, one that
belongs to you, and the cards will be stacked in your favor.*

PAT RILEY

Below are twelve simple reasons to lift weights commonly accepted by
sports professionals and the American College of Sports Medicine. Anytime
you feel like bagging a weight workout, make it a point to review this list
and maybe it will inspire you to change your mind.

1. *INCREASE HORMONES AND NEUROCHEMICALS THAT MAKE YOU
   FEEL GREAT, but also keeps you vital, physically and mentally. The
   good stress of lifting weights triggers the release of human growth
   hormone, lowers cortisol, and releases endorphins, dopamine, and
   endocannabinoids.*

2. *REDUCE MUSCLE LOSS: After the age of thirty you will lose about a
   pound of muscle every year. A pound of muscle burns about thirty
   to fifty calories a day at rest just for tissue maintenance.*

3. *INCREASE MUSCLE MASS: In a study of people lifting weights for
   twenty-five minutes three times a week, there was an increase of
   up to three pounds of muscle mass over an eight-week period. This
   is a huge return on investment. Weight lifting pays high dividends.*

4. *PREVENT METABOLIC RATE REDUCTION: Since lifting weights
   increases muscle mass, it prevents your resting metabolic rate
   from dipping. The more muscle you have, the more energy your
   body needs to sustain itself and the more it will turn food into fuel,
   not fat.*

5. *INCREASE METABOLIC RATE: The three-pound gain of muscle mass
   translates into an increased metabolic rate of 7 percent and 15
   percent of daily caloric intake. That means if you were eating a
   2,000-calorie-a-day diet, the three-pound muscle gain would
   translate into 250 calories more a day. When you create muscle,
   you use more calories all day long, even at rest. Your energy-
   intake-to-exertion equation gives you wiggle room, not jiggle room.*

6. *INCREASE BONE MINERAL DENSITY: Resistance training has the
   same effect on bone tissue as it does on muscle tissue. Significant
   increase in mineral density is stimulated by strength exercise.*

7. *IMPROVE GLUCOSE METABOLISM:* A 23 percent increase in glucose metabolism, which helps prevent the onset of adult diabetes, is associated with strength training.

8. *INCREASE GASTROINTESTINAL TRANSIT SPEED:* Delayed passage of food through your intestines has been linked to colon cancer. After twelve weeks of strength training an average 56 percent increased transit time was cited in people prone toward constipation who started lifting weights.

9. *REDUCE BLOOD PRESSURE:* Even in the absence of cardiovascular/ aerobic training, lifting weights alone considerably reduces blood pressure. When combined with aerobic exercise the improved results were seen in as little as two weeks.

10. *IMPROVE BLOOD LIPID LEVELS:* Blood lipid levels (cholesterol) can be improved after just several weeks of strength training.

11. *REDUCE LOWER BACK PAIN:* Lower back pain is a common ailment. Creating a solid core and strong lower back greatly reduces the impact of lower back pain. Do abdominal work and focus on strengthening your "Hercules girdle," the muscles of your lower abdomen that support your core, to help prevent onset of lower back pain.

12. *REDUCE OSTEOPOROSIS AND RHEUMATOID ARTHRITIS PAIN:* The impact of strength training creates endocrine and physiological changes that strengthen muscles, bones, and connective tissue that reduce swelling in arthritic joints.

AGING AND MUSCLE LOSS
DON'T BECOME A SHRINKING VIOLET

Old age is like a plane flying through a storm. Once you're aboard, there's nothing you can do.

GOLDA MEIR

I have to disagree with Golda Meir's stance on aging—weight lifting is one of the best things you can do to reverse the trends of getting older. As we age, we lose muscle mass, so the older we get, the more important it is to lift weights. In addition to the changes in muscle mass and metabolism, there are changes at an endocrine level that affect hormones and drain the fountain of youth. Strength training will trigger the increase of testosterone/ estrogen by lowering cortisol and increasing the release of HGH (human growth hormone)—a great anti-aging combination.

> *Grow old with me! The best is yet to be.*
> **ROBERT BROWNING**

Lifting weights is going to improve your physique by sculpting muscles. Weight lifting will change your veneer but will also modify your interior. Skeletal muscle accounts for about 40 percent of body weight in a medium-build, lean individual. The human body has more than 430 skeletal muscles; each muscle is made up of thousands of muscle cells. These cells are referred to as muscle fibers and are long and thin—roughly the thickness of a human hair—yet they can stretch as long as two and a half feet. You have two types of muscle fibers that lie side by side within each muscle, striated in a way that looks like light meat and dark meat when dissected. In general, endurance athletes use more Type 1 (slow-twitch) muscle fibers. Type 2 (fast-twitch) fibers would be associated with a sprinter. When you exercise, Type 1 muscle fibers are always activated first. When they become unable to do the job, Type 2 fibers are recruited. When you are lifting weights the Type 1s will exhaust first. All the benefit to strength training really lies in exhausting Type 2. The first eight reps are usually just getting you to that launching pad.

In a recent study, two groups of people ate the exact same diet and exercised for thirty minutes, three times a week. The first group did thirty minutes of aerobic exercise but did not lift weights; the other group did fifteen minutes of aerobic exercise and fifteen minutes of strength training each session. After eight weeks, the aerobics-only group had lost three pounds of fat and half a pound of muscle. The group that combined aerobics and strength training had lost ten pounds of fat and gained two pounds of calorie-burning muscle.

> *Character contributes to beauty. It fortifies a woman as her youth fades. A mode of conduct, a standard of courage, discipline, fortitude and integrity can do a great deal to make a woman beautiful.*
> **JAQUELINE BISSET**

Many people associate getting older with the downward spiral of growing weaker and less energetic. As we age, the pizzazz we had as a younger person often fizzles. Strength training is going to reverse this trend and give you more oomph. Lifting weights consistently will keep you feel and look youthful. If you want to remain stalwart and steady into your golden years, you have to make some type of weight training a part of your weekly routine. This is a mandate, not an option.

BASIC TRAINING TIPS

My motto was always to keep swinging. Whether I was in a slump or feeling badly or having trouble off the field, the only thing to do was keep swinging.

HANK AARON

Sets and Reps

A set is a group of successive repetitions performed without resting. A rep, or repetition, is the number of times you repeat the move in each set. Therefore, if your instructions were to do three sets of twelve (3 x 12) bicep curls, you would curl the weight twelve times in a row to complete the first set. Then you'd do two more sets, with thirty to sixty seconds of rest between each set.

Fast Twitch—Slow Twitch
Muscle Types 1 And 2

TYPE 1: These muscle fibers are typically referred to as slow twitch because it takes about 110 milliseconds to produce a twitch, one cycle of contraction and relaxation. These fibers suit aerobic or oxygen-dependent energy metabolism and are relatively resistant to fatigue. These are the first fibers enlisted when you lift weights; generally the first eight reps of twelve engage Type 1.

TYPE 2: These muscle fibers are referred to as fast twitch because they can produce a twitch in fifty milliseconds, twice as fast as the slow twitch. These fibers are more efficient in the anaerobic (sprinting) or oxygen-independent energy metabolism and use glycogen for fuel. These fibers are enlisted after you exhaust the Type 1 fibers. They tend to really burn when they are exhausted. Type 2 muscle provides the most important gain in muscle mass and strength, so bite the bullet and finish those final reps of every set.

Your goal with every set should be to exhaust muscle Type 1 first and then to completely exhaust Type 2 fibers. This is the key to *The Athlete's Way* strength-training program, and the most important thing to remember. Use low weights but completely exhaust the muscle group. This will release the highest amount of dopamine, endocannabinoids, endorphin, and serotonin.

Complete Range
No Half-Steppin'

Veni, vidi, vici.
JULIUS CAESAR

Full range of motion is an important component of proper form. Each exercise should be taken through the complete range of joint movement in a slow, controlled manner, with emphasis placed on the completely contracted position. If a weight is so heavy that you have to jerk, bounce, or swing to get it to the top of the movement, it's too heavy. Your form is compromised. Full range of motion movements contract and strengthen the muscle you're working (the prime mover, agonist) and stretch the opposing (antagonist) muscle.

The Flow Channel
Balanced Challenge

Do the one thing you think you cannot do. Fail at it. Try again. Do better the second time. The only people who never tumble are those who never mount the high wire. This is your moment. Own it.
OPRAH WINFREY

You want to find your flow channel and tonic level with weight lifting in order to lose yourself in it. Don't think about it strictly as a dry physical experience—create a state of flow. Remember to seek balanced challenge in weight lifting. You want to find the weight that is not overwhelming but also not so easy that you are bored. In general ten to twelve reps is the magic tonic level in terms of repetition maximum for strength. For endurance you could lower weights and extend your reps to twelve to twenty repetition maximum.

Overload Principle
Renew, Recover, Regenerate

Learn to labor and wait.
HENRY WADSWORTH LONGFELLOW

The overload principle is the basis of all training programs. In order to get stronger, you must overload the muscle by putting a heavier load on it than it is used to. The stress will break it down but stimulate it to rebuild— stronger, faster, bigger. You need to give your muscle time to rebuild. The key to overload is recovery. Without solid sleep the muscles cannot renew or regenerate. **Give yourself at least forty-eight hours between strength training a particular muscle group.** Do not consume mega doses of protein thinking it will make muscles grow faster; it won't. Eat a balanced diet, stay hydrated, get a good night's sleep, and the benefits of strength training are yours.

Learning to Count
Finish, Don't Fizzle

Pause, listen and count.
WALT WHITMAN

Lifting weights is ultimately a counting game. Each set of weight lifting should be broken down into two counting phases. If you are doing twelve reps, count up to eight and then count down from four to zero. This will guarantee you finish and don't fizzle. Be intuitive about when to start counting down. **Count up until you exhaust Type 1 fibers, then count down as you finish the set by exhausting Type 2 fibers.**

The key with lifting weights is to exhaust both Type 1 and Type 2 fibers. I like to think of each set as actually two sets in one. Most people tend to fizzle if they just keep counting up. One second you're chugging along counting up and lifting weights, but the second you engage Type 2s, everybody's first urge is to stop. The voices in your head change from saying, "This is easy," to, "I want to stop now," and down go the weights. That is why you must clean the slate after you exhaust Type 1s, regroup mentally, and set a new goal to exhaust Type 2s as you finish each set. Remember, exhausting Type 1s is just the launching pad.

Find the point at which you think you can squeeze out three or four reps and start counting backward to zero. The real results of working out are going to be in those final, most painful reps. Remember Arnold's hard-line quote: "The last three or four reps is what makes the muscle grow" and the one below. His advice on pumping iron influenced me as a teen, and these are important maxims to remember.

> *What we face may look insurmountable. But I learned something from all those years of training and competing. I learned something from all those sets and reps when I didn't think I could lift another ounce of weight. What I learned is that we are always stronger than we know.*
>
> ARNOLD SCHWARZENEGGER

Couple this counting method with proper form and technique and you are set for life in the weight-training department. Having good form in weight lifting is based on keeping your movements smooth and controlled. Anytime that you lift too much weight you are likely to cheat. Choose an amount of weight that you can lift at a speed between gravity and momentum. Target the muscle you are working by isolating it and keeping the use of other muscles to a minimum. You will notice that good form is mostly about not arching or straining in a way that puts added stress on any of your joints. Observe other people at the gym who lift weights with good technique and emulate them. Also, watch yourself in the mirror so that you can check your form.

Keep an Eye on the Clock
No Lollygagging

> *I never could have done what I have done without the habits of punctuality, order, and diligence, without the determination to concentrate myself on one subject at a time. . . ."*
>
> CHARLES DICKENS

Always start your stopwatch before you begin lifting weights. You want to be friendly and have friends at the gym, but don't do too much socializing on the weight deck. Do it before or after your weight lifting. You don't want to derail your train and lose momentum when you're working out. Working out with a partner is the best way to kill two birds with one stone. Just keep it peppy. You don't want to stretch your time out on the weight deck more than an hour. Keep your body moving and engaged. If you cool down too much between sets, each new set will be somewhat of a shock to the system. Keep the blood pumping.

You don't need to lift weights for more than forty-five minutes. Your muscles can't handle rebuild from the breakdown you overload them with in that time. You don't need as much rest between sets as people think. Give yourself about a thirty- to sixty-second break between sets to keep your heart rate up. Move quickly from station to station. **Go into the gym every time with a game plan and a mission. Accomplish it thoroughly and systematically.**

The Major Muscle Groups
The Exercises to Strengthen Them

When selecting exercises for your strength routine, it's important to choose at least one exercise for each major muscle group. This prevents muscle imbalances that can lead to injury. Let's take a look at the major muscle groups and a few of the exercises that target them:

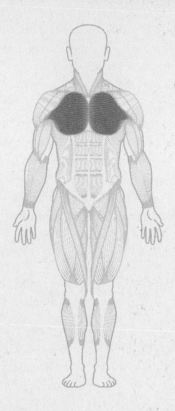

- *PECTORALIS MAJOR:* Large fan-shaped muscle (commonly referred to as "pecs") that covers the front of the chest. Exercises include bench press, chest fly, push-ups, chin-ups.

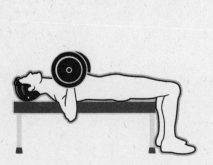 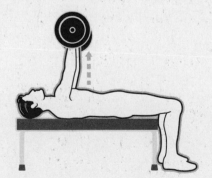

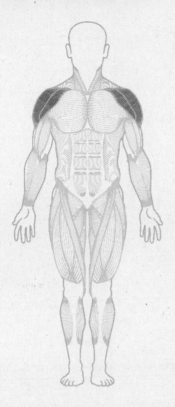 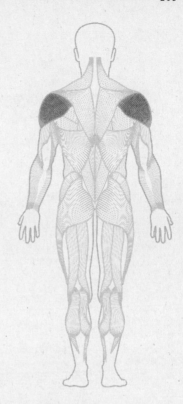

- *DELTOIDS: The cap of the shoulder. This muscle has three parts: anterior deltoid (the front), medial deltoid (the middle), and posterior deltoid (the rear). Different movements target the different parts. The anterior deltoid is worked with push-ups, bench press, and front dumbbell raises. Standing or seated shoulder presses target the medial deltoid. Rear dumbbell raises (done while seated and bent at the waist, or lying facedown on a flat bench) target the posterior deltoid.*

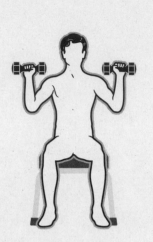
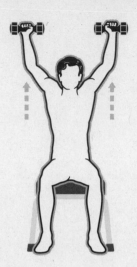
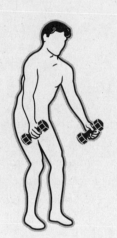
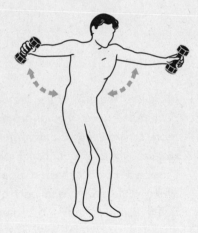

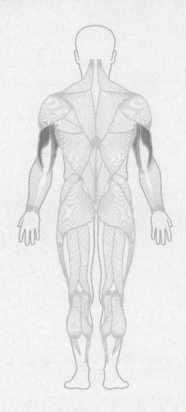

- *TRICEPS: The back of the upper arm. Exercises include pushing movements like tricep extensions, tricep kick-backs, overhead presses, and dips. The triceps also come into play during push-ups, the bench press, and the shoulder press.*

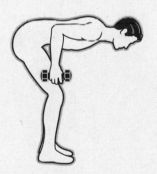 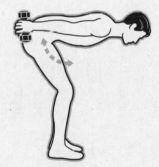

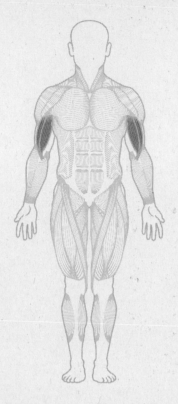

- *BICEPS: The front of the upper arm. Bicep curls are the fundamental exercise for the arms. They can be done with a barbell, dumbbells, or a machine. Other pulling movements like chin-ups and upright rows also involve the biceps.*

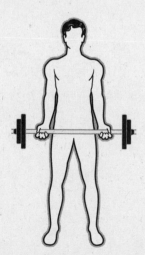 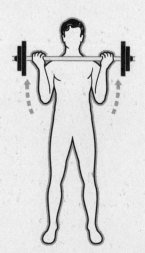

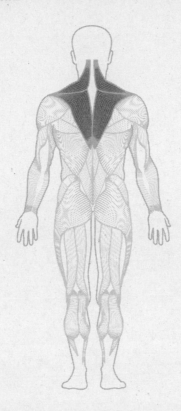

- *TRAPEZIUS: Upper portion of the back. The upper trapezius is the muscle running from the back of the neck to the shoulder. Exercises include up-right rows and shoulder shrugs with dumbbells.*

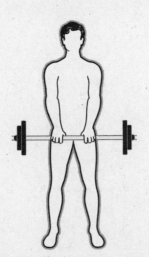 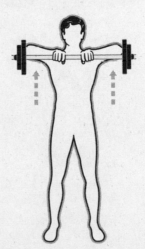

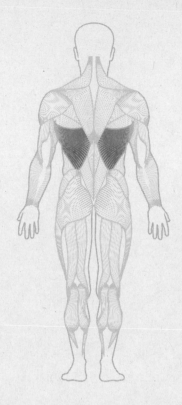

• *LATISIMUS DORSI: Large muscles of the mid-back (commonly reffererd to as "lats"). When properly developed they give the back a nice V-shape, making the waist look smaller. Exercises include pull-ups, chin-ups, one-arm-bent rows, dips, and the lat pull-down machine.*

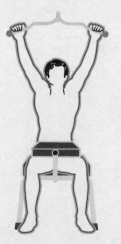 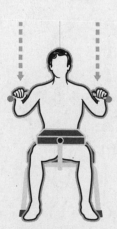

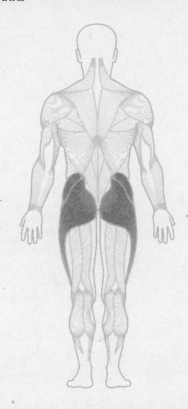

- *GLUTEALS: This group of muscles (commonly referred to as "glutes") includes the gluteus maximus, which is the big muscle covering your butt. Common exercises are the leg-press machine, lunges, and squats.*

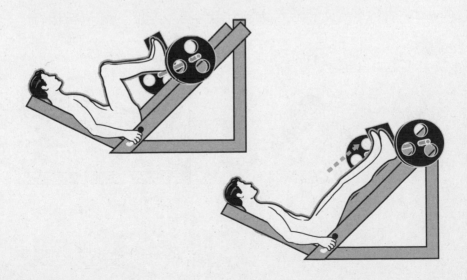

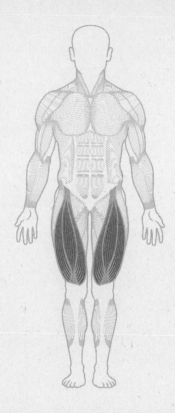

- *QUADRICEPS: This group of muscles (commonly referred to as "quads") makes up the front of the thigh. Exercises include leg-extension machine, leg-press machine, squats, and lunges.*

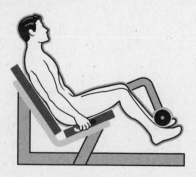 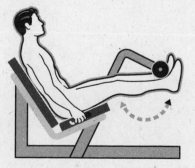

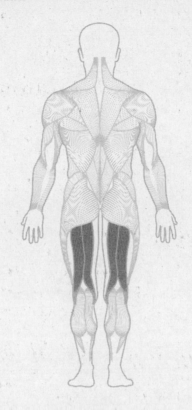

- *HAMSTRINGS: These muscles make up the back of the thigh. Exercises include leg-curl machine, squats, lunges, and leg-press machine.*

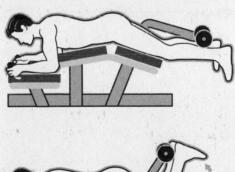

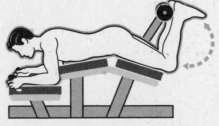

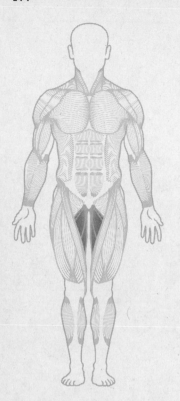 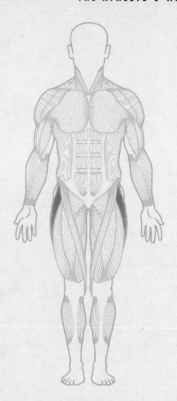

- *HIP ABDUCTORS AND ADDUCTORS: These are the muscles of the inner and outer thigh. The abductors are on the outside and move the leg away from the body. The adductors are on the inside and pull the leg across the centerline of the body. These muscles can be worked with a variety of multi-hip machines, side-lying leg lifts, and standing cable pulls.*

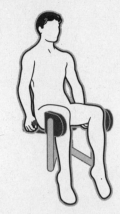

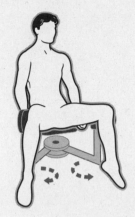

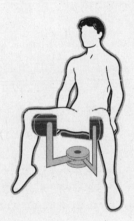

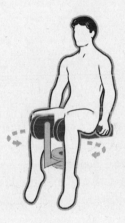

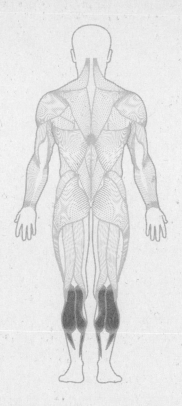

- *CALVES: The calf muscles are on the back of the lower leg. They include the gastrocnemius and the soleus. The gastrocnemius is what gives the calf its strong, rounded shape. The soleus is a flat muscle running under the gastrocnemius. Standing calf raises give the gastrocnemius a good workout, while seated or bent-knee calf raises place special emphasis on the soleus.*

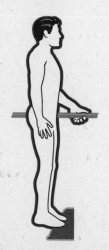 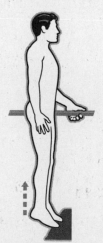 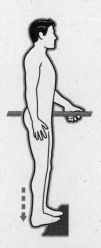

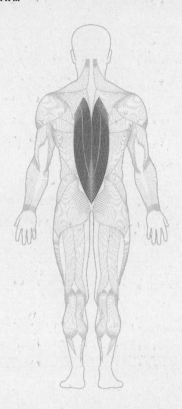

- *LOWER BACK: The erector spinae muscles extend the back and support good posture. Exercises include the back extension machine and prone back extension exercises. These muscles also come into play with almost everything you do. A strong stomach also leads to a strong lower back.*

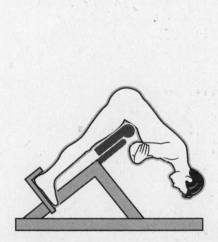 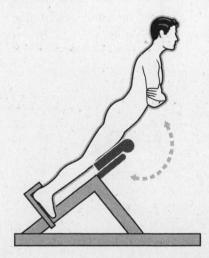

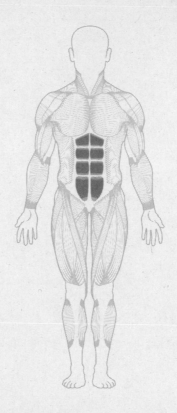

- *ABDOMINALS: These muscles (commonly referred to as "abs") include the rectus abdominus, a large flat muscle running the length of the abdomen, and the external obliques, which run down the sides and front of the abdomen. Exercises such as standard crunches and curls target the rectus abdominus. Reverse curls and crunches (where the hips are lifted instead of the head and shoulders) target the lower portion of this muscle. Crunches involving a rotation or a side angle work the external obliques.*

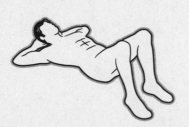 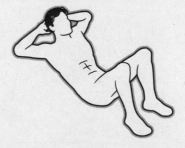

The Athlete's Way Gold Standard: "A Timeless Classic"

When I started lifting weights in 1983, I used Nautilus machines. Nautilus made specific machines for each body part and you moved from station to station doing a circuit designed to target all the major muscle groups. The protocol set up by Nautilius was based on the same principles used by weight lifters since the beginning of the physical culture; it is still the same today and is a timeless gold standard.

- *lift weights three times a week*

- *do two to three sets for each muscle group*

- *do eight to twelve reps in a full-body circuit*

The workout philosophy is exactly the same whether you are using free weights or machines. I tend to use both machines and free weights. Often, if a machine I need is being used I'll use free weights, or come up with another option to target the muscle I want to work.

I find that for 99 percent of people, this is a perfectly sufficient routine. If you want to train sport-specifically or have problem areas, you can target those, but my philosophy is very basic. Trends will come and go, but the gold standard below is tried and true. That said, you should always mix it up a little bit. Be creative to keep your body guessing. If you did this exact routine for the rest of your life, you'd stay in terrific shape. Tailor a program to fit your needs, and stick with it.

A BASIC GOLD-STANDARD FULL-BODY WORKOUT

1. *Leg press*

2. *Leg extension*

3. *Leg curl*

4. *Bench press*

5. *Shoulder press*

6. *Shoulder flies*

7. *Pull downs*

8. Upright rows

9. Biceps

10. Triceps

11. Abductor/adductor

12. Calves

13. Abdominals

THE KEY POINTS TO THINK ABOUT WITH STRENGTH TRAINING

- Have clear-cut goals.

- Use common sense.

- Establish your flow channel of balanced challenge: not too hard, not too easy.

- Keep a training log to chart progress.

- Keep moving—if a machine is taken do something else.

- Always start your stopwatch and be time efficient. Don't lollygag or spend more than thirty to forty-five minutes lifting weights.

- Focus on mind-set. Be mentally tough—focus to finish each set. Don't fizzle.

- For strength: do six to twelve repetitions. For endurance: do twelve to twenty repetitions.

- Completely exhaust Type 1 and Type 2 fibers each set.

- Count up to exhaust Type 1 and count down to exhaust Type 2.

- Heavy weights = injury. Choose a weight that you can lift with perfect form. Do not sacrifice form for heavy weight or you will injure yourself. Practice strict form. Bend your knees; don't strain your back. Stand centered.

- Lift weights at a slow and controlled rate between momentum and gravity. If you go too fast and throw the weight, momentum is doing the work, not your muscles. Likewise, if you drop the weight, gravity is doing all the work. Find the point in between these two.

- *Breathe normally in general. You can also try exhaling during the concentric (positive) as the muscle shortens to lift a weight and inhaling during the eccentric (negative) when you let the weight back down.*

- *Set up the gym like a Skinner box with each set a reward. See each set as a specific goal with a beginning, middle, and end. Break up each set psychologically into doable doses.*

- *Color-code exertion burn. A twelve-rep set would be coded 1 to 4 (yellow), 5 to 8 (orange), or 9 to 12 (red). Understand that each stage requires a different psychological approach. The last four reps should be very intense (code red).*

- *Rest for thirty to sixty seconds between sets.*

- *Do at least one exercise per body part.*

- *Start with large muscle groups, but ultimately the order doesn't matter that much, as long as you hit all the muscles at some point in the workout.*

- *Remember the comfort zone/comfort cusp point and surf that line. Find the perfect level of challenge/weight to match your skill/strength.*

GENETICS PREDETERMINES BODY TYPE
ONLY YOUR PARENTS CAN TAKE THE ACCLAIM

Nature gives you the face you have at twenty; it is up to you to merit the face you have at fifty.

COCO CHANEL

The type of body we have is predetermined to a large extent by our genes. Your body shape and physical appearance are genetically predetermined. There are three basic body shapes—a concept called *somatyping*—which were coined by Harvard psychologist William H. Sheldon in the 1930s and are still used today.

Ectomorphs tend to have a higher metabolism and a slender body with little fat. This body type has a lean frame, often with narrow hips, long legs, and a long neck. Think: beanpole. Ectomorphs have trouble gaining weight.

Mesomorphs tend to be short and stocky. Muscular mesomorphs look like bodybuilders, with wide shoulders, a narrow waist, and broad hips.

The weight they gain tends to distribute itself evenly, and they generally build muscle at a faster rate than either endomorphs or ectomorphs.

Endomorphs tend to be a combination of ectomorph and mesomorph and have typical "average" builds. They may put on pounds quickly, and they have to fight to keep off excess fat around their midsection. Without exercise, their body fat is tough to lose, even when they follow a healthy eating regimen.

It is important to understand that most people are a combination of all three body types to varying degrees. Technically, somatyping would rate each trait on a scale of one to seven and assign, say, a three-point score under each body type. Identifying your body type before starting this program will help you have realistic expectations and set attainable goals.

If you're an ectomorph, for example, an exercise and diet plan may change the amount of fat and muscle you have, but you might lose too much muscle mass if you lift weights, because your metabolism is high. You might have to increase calories. Some mesomorphs can lift weights for a week and see the inches begin piling up in their biceps. They require less work to build muscle. This is genetics. Ectomorphs could lift weights for a year and see little muscle gain. Even if you don't see the results, you are getting the benefits. Remember, the real benefits are under the surface.

BODY DYSMORPHIA
WARPED CONCEPTIONS OF SELF

Develop interest in life as you see it; in people, things, literature, music—the world is so rich, simply throbbing with rich treasures, beautiful souls and interesting people. Forget yourself.

HENRY MILLER

Body dysmorphia is a mental illness of misconception or preoccupation with an imagined physical defect that causes emotional distress and interferes with daily functioning. Most people have some type of body dysmorphia. The perfect example would be thinking that the zit on your nose is as big as Yankee Stadium and that it's all anyone is looking at. People commonly display dysmorphic attitudes about their bodies—"My thighs are fat," "My arms are skinny," "My butt is flabby," "My hair is thinning," "My breasts are lopsided." The media fuels these feelings of inadequacy by bombarding us with air-brushed perfection.

It takes more than just a good looking body. You've got to have the heart and soul to go with it.

EPICTETUS

The most important thing is to have the courage to "accept the things you cannot change and have the courage to change the things you can." Remember to be driven by intrinsic goals, not just extrinsic things like vanity. Be grateful for your body and all the things it does for you. Love and nurture it, and it will continue to provide you with the celebrations of life.

So much has been given me I have no time to ponder over that which has been denied.

HELEN KELLER

THINK OF YOUR JOINTS AS HINGES
AGONIST VS. ANTAGONIST

The doer alone learneth.
FRIEDRICH NIETZSCHE

Life is always going to be about opposing forces—and finding a balance between them. Muscles operate on the same principle. Movement of the skeleton occurs at the joint where two bones meet. Skeletal muscles work in push-pull fashion around the hinge of a joint. For example, the bicep contracts to pull your wrist toward your shoulder. To push it away, the tricep contracts. The agonist and antagonist principle makes it easy for you to figure out how to work a muscle if you slow down and think about how the joint moves and on which side you want the resistance to be.

You have six main joints you can think of as hinges to focus on when strength training: three upper—wrist, elbow, shoulder—and three lower—hip, knee, ankle. Get to know how each joint moves. Most muscles work in pairs called the agonist and the antagonist. As you sit there now looking over the list on page 219–20 touch each one and move the joint around to see where the push-pull would be and how you would resistance-train that muscle.

WHAT TO LOOK FOR WHEN JOINING A GYM

The towels were so thick there I could hardly close my suitcase.

YOGI BERRA

Walking into a gym for the first time as a teenager was a very intimidating experience. I was rail thin and felt completely gangly, like a ninety-eight-pound weakling. I put off joining for a few weeks because it brought up a lot of insecurities. I was clueless about lifting weights and thought that people would judge me, but I got over that.

If you have been putting off joining a gym for any reason, below are some points to think about when choosing a gym. Most gyms are busiest before people go to work and after work. Try to schedule a tour for when you will likely be working out so that you can get a sense of how crowded it is and a vibe of the people who tend to be there at that time.

I think paying more money to belong to a nice gym is a wise investment. I belong to Equinox, a premium gym here in New York, and worth every penny. If the price of a gym seems high, calculate the cost per day by dividing the monthly or annual fee by thirty or 365. In general even the most expensive gyms don't cost much more a day than a coffee from Starbucks. I have an all-access membership at Equinox, which allows me to go to any of their gyms here in the city, or across the country. I like the option of not getting stuck in a rut at the same gym day in and day out.

- *Convenience is probably the most important factor to consider. Join a gym that is close to your home or office and easy to get to.*

- *Is it a chain with other gyms that you can work out at?*

- *Number of machines. How long are wait times at peak hours?*

- *Is it well maintained and clean?*

- *Is the staff friendly and knowledgeable?*

- *Are there time limits posted on cardio equipment? If so, think about when you'll be working out and what your goals are. If you are training for endurance you might find a time limit restrictive. But if you are just trying to squeeze in twenty minutes of cardio before or after* work and have to be at the gym during rush hour, you might like that a rapid turnover on machines is guaranteed.

- Does it cater to your interests—classes, personal training, massage, spa?

- Is there free towel service?

- Does it have a good vibe? Clientele, acoustics, lighting.

- Do you feel self-conscious there, or like you'd fit in?

- Do they give you an introductory screening/fitness evaluation? Free training session?

- Do the classes you want fit your schedule?

- Do you feel comfortable in the locker room?

- Hours of operation, especially on weekends and holidays.

- Can you freeze your membership?

- Check the rules for canceling due to medical issues or relocation.

CHAPTER EIGHT

THE STRETCH PROGRAM

Ambition has one heel nailed in well, though she stretch her fingers to touch the heavens.

LAO TZU

THE FLEXIBILITY PRESCRIPTIVE

FREQUENCY: *Three to five times per week.*

TECHNIQUE: *Static stretching. Hold each stretch, without bouncing, for twenty to forty seconds. For improving balance, practice standing on one foot and other sobriety tests (See p. 240).*

TIME: *Ten to fifteen minutes per session of stretching. Three to five minutes for balance.*

TYPE: *Create a sequence of stretches that you do as a systematic routine.*

STRETCH YOUR NEURONS FROM HEAD TO TOE
DE-STRESS THE WEB OF BODY SNATCHERS

The human body is not a thing of given substance, but a continuous creation. The human body is an energy system . . . which is never a complete structure; never static; is in perpetual inner self-construction and self-destruction; we destroy in order to make new.

NORMAN O. BROWN (AMERICAN PHILOSOPHER)

This chapter is going to focus on flexibility and balance. *The Athlete's Way* is about the process of linking up body, mind, brain, and human spirit. The focus of stretching in this chapter is as much about stretching the cables of your nervous system, improving your state of mind, and getting in touch with your human spirit as it is about the flexibility of muscles and tendons. Stretching, and breathing deeply, is a great way to relax and decompress. It gets the kinks out of your nervous system. Think of stretching as a way to take a time-out from the hectic world and get yourself centered.

The focus of balance is on the cerebellum and plumping up your Purkinje cells. Balance is a use-it-or-lose-it system. This chapter will tell you how to practice using your balance system. You want to stretch a little bit every day, and get in the habit of discreetly balancing on one foot throughout the day, in line at the bank or waiting for the bus. Plan some time every week to do the balancing exercises in this chapter.

Stretching is a "tonic for your nerves and brain," my favorite tag line from Dr. Pemberton, who invented Coca-Cola. Remember that your nervous system is composed of more than one hundred billion cables entwined throughout your body from head to toe. You manipulate and invigorate this web when you stretch. **It is best to stretch when you're already warmed up. Stretch after you work out more than before**. And don't bounce or stretch till it really hurts. It should feel invigorating and maybe intense, like a deep Swedish massage, not painful.

The Hindu study of yoga, a discipline designed to promote the unity of the individual with a supreme being through a system of postures and rituals, began more than five thousand years ago. The ancient wisdom of yoga has evolved by means of empirical research. Yogis have a firsthand understanding of the nervous system that teaches us how to reap maximum neurobiological benefits with postures of movement, breathing, and thought. This chapter is not about teaching you yoga, but rather the simple principles of stretch, balance, and *The Athlete's Way*, which shares core tenets with yogic principles.

The wisdom of the yogic tradition is in keeping with modern neuroscientific discovery. The ancient wisdom of yogi sages created fine-tuned programs that trigger profound effects in our nervous system. Their approach was learned through trial and error, and the empirical evidence is as solid as anything science could deliver with modern technology. Although couched in terms of chakras and energy, yoga is as much about mind-body science and the nervous system as any spiritual system of belief. The wisdom and accuracy of the insights that yogis made long before we had MRIs and brain-imaging technology are valuable resources.

Stretching engages the network of neurons that is your nervous system and invigorates it—like a massage from the inside out. Neurons stretch from the back of your head to the tips of your fingers down your legs to the ends of your toes. When you bend over to touch your toes you are lengthening axons, elongating microtubules, and opening up the synaptic gaps that are the junctions of the billions of neurons woven throughout your entire body. Make waking up the nervous system and the benefits on mind, brain, and spirit your number one reason to stretch.

When you stretch your arms as wide as you can, you are elongating the axons that go from the base of your brain to your fingertips. Feel the electricity going through each neuron and in the synapses. The circuitry explodes when you stretch, because you are getting the electrochemicals and blood flowing into the nooks and crannies of the nervous system, which wakes it up. Breathe deeply and imagine sending oxygen and blood flow to those areas that feel tight.

Neurons need the nutrients delivered by blood flow and oxygen that stretching sends there. Visualize this when you stretch. Imagine every breath sending more blood flow and oxygen to the tight area. Feel the stretch as you hold it and breathe. Imagine that you are flooding that area with fresh nutrients and washing away the old stale toxins. This is a simple visualization that has worked for me every day for twenty years.

Your brain alone has enough energy to light a twenty-watt lightbulb, but there is much more energy than that in your entire nervous system. Your ability to tap the collective pool of energy in the universe is infinite. Imagine the kilowatts pumping through your nervous system and plug into it. Light up your spinal column.

BEND BUT NEVER BREAK ME
YOU ARE NOT A HUMAN PRETZEL

The bamboo that bends is stronger than the oak that resists.

JAPANESE PROVERB

You do not have to push the envelope when you stretch; there should be nothing competitive about. Keep it gentle and tonic feeling. The key to stretching isn't so much in learning the stretches. There are only so many ways you can bend each joint. The key, like everything exercise-related, is actually doing it. This chapter will give you reasons to want to stretch and practice balance. My goal is to motivate you. The emphasis of this chapter is to make stretching and balance work a part of your daily routine.

I stretch anywhere and everywhere I can. Though I recommend that you make specific time to stretch, do it anytime you have a few minutes to spare and some space. Also, sign up for a yoga class or rent a yoga DVD. I love to do yoga, but I often feel spastic in yoga classes so I understand how intimidating it can be to go into a yoga room for the first time. Take the plunge! Go with a friend. Wear comfortable clothes. Abandon rejection sensitivity. If a yoga instructor makes you feel self-conscious or "less than" in any way, find a different class or place to do yoga. Yoga, at its core, is the ultimate nonjudgment in a nurturing and accepting athletic/spiritual environment.

A SPA TREATMENT FOR YOUR NEURONS
STRETCH IS LIKE A MASSAGE FROM THE INSIDE OUT

I love to put on lotion. Sometimes I'll watch TV and go into a lotion trance for an hour. I try to find brands that don't taste bad in case anyone wants to taste me.

ANGELINA JOLIE

You need to stretch for your nervous system. Nothing lengthens and opens up your neurons like stretching. The benefits to muscles and tendons are secondary. Think of stretching as a spa treatment for your neurons and indulge in its therapeutic value. It feels really good. Many people who do cardio regularly have the best intentions to stretch after a workout, but time runs short and they regularly blow it off, just as they blow off lifting weights. Don't do it!

Stretching tends to fall to the bottom of the to-do list, because it seems superfluous. It's not. Make stretching a part of your weekly routine; be regimented about your relaxation. I know it sounds contradictory to be Type A about being Type B, but it's not. This is the high-wire act of *The Athlete's Way*—finding that balance. Stretching is invigorating and relaxing. This polarity is what makes it so dynamic. It wakes you up but makes you feel calm, grounded, and centered.

To be sensual, I think, is to respect and rejoice in the force of life, of life itself, and to be present in all that one does, from the effort of loving to the making of bread.

JAMES A. BALDWIN

Stretching and breathing reduce stress. They are also very sensual and rejoiceful experiences; relish in them. Soak it up. Because stretching and breathing calm the nervous system, you are flooding your body with calming anti-anxiety neurochemicals. Stretching the neurons that you activate will send the chemicals associated with a relaxed state of mind into the openings in the synaptic gaps.

THE STRETCH REFLEX
MUSCLE SPINDLES CAN LEARN TO LET GO

When you get in a tight place and everything goes against you, till it seems as though you could not hold on a minute longer, never give up then, for that is just the place and time that the tide will turn.
                                    HARRIET BEECHER STOWE

When you stretch, there is a mechanism called the *muscle spindle* that records the change in length. In order to prevent you from overextending a muscle, the stretch reflex is triggered in every muscle of your body to resist the change in muscle length by causing the stretched muscle to contract. The more sudden the change in muscle length, the stronger the stretch reflex will kick in. This basic function of the muscle spindle helps to maintain muscle tone and to protect the body from injury. Without the stretch reflex, our muscles would be like taffy. Your body would end up in a big puddle. Unfortunately, if you don't work past this initial reflex, your muscles will tighten over time.

With regular stretching, the spindle itself learns to relax, which is a key to flexibility. One of the reasons for holding a stretch for more than ten seconds is that as you hold the muscle in a stretched position, the muscle spindle and stretch reflex becomes accustomed to the new length and reduces its signaling to contract. Gradually, you can train your stretch receptors to allow greater lengthening of the muscles. This is the key to flexibility.

With regular stretching, the stretch reflex of certain muscles can be controlled so that there is little or no reflex contraction in response to a sudden stretch. While this type of control provides the opportunity for the greatest gains in flexibility, it also provides the greatest risk of injury if used improperly. You'll notice that dancers usually possess the ability to override the stretch reflex because they stretch so often.

The dynamic component of the stretch reflex, which can be very powerful, lasts for only a moment in response to the initial sudden increase in muscle length. This is why you should ease into a stretch. Give the spindle time to relax and send signals back to your spinal cord that it's okay to keep moving.

SYSTEMATIC AND METHODICAL PROCEDURES
ACTIVATE YOUR HABIT BRAIN

No matter how full a reservoir of maxims one may possess, and no matter how good one's sentiments may be, if one has not taken advantage of every concrete opportunity to act, one's character may remain entirely unaffected for the better. With mere good intentions, hell is proverbially paved.

WILLIAM JAMES

Stretching should be much more cerebellar than cerebral. Again, make it a ritual by doing it in the same place, and you'll be able to lose yourself and click into automatic performance more easily. You want to activate your habit learning and procedural memory housed in the down brain. This happens with repetition and practice.

Schedule times when you are going to relax, and use your stopwatch, hourglass, or kitchen timer (out of ticking range) just as you would for cardio or strength training. Don't use the timer to rush yourself; use it instead to block out time so that you can totally relax. Make sure that you have a cycle of stretching that you do in a particular order—one that has a beginning, a middle, and an end. Choose ten to twelve stretches and do them in a cycle.

I provide twelve stretches as a starting point, but do some more research on stretching. Draw stick figure sketches in your workbook, and follow the personalized sequence you like. Stick with it for a while, until you master it. If you get bored, mix it up. The stretches here cover the basics and can be done in ten to fifteen minutes. See how long it takes you to do the sequence, but don't rush. If you take a yoga class, remember the sequence there. Write down the order of stretches and make thumbnail figure sketches in your workbook. With stretching, as with everything, consistency and contiguity are key.

To whom it may concern: it is Springtime. It is late afternoon.

KURT VONNEGUT

Make stretching a ritual—same mat, same sequence, same time of day. By shutting down the cerebrum and operating from cerebellum when stretching, you can better create a default state. The cerebellum won't have to work overtime with the proprioception of sorting out the details of your surroundings. Clearing your mind when you stretch is important. It should become a procedural memory. You want to lose yourself when you stretch. Remember that deep breathing and stretching lower cortisol (the stress molecule).

KEYS TO STRETCHING
DAILY PRACTICE

You are either part of the solution or part of the problem.
(LEROY) ELDRIDGE CLEAVER

Stretching is a skill. It takes practice. Give your body time to get used to it. During the first eight weeks, you will begin to master it, I guarantee. Stay dedicated to your daily practice. Squeeze in stretching at all points through the day, and remember to breathe deeply.

- *Use the same mat and stretch in the same place. This allows your cerebellum to let go of some of its proprioception (body position) duties by being still and familiar in space.*

- *Do each stretching cycle as a sequence, in the same order every time.*

- *Remember the electricity of the nervous system, quiet but invigorated. Humming.*

- *Relax tonis (muscle tension) in your mouth and throat by touching the tip of your tongue to the back of your top teeth, breathe deeply, and fix your eyes on a pinpoint of an object to tap the cerebellum and create a reverse REM/VOR default state. (Practice this meditative technique of focusing your eyes on a fixed point and breathing deeply during cardio and strength training, too.)*

- *Imagine blood flow and oxygen going through every muscle into the belly of the stretch.*

- *Hold each stretch for fifteen to twenty seconds, or three to five breaths.*

- *Try tensing groups of muscles in your face and body and then releasing them. Move systematically from top to bottom and up again.*

- *Imagine neurons firing and elongating, and oxygen and blood flow filling muscles with every inhale and exhale. Deeper and deeper.*

- *Stretching might cause a minor feeling of discomfort but should not cause pain. If it hurts—I mean really hurts—stop.*

A STRETCHING STARTING POINT
TWELVE BASIC EXERCISES: SIX STANDING, SIX ON THE FLOOR

Her body calculated to a millimeter to suggest a bud yet guarantee a flower.

F. SCOTT FITZGERALD

The following are examples of general static stretching and mobility exercises that could form part of the cooldown routine at the end of a training session, or at any time of day. The aim is to relax the muscles and facilitate an improvement in maximum range of motion. Ultimately, the goal is to reduce stress and invigorate the nervous system. This is a starting point; do more research for stretches that suit your needs.

STANDING STRETCHES

1. SHOULDER SHRUGS (ten times each)

   a. Roll shoulders forward

   b. Roll shoulders back

   c. Lift shoulders up toward ears and release.

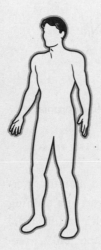 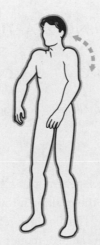 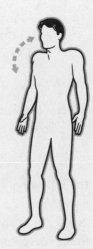

2. TOE TOUCHES

   a. Bend forward and let your torso hang gently, touching the floor
   with your hands.

   b. Try same exercise with your arms locked and hands clasped
   behind your back. Feel the hamstring stretch.

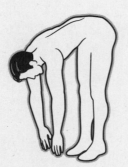 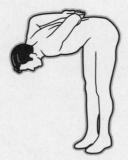

3. SIDE BENDS

    a. Bend to the right, reach for the wall. Hold to one side. Feel the side of your body open up like a bow from ankle to wrist.

    b. switch sides and reach for the other side.

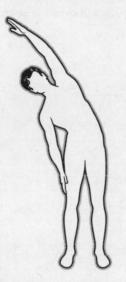 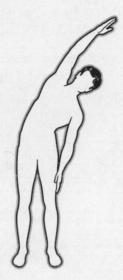

4. CALF STRETCH

    a. Place your hands against a wall, one foot back, heel to the ground.

    b. Lean forward. Feel the calf stretch in a straight line from ankle to butt.

    c. Bend the knee of back leg and feel the stretch lower in your leg toward your Achilles tendon.

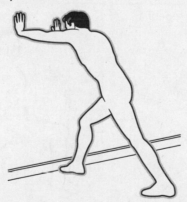

5. QUAD STRETCH

   a. Stabilize yourself with a chair or rail.

   b. Grab your foot and bring it toward your butt. Keep your knees parallel; the lifted leg should stay perpendicular to the ground. (Pulling the leg you are stretching back moves the stretch into the hip, and out of the quad.)

   c. Switch legs and repeat.

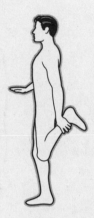

6. LUNGE STRETCH

   a. Lunge forward with one leg. Keep the knee above the ankle at a right angle. Feel the stretch in the groin.

   b. Straighten the forward leg and feel the stretch in the hamstring.

   c. Flex and point your toes and feel the stretch in your lower leg.

   d. Switch legs and repeat.

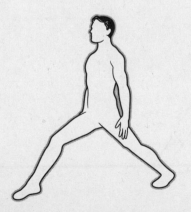
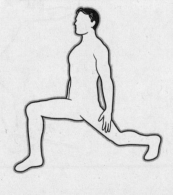

FLOOR WORK

*(Use a mat and a small towel to hook around your feet to elongate the
    stretch)*

7. HAMSTRING STRETCH

   a. *Sit on the floor and place your feet directly in front of you.*

   b. *Bring your chest toward your knees, keeping your back straight.
      Wrap a towel around your feet and use it to pull your chin gently
      toward your shins.*

   c. *Breath deeply and relax. Go deeper into the stretch with each
      exhalation.*

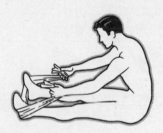

8. SEATED SIDE STRETCH

   a. *Make a V with your legs. Reach straight ahead and feel your
      groin and lower back open up.*

   b. *Sit upright and bend over to the right side toward your toe. Feel
      your sides open up.*

   c. *Repeat on the other side.*

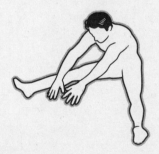 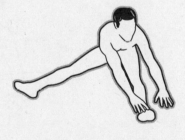

9. *SPINE SUPINATE STRETCH*

    a. *Sitting upright, place your legs straight in front of you.*

    B. *Place your right foot to the outside of your left leg and lock your right arm against the right knee.*

    c. *With a straight arm gently twist your torso, creating "torque" as you twist your torso to the left.*

    d. *Switch legs; repeat.*

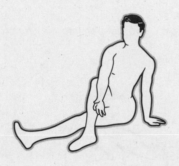

10. *GROIN STRETCH*

    a. *Put the soles of your feet together. Bring your heels toward your groin, knees toward the ground.*

    b. *Cup your feet with your hands and lean forward.*

    c. *Breathe deeply and feel the breath going deeper and deeper into the muscles you are stretching. Imagine air bubbles filling each stretch.*

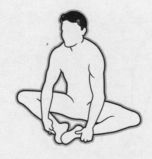

11. FETAL POSTION

a. Lying on your back, bring your knees to your chest and curl up into a fetal position.

b. Rock gently like a rocking chair.

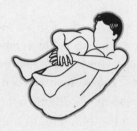

12. STOMACH STRETCH

a. Lying facedown on the floor, push your torso up away from the ground.

b. Gently roll your head back and look at the ceiling. Lock your arms and pretend you're a cobra.

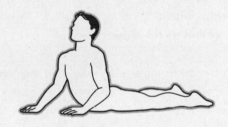

BALANCE WORK
BUILDING A BIGGER CEREBELLUM

Life would be infinitely happier if we could only be born at the age of eighty and gradually approach eighteen.

MARK TWAIN

Practicing your balance every day keeps the cerebellum big and strong. Our cerebellum shrinks as we age, which is one reason older people wobble and fall down and break bones. People who are bedridden for more than six months can lose up to 23 percent of Purkinje cell (muscle memory) volume. Many senior citizens have a fear of falling to the point of avoiding getting up, which increases their odds of falling when they actually do get up.

You should try a sobriety test daily. Walk a straight line heel to toe down the sidewalk or touch your nose while standing on one foot. When police officers test for sobriety, they are testing your cerebellum, which is the first part of the brain affected by alcohol. These exercises will keep your Purkinje cells in the cerebellum bulked up. New hospital techniques involve vibrating/shaking bedridden people to stimulate brain cells that atrophy when they don't move. As we get older, and move less, balance work becomes much more important.

Stand on one foot and try these exercises:

1. Hold on to a chair or table with hand, and then one finger.

2. Let go and balance.

3. Close your eyes and hold the pose (if you can).

4. Repeat with other leg.

Trying to balance with your eyes closed is one of the best ways to feel the gyroscope/balance effect of the cerebellum and wake up your sense of proprioception.

Sobriety Tests for Balance
Think Like a Wire Walker

• *Walk a straight line forward and backward: Take nine to twelve heel-to-*

toe steps along a line moving forward; turn and take nine to twelve toe-to-heel steps backward.

- *One-leg stand: Stand with your heels together, arms at your side, and then raise one leg at a time six inches off the ground while counting to fifteen.*

- *Finger-to-nose: Stand on one foot with your arms to the side and alternate bringing the index finger to the nose with eyes opened and closed.*

The Ancient Martial Arts
Tai Chi and Neurobiology

Clay is molded to form a cup, but it is on its non-being that the utility of the cup depends. Doors and windows are cut out to make a room, but it is on its non-being that the utility of the room depends. Therefore turn being into advantage, and turn non-being into utility.

LAO TZU

If you have access to studying any type of Tai Chi or martial arts I recommend signing up for a class. The traditional martial arts are a terrific way to stretch and strengthen your nervous system and practice the mental skills of creating flow. Csikszentmihalyi, the author of *Creativity: Flow and the Psychology of Discovery and Invention*, states:

> The warrior strives to reach the point where he can act with lightning speed against opponents, without having to think or reason about the best defensive or offensive move to make. Those who perform well claim that fighting becomes a joyous artistic performance, during which the everyday experience of duality between mind and body is transformed into a harmonious one-pointedness of mind.

I see this presence of mind linking up with brain and body in people doing Tai Chi in the courtyard of my apartment complex, and along the East River, every morning. Tai Chi movements sum up fluid performance and the act of systematically stimulating your nervous system. The ancient physical art forms were mastered over centuries by sages who figured things out that brain imaging can now verify. The medical world has proven again and again the ability of these practices to improve your overall state of well-being and mental health.

CHAPTER NINE

THE NUTRITION PHILOSOPHY

To safeguard one's health at the cost of too strict a diet is a tiresome illness indeed.

FRANÇOIS ROCHEFOUCAULD (*SENTENCES ET MAXIMS MORALES*)

We are not what we eat. We are what we think and do. Experts are convinced that making the right dietary choices can improve health and protect us from certain diseases. Unfortunately, no one can seem to agree on what the exact choices should be for every circumstance. When it comes to what people should eat, there are lots of opinions and little certainty. Nutrition is a potentially confusing and often misunderstood field. Therefore, the nutrition prescriptive set forth in this chapter is: use common sense, eat intuitively, keep track of calories in/calories out, stay hydrated, and eat a variety of foods. You also want to avoid food fads. Don't make dietary choices based on newspaper headlines, and avoid making any foods taboo. That's it in a nutshell. Food should be a source of joy, not neurosis.

I want this chapter to convince you to lighten up about food. Worrying or obsessing about what you eat is counterproductive and will create a stressed-out chemical environment in your brain and body, which is more toxic than any food you could ever ingest. This book looks at your body as a wonderfully resilient and adaptable system. You respect it by treating it well and nourishing it, not by being obsessive or depriving it.

Food is life. Food is love. Food is delicious. Enjoy it. Just don't be a glutton. No energy source, fossil or caloric, should ever be overconsumed. That is *The Athlete's Way*. Take only what you need. Think like a Spartan. Give thanks and relish in it. Be grateful for food. More than eight million people die every year from starvation worldwide. We are the lucky ones.

The richest 1 percent of the world's population owns 40 percent of total global assets, while the poorest half of the world's population shares less than 1 percent of these global assets. In the United States, the richest 1 percent of the nation's population holds over 50 percent of total household wealth.

WORLD INSTITUTE FOR DEVELOPMENT ECONOMICS RESEARCH

There are no menus or food plans to follow here. This chapter offers facts and philosophy on food and gives nutritional advice for athletes, which is basically the same as it is for everybody else. Maintain energy balance and stay hydrated. I cover a lot of the basics of nutrition so that you can make informed decisions, but I don't perpetuate myths. There are no great secrets here about nutrition for sport or otherwise because they don't exist.

The most important thing to remember is caloric intake and expenditure. Get to know how many calories are in the foods you eat and then make educated decisions about the quantities you consume. This especially holds true in sports, which is about translating nutrition into power and stamina.

DON'T BELIEVE THE HYPE
AGELESS PRINCIPLES SURROUNDING FOOD

'Tis superstition to insist on a special diet. All is made at last of the same chemical atoms.

RALPH WALDO EMERSON

Unless you are competing in endurance sports or racing, you don't need to make too many changes to your diet. There is a lot of hype surrounding sports nutrition, and I don't buy it or preach it.

If you believe that a specific nutrition strategy is going to change your life and make you a better athlete, it actually might. I don't deny the placebo effect. I'm not going to give you any secret food combinations. My research and experience does not confirm these to exist. People hate to hear that. I always say focus on who are and what you do, how you think, feel, and behave, not on what you ingest. You are going to find long-term success in your willpower, passion, and motivation, not in a bottle of Gatorade or Red Bull. I love going to McDonald's after races. I do it in every country around the world as a ritual. In Kona, you pass the Golden Arches about a quarter mile from the finish line. I actually think of them as the gateway to the end of the race and then go back and eat a Big Mac and cheer others in the homestretch.

Fad diets will always come and go. When I started running, I went on what George Sheehan, the author of *Running and Being*, refers to as the Tab and cottage cheese diet. He was a mentor to me and a great writer, and when he wrote his book in the late seventies, Tab and cottage cheese was it. Then it was all carbs and no protein on the *Eat to Win* diet of the mid-eighties. Then it was no carbs and all protein on Atkins. You get the point. Use common sense. And listen to your body. **Eat when you're hungry; stop before you're full.**

Strict diets tend to ignore the realities of life and set up a cycle of denial, guilt, craving, and binging, which takes all the pleasure out of food. Instead of being really strict about counting calories, just get to know how many calories are in the foods you eat. Enjoy a variety of foods and avoid being neurotic or obsessive about food.

I encourage you to delete the idea of going on a diet from your mind-set. Diets are based on a mentality of deprivation; they don't work. The trick is to eat foods that you enjoy and strive to practice portion control by learning to pay attention to the feeling of true hunger and satiety. By not forbidding certain foods, you will crave them less.

The nutritional foundation of *The Athlete's Way* is to identify your own personal relationship to food, understand what motivates you, and then change your mind-set and behavior. Mind-set, just as in sports, will be cerebral—you think and decide what to eat. In your cerebellum, in your habit brain, you will create new habits.

ENERGY BALANCE: CALORIES IN/CALORIES OUT
ENERGY IS NEITHER CREATED NOR DESTROYED

The sun, with all those planets revolving around it and dependent on it, can still ripen a bunch of grapes as if it had nothing else in the universe to do.

GALILEO GALILEI

Fat is stored fuel. Everything you eat with a caloric (energy) value needs to be burned up through work or used to build your body. All the excess has nowhere to go except to turn to fat. Since energy cannot be created or destroyed, but can only be changed from one form to another, all the energy that we consume in the form of food originated from the sun and traveled to

earth in the form of solar energy. The sun's energy literally fuels every physical movement an athlete or an animal makes. Living plants are able to convert solar energy to chemical energy by a process called photosynthesis.
This chemical energy is used to make other substances such as carbohydrate, fat, and protein, all of which provide energy—as well as the protein
amino acids necessary for growth and repair. Animals cannot use solar energy directly, therefore we convert the chemical energy contained in food.

The glycogen that fuels our cells and builds our bodies is energy that
originated on the surface of the sun. Not only does the sun's energy allow
you to move, it is what has allowed you to grow muscles and bones and is
stored as fat. You don't want to carry around the sun's energy; that would be
hogging it. You want to put it back out there. This is my philosophy on calories in, calories out, and energy balance. Never be a glutton with any fuel
source. Take only what you need.

Three ways the energy we consume is used:

- *To maintain body functions—to keep the heart beating, to breathe, to
  keep the body warm.*

- *For physical movement—muscle contraction.*

- *For growth and repair, which require new tissues to be made.*

When energy is burned during exercise, heat and motion are generated.
Sweating is the process of your body cooling itself when you burn energy
through movement. The food we eat is energy that is measured in calories.
A calorie (cal) is defined as the energy needed to raise the temperature of
one gram of water from 14.5° to 15.5° C.

When you eat a bowl of pasta, you convert that energy into glycogen
and then into motion and heat. If you consume more energy than you use, it
has nowhere to go but to be stored in your body in the form of fat. Glycogen
is the main source of fuel used by the muscles to enable you to undertake
exercise. If you train with low glycogen stores, you will feel tired constantly,
training performance will be lower, and you will be more prone to injury
and illness.

QUID-PRO-QUO EATING (THIS FOR THAT)
BE PRAGMATIC AND INTUITIVE

Give a man a fish and you feed him for a day. Teach a man to fish and you feed him for a lifetime.

CHINESE PROVERB

The goal of *The Athlete's Way* nutrition program is to learn how to listen to your body, to recognize what your body wants, and to regulate how much you eat based primarily on hunger and satiety. The eating plan is based on what nutritionists call intuitive eating coupled with the idea of what I have coined *quid-pro-quo eating*, meaning that you are pragmatic about the energy exchange of calories in, calories out. Quid pro quo is not about being extreme. It is about balance. Do not monitor your calories obsessively. Eat when you're hungry, and stop before you're full.

Consciously make deals based on a quid pro quo, the energy exchange of food in, energy out. Your body is an energy-driven machine. The fuel we run on is consumed in the form of calories. Excess fuel is stored as fat. Whatever you don't burn in a given day is held in reserve. In days of feast and famine, this was a generous biological design. Now that food is plentiful and we move less, there is a double whammy occurring that has led to an obesity epidemic.

Take inventory of how many calories you need to fuel the activity level and metabolic burn rate of your life. If you are sedentary, eat less. Remember the key to revving your metabolism is combining cardio and strength training. The energy required to rebuild muscle pays high dividends beyond the parking meter aspect of time spent burning calories doing cardio. Get to know your body and the amount of energy in, energy out that creates weight loss. If you want to lose weight, create a slight caloric deficit every day and watch the pounds melt away over the months. Learn to make deals—I want the chocolate cake for dessert, but I'll burn it off in the morning. You can do this without being an exercise bulimic. Be a bean counter of sorts by keeping tabs on calories in and calories out in a casual way. It is an art to a degree; you have to learn to walk the line.

Only dull people are brilliant at breakfast.

OSCAR WILDE

One aspect of intuitive eating that is initially counterintuitive for people conditioned to restrictive dieting is the concept that there is a place for every food. There is no food you can never have. Never make a food you love taboo. Dieting triggers psychological and physiological urges to binge on taboo foods. If you eat intuitively you are less likely to binge because you know that the forbidden food is no longer taboo. You can have a little bit of it today and a little bit tomorrow, for the rest of your life. Once the foods are no longer forbidden, people tend to lose interest in overconsuming them.

To eat intuitively, it is important to know what's in the foods you eat and to know how many calories they have so that you can make educated choices. You want to be intuitive *and* educated.

THE HABIT BRAIN CRAVES AND BEHAVES
THE THINKING BRAIN GUIDES AND DECIDES

Habit is necessary; it is the habit of having habits, of turning a trail into a rut, that must be incessantly fought against if one is to remain alive.

EDITH WHARTON

Remember to guide the cross talk between the cerebrum (up brain) and cerebellum (down brain) about nutrition just as you would doing cardio or strength training. You want to create a new mind-set and system of belief cerebrally and implement it with new habits and behavior acted out by the cerebellum, your intuitive and often impulsive animal brain. Most animals eat for instant gratification. We are one of the few animals who can delay gratification, but instinctively we are wired to want to eat all food available to us in a feast-or-famine way. Animals in the wild fill up or graze all day, since they never know for sure when the next meal will appear. The human animal will always have a struggle when it comes to food. You must practice some restraint.

Learn to guide the cross talk in your head in a constructive way. Down brain says what it wants to eat, and up brain says what it should eat. This is classic executive function versus animal impulse between your two brains that begins the minute you wake up.

Remember that your large prefrontal cortex is what allows you, as a human, to delay gratification and exercise free will unlike other animals.

Learn to step back and understand that you are the big boss ultimately, but also learn to listen to the cravings and desires coming from down below, from your cerebellum. Create good habits and they will be reinforced at a neural level.

> *Whenever you are angry, be assured that it is not only a present evil, but that you have increased a habit.*
>
> EPICTETUS

You want to listen to your body because oftentimes the cerebellum knows what your body needs, but be aware that it is also an impulsive brain. If the smell of cheese pizza stirs a craving, there may be something in the craved food that you need. Trust your instincts, but also use common sense.

The key to eating intuitively is about eating when you're hungry and stopping when you're full. It's also about bartering occasionally. You need to practice some executive function, but bow to your cravings. For example, you may tell yourself, "You can have another slice of pizza, but you have to run an extra ten minutes tomorrow." Again, you can make deals about energy intake and expenditure without being an exercise bulimic. It's just about common sense and accountability. The sky is not the limit in either direction. Don't eat ten bags of cookies and run ten hours. Find your middle way. When it comes to diet and nutrition, moderation and variety are key.

> *An empty stomach is not a good political adviser.*
>
> ALBERT EINSTEIN

TAKE ACCOUNTABILITY FOR YOUR CONSUMPTION
PORTION SIZE MATTERS MOST. KNOW YOUR UNITS

> *Character—the willingness to accept responsibility for one's own life—is the source from which self-respect springs.*
>
> JOAN DIDION

A unit serving is much smaller than you think. Make choices about how much you eat by knowing unit sizes and recognizing volume and weight.

I really can't tell with the single serving bags of chips I eat at lunch how much is air, but they're all different, and I don't count chips. I do look at ounces

and do the math. You won't quite know how many chips are inside the silver foil bag unless you read the label. A single serving unit of potato chips
can vary from one ounce to two ounces. Be on the lookout for unit sizes in
your day-to-day life.

When it comes to units, for example, I would never cram three English
muffins into my toaster in the morning, but I will wedge the same number
of calories held in one dense New York bagel into my toaster and consider it
a single unit. Since I am cognizant of unit size, I eat just half a bagel with
fruit and yogurt, and freeze the other half for the next day. That is the unit of
carbs that I should eat at breakfast, and that is educated, intuitive eating.

Nutritionists have discovered that consumers will often finish a unit of
food despite the quantity in relation to how hungry they are. The term used
to describe portion subjectivity is *unit bias*. People in other countries,
France, for example, have smaller portions across the board. Their unit bias
leans toward a serving that is much smaller than an average American
would consider.

Andrew B. Geier, a graduate student in Penn's department of psychology who studies obesity, said, "We have a culturally enforced consumption
norm, which promotes both the tendency to complete eating a unit and the
idea that a single unit is the proper amount to eat. In terms of food, unit bias
applies to what people think is the appropriate amount to consume, and it
shows why smaller portion sizes can be just as satisfying."

EXERCISE BURNS LESS THAN YOU THINK
DON'T WORK OUT, THEN PIG OUT

And gain is gain, however small.
ROBERT BROWNING

I feel bad using the wonderful and inspiring Robert Browning quote "And
gain is gain, however small" in a nutrition chapter. It has much more significance than gain of ounces on your derriere. I use his words here to make
the point that we get fat gradually over time. It is the two teaspoons of sugar
adding up to thirty-five calories a day that becomes a pound of fat every one
hundred days, and three pounds over the course of a year, and thirty
pounds in a decade. The ability to burn a few extra calories a day is the energy balancing power of exercise. Burning just 250 calories a day with exercise over a year could result in twenty-six pounds of weight loss in a year!

Small increments on both sides add up. Unfortunately most people go to the gym, work out, then get home and say, "I am a calorie-burning machine," and proceed to consume more calories than they burned. This is why people often don't see results in the weight-loss department when they start exercising. To lose weight, keep intake the same and increase exertion. It's simple.

> *He had not an ounce of superfluous flesh on his bones, and leanness goes a great way towards gentility.*
>
> ELIZABETH GASKELL *(WIVES AND DAUGHTERS)*

Some people think that athletes can eat whatever they want and not get fat, but that is not true. The key in most sports, especially cycling, is power-to-weight ratio. You want to be lean and strong. "Fat don't fly" is a common saying. The trick to maintaining a lean body weight is to avoid making foods taboo and to learn the art of making educated decisions without feeling deprived or being neurotic. I will expand on some ways I keep myself lean without being ascetic.

AVOID THE OSTRICH APPROACH:
READ AND DIGEST FOOD LABELS

> *Some books are to be tasted, others to be swallowed, and some few to be chewed and digested: that is, some books are to be read only in parts, others to be read, but not curiously, and some few to be read wholly and with diligence and attention.*
>
> SIR FRANCIS BACON

I always get a sweet tooth after biking in the cold. There is nothing better than hot coffee and one of those pecan rolls from Au Bon Pain on blustery, cold afternoons after riding in the park. After years of a "hear no evil see no evil" approach as I ignored the nutritional information, I realized I should practice what I preach and look at the information on their computer. Knowledge is power, because I found out that the roll has more than 500 calories. Basically an hour of intense cardiovascular exercise could be negated in about four minutes of scarfing that thing down. Instead of depriving myself of the pastry altogether, I have half in the afternoon and the other half for breakfast with some yogurt and fruit. Be pragmatic.

YOUR BODY IS NOT A TEMPLE
IT IS A WARHORSE

It was not her sex appeal, but the obvious relish with which she de-
voured the hamburger, that made my pulse begin to hammer with
excitement.

RAY KROC (FOUNDER OF MCDONALD'S)

The body is an incredibly resilient machine. I think of my body as an ancient
Viking warhorse that is incredibly adaptable and resilient. My Scandinavian
ancestors survived long winters on some meat and potatoes, a sprig of pars-
ley, and lots of Aquavit, and still had the stamina to go out and rape and pil-
lage the world in their Viking ships. I live in a modern civilization with
fruits and vegetables full of nutrients flown in from all over the world year-
round. Food is bountiful. There is no need to fret about exact combinations
of nutrients if I use common sense and eat different-colored foods every day.
I'll be fine and will have more energy than my ancestors to go out and conquer the world.

I spent a decade of my life obsessed with eating healthy and was no fun
to be with. Early in my athletic career, I bought into the idea that my body
was a temple, and it became its own kind of eating disorder. The stress associated with worrying about the food you're eating is worse for you than any
trans fats or preservatives in a Ring Ding or Fritos, in my opinion. That said,
use common sense and feed your body well. Respect it. Make healthy
choices, and you will feel better and be healthier. The objective is to make a
healthy choice when you can, but not to forbid foods you like.

SMART FOOD CHOICES
THESE ARE THE SIMPLE GUIDELINES

Eat a diet rich in fruits, vegetables, whole grains, low-fat dairy products,
lean meats, and fish, and drink plenty of water.

As you can see, eating healthy can be summed up in two lines. We all
intuitively know what foods are healthy. Don't make it a big deal.

I was a very strict vegetarian and macrobiotic eater for much of my time
in college. Although some people can eat that way without feeling deprived,
I was in a constant tug of war between my cravings and my rigid dietary

guidelines. I was neurotic about what I ate and the food had all the power. It dominated my life. When the floodgate opened, instead of eating one unit of a forbidden food like a brownie, I would eat a whole tray of brownies. It set up a dangerous minefield. I was constantly wracked with guilt. Now, if I want a brownie, I eat a brownie or half a brownie because it is not taboo or forbidden.

> Fear less, hope more;
> Eat less, chew more;
> Whine less, breathe more;
> Talk less, say more;
> Hate less, love more;
> And all good things are yours.
> SWEDISH PROVERB

STAY HYDRATED
THE WATER BEARER

Cerebrospinal fluid is 99 percent water.

Water is an essential nutrient. In fact, it is in many ways the most essential nutrient. A human being cannot live for more than seven days without water or eleven days without sleep, but can survive for almost two months without food. There have been reports that too much water may be as dangerous as too little during long-distance athletic events, but overhydration may be dangerous in all sports. The problem lies in diluting the amount of sodium in your body with too much water and causing hyponitremia, which is an electrolyte imbalance that can kill you.

I recommend sipping water all day long. I am reluctant to give specific guidelines regarding quantities of fluids because so much can depend on weather conditions. Once again, use common sense. Listed below are some tips from Catherine O'Brien and Samuel N. Cheuvront, who have done extensive research on hydration and sports on U.S. Army recruits and give the following advice:

COMMON SENSE TIPS ON HYDRATION

- The Boy Scout adage still holds: "Check urine color. It should be relatively clear. If it's dark, you need to drink more," O'Brien says.

- "The recent Institute of Medicine report on water and electrolytes established an adequate intake for water of 3.7 liters per day for a normal adult male, but there is wide variation. Importantly, that 3.7 liters includes water from food and drink, including beverages like coffee or tea," Cheuvront says.

- Exercise fluid intakes should result in neither weight gain nor excessive weight loss (more than 2 percent of body weight). "Weighing oneself nude before and after exercise is the best way to gauge success around this recommendation."

- Don't drink too much, even in the heat: "We have this mistaken belief that more water is better. Not true. The Army has actually reduced the amount of water it gives in the heat," says O'Brien.

THE NUTRITION BASICS

- CARBOHYDRATES: Our main source of energy.

- PROTEINS: Essential for growth and repair of muscle and other body tissues.

- FATS: A source of energy and important in relation to fat-soluble vitamins

- MINERALS: Inorganic elements occurring in the body that are critical to its normal functions.

- WATER: Essential to normal body function as a vehicle for carrying other nutrients and because about 70 percent of the human body is water (85 percent of the brain is water).

- ROUGHAGE: The fibrous, indigestible portion of our diet essential to the health of the digestive system.

A BALLPARK RATIO OF NUTRIENTS FOR THE AVERAGE PERSON

- 55 percent carbohydrates (starches, rice, potatoes, bread; fruits and vegetables; desserts, candy, and cakes)

- *25 percent fats (butter, oil, saturated, unsaturated)*

- *20 percent protein (meat, poultry, fish, eggs, dairy)*

ENERGY YIELD PER GRAM

- *Carbohydrate = four calories*

- *Protein = four calories*

- *Fat = nine calories*

WHAT IS YOUR BODY MADE OF?

On average 70 percent water, 20 percent fat (slightly less for men) and 10 percent of mostly protein-plus carbohydrates, minerals, vitamins. Based on these percentages a 140-pound person's weight could be broken down into:

84 pounds of water

28 pounds of fat

25 pounds of protein

7 pounds of minerals

1.4 pounds of carbohydrates.

Trace vitamins

TEN NUTRITION TIPS FOR EATING THE ATHLETE'S WAY

1. Know Your Caloric Densities and Nutritional Values

The key to maintaining a healthy weight comes down to energy balance, calories in, and calories out. In order to know how many calories you're taking in, you need to know the caloric density of the foods you eat. When you are eating intuitively, you want to make smart choices, and you need the basic nutritional value. Keep it simple. For example, if you have eaten a lot of starch for breakfast (bagel) and lunch (pizza), don't have a starchy supper (pasta). Have a protein-based dinner. This is common sense. Keep tabs as you go through the day. If you learn to listen to your body, it will guide you. Don't stop eating starch altogether, just make informed decisions on how often and how much as you go through the day.

Go to www.theathletesway.com for links to calorie-counting resources to find out how many calories are in the foods you eat and to calculate the daily consumption of the fuel you take in, and the fuel you burn.

2. Moderate Portion Control

More important than what you eat is how much you eat. Practice eating smaller portions and get in the habit of making the serving size of a unit smaller.

3. Slow Down—Chew Your Food

Slow down. I am someone who eats really fast. I inhale food. In life and in eating, I am constantly reminding myself to slow down. I say, "Where's the fire? What's the hurry? Slow down. Look up from your life, Chris." whenever I go into a feeding frenzy. Don't be a chain eater. Many, like me, tend to take one bite while they swallow the one before. Slow down, savor what you're eating, and taste the food. Eating more slowly will give your brain a chance to signal satiety and decrease the tendency to overeat.

4. Do Not Forbid Any Foods

Anytime you forbid yourself to consume a food you love, you are going to crave it. Eat small quantities of the foods you enjoy and focus on portion control instead of forbidding foods. No food should be taboo.

5. Combine Cardio with Strength Training

Increasing your activity level translates to increased metabolism. Weight lifting is as important as cardio training; don't neglect it. Strength training will especially increase your metabolism by adding energy-burning muscle to your frame. Remember, a pound of muscle burns thirty to fifty calories a day; a pound of fat burns two. A pound of fat is 3,500 calories. Create a caloric deficit of 350 calories by combining exercise and diet and lose a pound in ten days.

6. Eat When You're Hungry, Stop Before You're Full

Most people forget what it feels like to be hungry. The key to eating only when you're hungry is to avoid getting so hungry that you binge. Find a balance between allowing yourself to get hungry and not overindulging. Some tricks for eating less and signaling the end of a meal:

- *Eat on smaller plates with smaller utensils.*
- *Place knife and fork side by side on top right side of plate, at a 45-degree angle, signifying that you are finished eating.*
- *Order a hot tea or coffee and have a little something sweet.*
- *Ask for a doggy bag in restaurants.*
- *Brush your teeth.*

7. Get Enough Sleep

Most adults need eight hours of uninterrupted sleep per night. Not getting enough sleep will disrupt your hormonal balance and cause you to eat more and gain weight. Many people eat when they're tired, subconsciously thinking that it will increase their energy. Remember, not sleeping makes you tired, stupid, fat, and sick. It sounds harsh, but it's true. Lack of sleep exhausts you, retards your learning and memory, slows metabolism, and lowers immune function.

8. Limit Snacking

I think everyone has an oral fixation to some degree. The easiest way to eat less is to have tricks to satisfy an oral fixation or to ingest something that is satisfying and low calorie. Gum is America's favorite snack food. Although people spend more money overall on chocolate, it is second on the list. Fresh fruit is third. Neither of those comes close to the number of times people reach for gum on a daily basis, according to Harry Balzer of the NPD (National Purchase Diary) group, which has been collecting data for twenty years on what people eat between meals.

With people trying to put fewer calories and fewer cigarettes in their mouths, gum is a perfect substitute. I use gum throughout the day to satisfy a need to chew on something. I also recommend ice water, hot beverages (coffee or black and herb teas). Seltzer and caffeine-free diet soda also feel like a snack but are calorie free. Grazing all day is not a good idea. Find low-calorie substitutes to satisfy a food craving, and make them part of a healthy, active lifestyle and a balanced diet. Ideally you should listen to your body and eat only when you feel hungry.

9. Weigh Yourself

To weigh or not to weigh? That has been an ongoing question for dieters, nutritionists, and coaches The latest research has shown that weighing yourself helps people trying to lose weight, because it provides instant feed-back. Statistically, people who weigh themselves daily are most likely to lose weight. But there are pitfalls to weighing yourself daily, the primary one being that weight fluctuates from day to day, not just based on percentage of body fat. Remember that water loss can contribute to as much as six pounds a day in weight loss or gain. The key to weighing yourself is to look for trends over the long term, like watching the stock market.

Keep track of your weight in your journal and look for the trajectory of gain or loss over the course of a few weeks. I recommend trying daily weigh-ins to see if you respond well. Everyone is different. See if weekly weigh-ins (or not using a scale at all) are better for you. Even if you do use a scale to gauge weight, also pay attention to how your clothes are fitting and how you look and feel. If you do weigh yourself daily, do it at the same time of day on the same scale. If you notice that you are gaining weight, do something about it.

10. Set Intrinsic Goals (Lose Weight for Health and Esteem, Not Vanity)

When making decisions about food do it for reasons of feeling better physically and mentally. Don't focus on purely external reasons for wanting to eat right and keep a healthy weight. The natural mechanisms that regulate weight and energy balance work to keep your set-point weight in a relatively narrow range. In the long term, intrinsic motivations will help keep your weight to the lower end of your set point.

RIMONABANT (ACOMPLIA/ZIMULTI)

New Obesity Drug Blocks Endocannabinoid "Pleasure Circuit"

Endocannabinoids are the focal neurochemicals of this book and the cannabinoid system is at the root of a new line of obesity drugs that literally get rid of the munchies. Be on the lookout for a new family of drugs that will target the cannabinoid system and reduce food craving by taking some of the pleasure out of eating by blocking the CB-1 cannabinoid receptors. Rimonabant, trade name Acomplia in Europe and Zimulti in the United States, is the first in the family of drugs that was slated for release in 2007. It was rejected by the FDA but is up for appeal.

The idea of blocking the cannabinoid pleasure receptor, CB-1, offers a new approach to treating compulsive behavior and obesity, but nobody knows what else endocannabinoids do or the long-term effects of tampering with this system. At this writing the drug is currently undergoing clinical testing. Other drugs linked to the endocannabinoid system for depression and bone density are the future.

FOOD AND MOOD

Don't Be "Hangry"

I have eaten
the plums
that were in
the icebox

and which
you were probably
saving
for breakfast

Forgive me
They were delicious
So sweet
And so cold.

WILLIAM CARLOS WILLIAMS ("THIS IS JUST TO SAY")

One of the first things you learn as an athlete is that when you are hungry, your inner dialogue changes. My friends and I call it being *hangry*—hungry and angry. Usually if I start to have negative cross talk at any point during a race or training and utter things like "This is so pointless," "I am miserable," I'm never doing one of these races again," inside my head I know it's time to eat. Within ten minutes of eating a PowerBar, the world seems better again, and my inner dialogue reflects this. Remember **food = mood**. If the voices in your head are cranky, you might just need a snack, in life and especially inside the athletic process.

REFUEL AND REHYDRATE
THE PUMPING STATION

For a certain amount of money, you'll eat Alpo.
REGGIE JACKSON

There is a lot of hype surrounding supplements and sports beverages, but only a very small percentage of people actually need to use these products. In general the use of sports beverages and sports bars is not necessary for the average person doing less than sixty minutes of exercise a day. Of course it depends on the conditions and level of intensity. For the most part, these specialty products are just loaded with sugar, and you could get better nutrition from eating real foods. You should look at these sports foods as an additional source of calories, protein, and electrolytes, depending on your sport, never as a substitute for real food.

If you are trying to lose weight, be very careful about consuming more calories in the form of a sports beverage or food than you are burning in the workout. Most sports bars or drinks average about 250 to 350 calories for a full serving, which calorically can negate a good thirty minutes of intense cardio. Use common sense when keeping blood sugar high, but don't over-fuel, either.

BASAL METABOLIC RATE
THE ENERGY YOU BURN

Banging your head against a wall uses an estimated 150 calories an hour.

UNKNOWN

Your basal metabolic rate is the energy used by your body to maintain life functions including cell turnover, resting heart rate, respiration, body warmth, and digestion. Typically anywhere from 50 to 75 percent of a person's total energy expenditure goes to basal metabolic rate. The most metabolically active parts of your body are your heart, brain, lungs, and kidneys. Although they account for less than 5 percent of your body weight, they account for 50 to 60 percent of your energy intake. The brain alone is 2 percent of body weight but consumes 20 percent of the body's energy.

To tip the scale of energy balance in favor of weight loss, start by determining how many calories you should consume each day by checking out the links on my Web site. You want to create a caloric deficit every day. To do so, you need to know how many calories you need to maintain your current weight. Also, don't get discouraged if you don't lose weight initially by exercising. Think of long-term caloric shifts in energy balance. Try to make your key motivations intrinsic, based on self-esteem, achievement, mental, and physical health, not just outward appearance or weight loss.

According to Brian Duscha of Duke University, who studies exercise and weight loss, "The participants in our study received the fitness benefits without losing any weight. Many people exercise to lose weight, and when that doesn't occur, they stop exercising. Remember, that you can improve cardiovascular fitness and reduce the risk of heart disease by exercising without losing weight."

SLIGHT INCREASE OF OUTPUT
SLIGHT DECREASE OF INTAKE

Patience and tenacity of purpose are worth more than twice their weight of cleverness.

THOMAS H. HUXLEY

Though this book is not promoting the body beautiful as the ultimate goal, being overweight is bad for your health. If you are overweight you should lose weight. Obesity has reached epidemic proportions in the United States. According to recent figures, about 65 percent of adults are overweight, and of these 50 percent of overweight people are considered obese. Although the diet and weight-loss industry has exploded, Americans have continued to gain weight. If the goal of dieting is for us to reach and maintain a healthy weight, it is obviously not working. **The key to weight loss is energy balance, portion control, and combining strength training with cardio to burn calories and keep metabolism high**.

To lose one pound, you need a caloric deficit of 3,500 calories. The objective: create a deficit by exercising and cutting back on calories. The number of calories you'll burn during exercise is affected by your body weight, the intensity of your workout, your conditioning level, and your metabolism, so burn rates are going to be only an estimate. But the 3,500 rule is a good benchmark. Use the calculators on my Web site to help estimate how much energy you're burning every day.

KEEP YOUR METABOLISM REVVED UP
NOT EATING SIGNALS FAMINE RESPONSE

Hunger is power.
IVANA TRUMP

The truth is, hunger is weakness. Real hunger causes a slow metabolism. You never want to let yourself get too hungry, because your starvation response will kick in and you will slow your metabolism. On the flip side, you should feel a little hungry before you eat. You want to feel a slight pinch of hunger as a Spartan would every day and then eat.

If one person cut back on calories without exercising and another person increased exercise without cutting back on calories, the first person would lose weight more quickly in the short term. That's because it's easier to cut 500 calories from your diet than it is to burn 500 extra calories through exercise. You'd have to walk or run about five miles a day, or thirty-five miles a week, to lose one pound of fat. In the long term, if you cut back only on calories, you are more likely to regain the weight you lose. The body reacts to weight loss as if you were starving and, in response, slows its metabolism to conserve what it assumes is a limited food supply. When your metabolism slows, you burn fewer calories, even at rest.

A regular schedule of exercise raises not only your energy expenditure while you are exercising but also your resting basal metabolic rate. Resting energy expenditure remains elevated as long as you exercise at least three days a week on a regular basis. Because it accounts for 60 percent to 75 percent of your daily energy expenditure, any increase in BMR is extremely important to your weight-loss effort.

BE ON THE LOOKOUT FOR SUGAR WATER
HIGH-FRUCTOSE CORN SYRUP IS BAD NEWS

When you go in search of honey you must expect to be stung by bees.

KENNETH KAUNDA (ZAMBIAN FREEDOM FIGHTER)

Sugar in beverages is the main source of calories in the American diet, according to a recent Tufts study. The leading source of calories in the American diet used to be white bread. America is now drinking those calories instead, and it's making us obese. According to Odilia Bermudez, Ph.D., "More than two-thirds of people surveyed drink enough soda and/or sweet drinks to provide them with a greater proportion of calories than any other food." A 24-ounce fountain Coca-Cola has 280 calories. If you drank one 24-ounce Coke every day for a year, and did not adjust your energy expenditure, you would gain twenty-nine pounds. That would be almost a one-hundred-pound weight gain in three years.

Be on the lookout for fructose-sweetened beverages. They are not metabolized by the body the same way as glucose and can make you put on fat. Magnetic resonance technology was used to monitor body fat in mice. Total caloric intake was lower in the mice that consumed the fructose-sweetened water than in the other groups, except for the control animals provided with water only. "We were surprised to see that mice actually ate less when exposed to fructose-sweetened beverages, and therefore didn't consume more overall calories," said Dr. Tschöp. "Nevertheless, they gained significantly more body fat within a few weeks." Be on the lookout for hidden sugar in beverages—especially high-fructose corn syrup—and pay attention to hidden calories in beverages you drink.

CAFFEINE
JACK YOUR BODY

We have two ears and one mouth so that we can listen twice as much as we speak.

EPICTETUS

We are a Starbucks nation. I love coffee and I love the coffee klatsch. Though people have been ingesting caffeine for millennia, not until 1820 was the chemical structure of caffeine, the stimulant in coffee and tea that inspires devotion, and addiction, finally identified. Only in the last 200 years have we come to have anything close to a true grasp of how this casually consumed drug radically affects our body and brain. Do you remember how potent the first cup of coffee you had was? I had my first cup of coffee in college. I got so amped up I had to go run twice as far as I had ever run in my life until then. I am a regular coffee drinker now, but have cut back on my caffeine intake after researching this book.

Caffeine is a rather lumpy molecule that, unlike alcohol, tends to attach itself to very few molecules in the body. When an attachment is made, the fit is tight, and the interaction per milligram is much stronger than that of alcohol, which is shaped in a way that makes it fairly indiscriminant about what it binds to. This is why one small cup of coffee—which contains about 100 milligrams of caffeine (a large, sixteen-ounce cup has 1,000 mg)—can have a physiological effect on the body that is as powerful as one beer, which holds about 14,200 milligrams of alcohol.

Caffeine increases dopamine levels in the same way that amphetamines do. Heroin and cocaine also manipulate dopamine levels by slowing down the rate of dopamine reuptake. Obviously caffeine's effect is much lower than that of amphetamines, but it taps the system of reward. It is suspected that the dopamine connection contributes to caffeine addiction.

The Three Main Reasons That Caffeine Gets Us Hooked

- *Caffeine blocks adenosine reception so you feel alert.*

- *It injects adrenaline into the system to give you a boost.*

- *It manipulates dopamine production to make you feel good.*

The more caffeine you ingest, the more it takes to get the adrenaline going again. The long-term effects of caffeine tend to compound. For example, once the adrenaline wears off, you face fatigue and lower mood. Having your body in a state of emergency all day long isn't very healthy, and it also makes you jumpy and irritable.

The half-life of caffeine in your body is about six hours. The most important long-term problem is the effect that caffeine has on sleep. Adenosine reception is important to sleep, especially to deep sleep. If you consume a big cup of coffee with 400 mg of caffeine at 4 P.M., then by 10 P.M. about 200 mg of that caffeine is still in your system. You may be able to fall asleep, but your body probably will miss out on the benefits of deep sleep. That deficit adds up fast. The next day you feel worse, so you need caffeine as soon as you get out of bed. The cycle continues day after day. I have a 4 P.M. cutoff for consuming caffeine and drink herbal tea as a substitute hot beverage.

Once you get in the cycle of having caffeine, you have to keep taking the drug. Ninety percent of Americans consume caffeine every day. Even worse, if you try to stop having caffeine, you get very tired and depressed and you might get a terrible, splitting headache as blood vessels in the brain dilate. If you consume huge quantities, try to monitor it, not by stopping altogether but curbing it.

YOU ARE THE SALT OF THE EARTH
A GEOLOGY ALLEGORY

The cure for anything is salt water: sweat, tears or the sea.

ISAK DINESEN

THE COMPOSITION OF SWEAT:
Sodium 1,200 mg/l Chloride 1,000 mg/l Potassium 300 mg/l Calcium 160 mg/l Magnesium 36 mg/l Sulphate 25 mg/l Phosphate 15 mg/l Zinc/iron 1.2 mg/l each

Sodium and potassium are the two most important electrolytes in your body. You lose both when you sweat, as you can see by looking at the composition of sweat above (sodium + chloride = salt). Sodium is a soft, silvery metal that is essential for the movement of all electrical impulses in the nervous system. Without sodium there would be no action potential in your neurons; synapses would not fire.

When you sweat make sure to replace these crucial electrolytes by getting some sodium and potassium back into your body using sports nutrition or regular food. Sodium is easy to find in almost any prepackaged foods; it's tough to avoid and odds are you have plenty of it. People who suffer from hyponitremia are often on sodium-restricted diets. If you are sweating, don't overly restrict your sodium or potassium intake. These are the most important electrolytes. Great sources of potassium are bananas, orange juice, and chicken broth, which is why these foods are often served at finish lines of endurance events.

The earth is 4.5 billion years old. The crust of the earth has contained all of the same actual chemical elements we have today. They have all been trapped here. The sodium from 4.5 billion years ago is the same sodium that you shake on your french fries, or wipe crusted from your nose after a workout. It is a very tough chemical and hard to break apart. It is generally neither created nor destroyed, just passed along. Sodium will always be sodium. And the same sodium molecules that pass through your body today could pass out of you . . . into a river near your house and end up in a fish, eaten by another person, or end up on a pretzel sometime later this century. Sodium goes around and around and is recycled.

I have a sweat fetish. I admit it. I love to sweat. I love the word. I love the feeling. I even love the smell. Breaking a sweat is my daily practice. I like to stretch after I work out and wait for the sweat to dry as I cool down before I get in the shower. When it is dried and crusty in ridges on my brow, I wipe dried sweat from my temples or nose, rub it between my fingertips, and remind myself, these grains are 4.5 billion years old, and then I lick it off my thumb.

Reingesting the salt you sweat may seem gross. But it is an animal instinct. It represents the salt coming and going out again. It completes the circle and makes me feel connected to 4.5 billion years of earth inside me, the same earth that is all around me. It's as close to reincarnation, or God, I imagine I'll ever get.

> There are two ways to look at life.
> One is as though there are no miracles.
> The other is as though everything is a miracle.
>
> ALBERT EINSTEIN

Every time I exercise, one goal I have is to pull a grain of 4.5-billion-year-old sodium through my pores and bring it back to the open air. I like to wear gray cotton tank tops when I run so I can see the sweat release to make a dark V, knowing it brings out the sodium with it. That idea motivates me. Some days if I don't feel like working out I say, "But you won't be pulling out the salt, Chris—it won't be surfacing today—you'll be breaking the cycle." The thought of sodium molecules coming out of my skin actually motivates me, and then when I lick my thumb as if it's a salt lick in a horse corral. It becomes a reward. Maybe the notion of 4.5 billion years at your fingertips will motivate you some day, too. You need as many tricks up your sleeve as possible.

USE ENERGY TO CREATE ENERGY
EXERCISE MAKES YOU MORE ENERGETIC

Zen does not confuse spirituality with thinking about God while one is peeling potatoes. Zen spirituality is just to peel the potatoes.

ALAN WATTS

One reason I believe that exercise is a quantum experience is that the human machine is the only vehicle I know that actually creates energy by using energy. For example, when I ran the 154-mile treadathalon I consumed a total of only 8,000 calories, yet the effort required 20,000 calories. The extra energy would have required four pounds of fat, which I did not have at the time. I know that the energy moving me was something more than calories in, calories out. There is something both quantum and pragmatic about that.

GO ON A LOW-CARBON DIET
NOT LOW CARBS

What makes the engine go?
Desire, desire, desire.

STANLEY KUNITZ ("TOUCH ME")

Don't spend too much time worrying about food; instead use food to fuel your life and achieve your dreams.

Consider the global impact and good fortune of your nutritional choices. We are so lucky to have the luxury of getting fat. Give thanks and take only what you need. Use your energy as fuel. Seek transportation alternatives as part of your commitment to energy balance. Save money, resources, and the ozone. This is *The Athlete's Way.*

Don't go on a low-carbohydrate diet, go on a low-carbon diet. All fossil fuels, whether they be oil, gas, or coal, create carbon dioxide (CO_2), a greenhouse gas, when they are burned for energy. Your carbon footprint is the amount of CO_2 that your energy consumption emits into the atmosphere. As the Dakota proverb goes, "We will be known by the tracks we leave behind."

Make treads with your sneakers, not steel-belted radials, and the only CO_2 you'll be emitting is that which you exhale. Use your own energy for locomotion—buy a bike, walk to work if you can, use your caloric power and stored fuel (aka fat) for the commute. Save time, money, resources, and the environment. In general Americans produce twice as much CO_2 per capita (about twenty tons) compared to Europeans. Do not be an energy glutton.

All philosophy lies in two words; sustain and abstain.

EPICTETUS

CHAPTER TEN

STICKING WITH IT

The greatest discovery of my generation is that a human being can alter his life by altering his attitudes of mind.

WILLIAM JAMES

CHANGING ATTITUDES AND PATTERNS
OF BEHAVIOR
REWIRE YOUR BRAIN. REARRANGE YOUR MIND

Now that we've covered the basics of training and eating right, this chapter focuses on rewiring your brain by reprogramming mindset and changing behavior to make it easier to stick with this program. To do this we take a two-pronged approach by focusing first on changing your actions, and second on changing your thinking.

The principle of *The Athlete's Way* philosophy is that all human behavior is learned and therefore can be unlearned. Your objective in reading this section should be to imagine ways in your day-to-day life that you could implement these changes. After familiarizing yourself with the four methods of conditioning, play around with what fits best into your workouts. Spend the next eight weeks experimenting with the methods to which you best respond. Behavioral therapists agree that different people respond better to different types of training and conditioning methods. Use the references here to personalize a combination that works for you.

The focus of behaviorism is on what an animal does, not how it thinks. The behaviorist looks at learned habits and tries to make them extinct by shaping new behavior. I link this type of therapy to the cerebellum. To retrain the brain, you will be using the four basic methods of behavioral conditioning: classical conditioning, reward conditioning, contiguity theory, and token economy.

To change behavior, we will tackle the cerebellum as your habit-learning brain and use behavioral conditioning methods to break old patterns of behavior. To change habits you will learn to identify, describe, predict, and control your behavior.

Imagine for yourself a character, a model personality, whose example you determine to follow, in private as well as public.

EPICTETUS

You have your own existing unique way to see and do things, but your brain is also something of a tabula rasa (clean slate) on which you can imprint ideal character traits, behaviors, and ways of thinking. By repeatedly doing so, you will become what you aspire to be. This will happen on a psychological and synaptic level. The key to reprogramming the brain is based on the fire-and-wire principle of synaptic plasticity: the cells that you use will get wired together.

As an athlete, I have always used my imagination and been resourceful choosing character traits and sources of inspiration when molding my athletic mind-set. I encourage you to do the same. Use anything to help mold your alter ego and make it your own. Remember always to be true yourself and incorporate new traits into your true self.

When I examine myself and my methods of thought, I come to the conclusion that the gift of fantasy has meant more to me than my talent for observing positive knowledge. . . . After a certain high level of technical skill is achieved, science and art tend to coalesce in esthetics, plasticity, and form. The greatest scientists are always artists as well. All religions, arts and sciences are branches of the same tree.

ALBERT EINSTEIN

FADING PAPERS IN THE SUN
OPENING THE MEMORY BOX

We think too small, like the frog at the bottom of the well. He thinks the sky is only as big as the top of the well. If he surfaced, he would have an entirely different view.

MAO TSE-TUNG

When you open any memory it is forever changed both chemically and electrically; this happens at a neural level. New proteins that bond synapses between neurons are constantly forming and reconfiguring the existing network. This system of recall and reshaping is an evolutionary survival mechanism. It allows us to remember when someone we thought was a friend betrayed us and became a foe, or if our daily watering hole has turned toxic. The good news is that the same system works in reverse. You can change associations to a place you used to associate with pain and drudgery (like the gym) to being a place you enjoy, which is what this chapter will show you how to do.

Most people who don't like to exercise clump everything about exercise in a "disagreeable" memory box. You could brainstorm exercise to be: painful, intimidating, boring, torture, and tedious, or you could associate it as being exhilarating, rewarding, relaxing, therapeutic, and blissful. Your job is to get inside the athletic process and systematically begin to make new associations one by one. Each time you go into the experience, lay down new thinking and behavior. Over time you can delete all the negative associations of thinking and negate patterns of behavior.

THE EARTH IS FLAT
ROSE TINT MY WORLD

Life has no other discipline to impose, if we would but realize it, than to accept life unquestioningly. Everything we shut our eyes to, everything we run away from, everything we deny, denigrate, or despise, serves to defeat us in the end. What seems nasty, painful, evil, can become a source of beauty, joy, and strength, if faced with an open mind. Every moment is a golden one for him who has the vision to recognize it as such.

HENRY MILLER

You can make the world any color you want it to be—dark and gray, or light and green. You can choose to look on the bright side of any situation, or you can decide to be a pessimist. You can look at the world through rose-colored glasses, orange-colored glasses, or you can look at it through a cynical, jaded lens. They all become habits. The sights, sounds, and images that flood into your brain are as much based on your previous experience and subjective perceptions as on reality. If you think that exercise is a disagreeable experience, slow down, back up, and begin to take a different point of view.

> *An optimist may see a light where there is none, but why must the pessimist always run to blow it out?*
>
> RENÉ DESCARTES

You change your preconceived notions by opening up the memory or experience and laying down a new thought pattern that overrides the old one. This is how we reprogram our minds. We have to bring up the state-dependent memories in order to reshape them, and we need to form new ones. You have to go inside the memory or experience and relive it in order to change old habits and learn new ones.

> *Our deepest fear is not that we are inadequate.*
> *Our deepest fear is that we are powerful beyond measure.*
> *It is our light, not our darkness, that most frightens us.*
>
> MARIANNE WILLIAMSON

There is always going to be cross talk between your up brain and your down brain. The input of stimuli usually enters the primitive brain first for immediate visceral responses. Our reflex brain senses everything and shoots stimuli up via the Purkinje cells in the cerebellum to the cerebrum; this is called bottom-up processing. It is what behaviorism tackles. Cognitive therapy tackles the intellectual reactions to the gut instincts that the cerebellum senses, but might not send them upstream.

Ideally, top-down and bottom-up processing will match up inside the athletic process. That is why you need to practice flexing your psychological mind-set and behavior mind simultaneously.

> *Out of damp and gloomy days, out of solitude, out of loveless words directed at us, conclusions grow up in us like fungus: one morning they are there, we know not how, and they gaze upon us, morose and gray. Woe to the thinker who is not the gardener but only the soil of the plants that grow in him.*
>
> FRIEDRICH NIETZSCHE

The next time you feel a negative thought take hold, imagine it as an actual neural network in your brain. Let it go. Picture it breaking apart. The links will literally dissolve. Allow your thoughts to travel only on those trails you have selected. Get in the habit of guiding and sifting your thoughts by viewing them as something tangible. Engage or dissolve them by holding on or letting go. Patterns of thought will become a habit as they literally carve ruts into your brain. Consciously change the way you think and your brain will reshape itself.

> When I was a child and the snow fell, my mother always rushed to the kitchen and made snow ice cream and divinity fudge—egg whites, sugar and pecans, mostly. It was a lark then and I always associate divinity fudge with snowstorms.
>
> EUDORA WELTY

BURN, BABY, BURN
LEARNING TO INCINERATE NEGATIVITY

> We say pulling out the weeds will give nourishment to the plant. We pull the weeds and burn them near the plant to give it nourishment. So, even though you have some difficulty in your practice, even though you have some waves (obstacles), those waves themselves will help you. . . . You should rather be grateful for the weeds, because eventually they will enrich your daily practice. If you have some experience of how the weeds in your mind change into mental nourishment, your practice will make remarkable progress. You will feel the progress. You will feel how the weeds change into self-nourishment. Of course it is not so difficult to give some philosophical or psychological interpretation of our practice but that is not enough. We must have the actual experience of how our weeds change into nourishment.
>
> SHUNRY SUZUKI

Buddhist monks are sages of the nervous system. The weeds in the Shunry Suzuki quote above can be viewed as helpless or pessimistic neurons, and the daily act of removing them is part of the learned optimism and is a perfect metaphor for neural Darwinism. Visualize the neurons as weeds that burn as fuel to create light inside your head, making your other neurons stronger. Consciously incinerate the neurons that feed into negativity and

hear them sizzle like documen   ur computer's trash can. Picture a
bonfire in your brain as the circ   lodes.

Consciously cut off negati   hts from any irrigation and let them
dry up in the sunshine like w   ines on a hot summer day. A happy
brain is wet and lush like a rain___. A jungle of joy, with all the vinelike
neural nets wrapping and twisting to create a dense state of rapture. A con-
spiracy of happiness.

FIVE-FACTOR PERSONALITY MODEL
YOUR WHEEL OF LIFE NEEDS BALANCED SPOKES

*We continue to shape our personality all our life. If we knew our-
selves perfectly, we should die.*

ALBERT CAMUS

The five-factor character-trait theory is the gold standard for assessing personality; it states that we are all a unique blend of five traits.

As you look at these **big five factors,** think of your own personal tendencies, and rate each one on a scale of one to seven:

1. *NEUROTICISM: Anxious, self-conscious, depressive, hostile,
   impulsive, vulnerable.*

2. *EXTROVERSION: Outgoing, positive emotions, assertive, full of
   energy, excitement-seeking, warm.*

3. *OPENNESS TO EXPERIENCE: Rich fantasy life, action-oriented, novel
   ideas, eccentric, adventurous.*

4. *AGREEABLENESS: Trusting, straightforward, compliant, modest,
   tender-minded, altruistic.*

5. *CONSCIENTIOUSNESS: Competent, orderly, dutiful, self-disciplined,
   deliberate, achievement-oriented.*

These five traits are the core personality factors that shape a person's
mind-set and behavior. Evolutionary theorists contend that these traits
emerged as an important feature for guaranteeing our evolutionary
progress. We developed a sensitivity to stress (neuroticism), the need for

company for protection and mating (extroversion), the ability to problem solve (openness to experience), the aptitude to cooperate and work collectively (agreeableness) and an obligation to meet social and moral needs of community (conscientiousness). The final four have positive neurotransmitter associations, while neuroticism has the biggest chemical enemies at its heart.

As an athlete, I use these traits as a checklist for shaping my ideal athletic mind-set, credo, and code of conduct. I aspire daily to eliminate all forms of neuroticism and find a perfect balance between the other four cardinal traits. Being uptight/neurotic is an addictive and toxic state of mind. Don't let it become a habit. I visualize mind-set as a bicycle wheel with four spokes, the cardinal traits that form an X. Work to find a perfect balance by using this checklist to identify areas you need to focus on.

In biking, as in life, you want all the spokes on your wheel to have the same amount of tension. You want a wheel that doesn't wobble and rolls smooth and fast. In bike world, it is called "trueing your spokes." Using the bike-wheel analogy, neuroticism doesn't deserve a spoke.

Neuroticism should never be a part of your game or a part of your life. Strive to eliminate it, because it is the key trait associated with rejection sensitivity and fear of failure. It raises cortisol and lowers serotonin, which is the most lethal combination to have pumping through your system. Strengthening the other four cardinal traits will boost serotonin (confidence), dopamine (achievement), anandamide (the bliss molecule), and vasopressin/oxytocin (connectedness), while lowering MAOs (serotonin-eating Pac-Men) and lowering cortisol (the stress hormone).

You cannot have a proud and chivalrous spirit if your conduct is mean and paltry; For whatever a man's actions are, such must be his spirit.

ARISTOTLE

People with neurotic tendencies tend to hold on to a bad mood longer than other people. Extroverts tend to stay in a positive mood longer than average people. Scott Hemenover, an assistant professor of psychology at Kansas State University, performed a study that found that people with different personality types have different rates of mood decay.

"Maintaining a negative mood for a long period of time is harmful to your health. People think that getting stressed and anxious is bad for you. The key isn't how stressed you are, but how long you are stressed," he says.

"Staying stressed for a long time can impair your immune and cardiovascular functions."

The pitcher has got only a ball. I've got a bat. So the percentage in weapons is in my favor and I let the fellow with the ball do the fretting.

HANK AARON

People who tend to stay in a bad mood for a long time can learn strategies to help them snap out of it faster. "Neurotics see the world as a nasty place. If you teach them to view the world in a positive way, and to think their way out of feeling bad by rephrasing things in a positive way, it can help their health," Hemenover says. The bottom line is to change the script in your head. Picture the neural networks inside your head and disengage the neurotic ones.

GETTING MUGGED BY THREE GUYS IN NEW YORK CITY
A TESTAMENT TO ATHLETIC MIND-SET

It's just a job. Grass grows, birds fly, waves pound the sand. I beat people up.

MUHAMMAD ALI

The following recounts the events and lessons I learned when I was jumped by three guys and got beat up pretty badly. I tell this story as a lesson about resilience and the athletic mind-set in action when faced with an unexpected blindsiding—learned optimism, collectivism, reaching out for help, dealing with fear conditioning, and avoidance learning—and using something terrible as a springboard for better things.

I was walking home from dinner at Pete's Tavern on Gramercy Park on an August night in 2003 at around eight o'clock when my life took a turn. The sun had set but the sky was still glowing. Everything had taken on a pinkish-orange iridescent hue. I was walking home slowly in my flip-flops and talking on my cell phone. I had just enjoyed a great dinner with my friend Julia, who lives around the corner from Pete's Tavern.

I was in such a carefree mood that night. I always walk home from Pete's on the same route—down Irving Place to Sixteenth Street, drop Julia at her house, head straight east through Stuyvesant Park to my apartment on Avenue A. I was on the familiar route and on autopilot, walking and talking on my cell phone.

As I entered the gates of Stuyvesant Park, three kids hanging out asked me, "Excuse me, sir, do you know what time it is?" in an overly genuine and earnest tone that made my ears perk up. I remember thinking how strange it was that they called me sir, because I was dressed like a total slob. A little street smarts voice in my head said, "That's strange," and I debated in a flash whether to ignore them and keep walking or be polite and give them the time. I decided to be polite.

> *There's nothing that cleanses the soul like getting the hell kicked out of you.*
>
> **WOODY HAYES**

I pulled my phone away from my ear for a second, looked at the time on the display, and said, "It's around 7:45." I took about twelve more steps when I sensed that something very strange was happening. There was a sudden burst of energy behind me, and then *whoosh—voom-bam*. I thought that a branch had fallen or maybe a bomb had gone off, because I felt like a cartoon character defying gravity and reality.

Pop! Pop! Bam!
Cinderella Man

> *Pain is inevitable. Suffering is optional.*
>
> **M. KATHLEEN CASEY**

My face was against the pavement in a millisecond. I couldn't sort out what had thrown me down. I remember hitting my chin on the ground and thinking, "Oww, that hurt. Did I lose any teeth?" My brain had been this disoriented only once before in thirty years and I had cerebellar flashbacks to a bike crash. I would flash back to this new incident, though, when I found myself knocked down and smashed into a brick wall months later during the Treadathalon.

I was too disorientated to think clearly. One second I had been standing upright walking, and by the end of that same second, my eyes were a centimeter from the ground. It happened lightning fast. Within the next second, the kicking and punching started. Surrounded by three guys who had obviously followed me from the gate, I was like a punching bag at their disposal, facedown at first and then curled up in a fetal position, getting kicked primarily in the torso and head. The feeling was unlike anything I had ever experienced. It felt like being in an industrial washing machine with about eight cinder blocks.

Your whole life really does flash clearly before your eyes when you think you're going to die. I think it's the cerebellum opening the floodgates into the cerebrum to put every survival mechanism it has ever stored at your disposal to stay alive. I kept wondering why three guys would gang up on one. It seemed so cowardly and unsportsmanlike. If you want to beat me up, at least give me a fighting chance. The odds were clearly not in my favor. The only way to fight back would be self-defense and not giving in.

Ultra-running has often seemed like a boxing match to me. The runner who can pound himself into the ground, stay standing, and keep moving forward, wins. Runners deliver punches to competitors by pushing themselves harder and forcing their rival to respond. There is something masochistic (and sadistic) about it that makes you very tough. The times I've collapsed when running are always best captured in the knockout scenes of a boxing movie. Now I felt like I was in the ring for real. The prizefighter instincts I'd learned as a runner kicked in even amid the continued pounding, blurry vision, and disorientation.

I tried to get up on all fours again and again as if there were a referee countdown. Being on the ground was the last place I wanted to be. With every blow to my head, I thought my skull must be cracking. I could see blood all over the ground and on my hands, sweatshirt, and jeans. The words that echoed from the back of my head were, "I am going to be a statistic." That is what echoed in my head—"I am becoming a statistic." I tried to block as many blows to my head and my organs as possible. And kept saying, "Just get back on your feet, Chris. Get back on your feet." I really did see my old life vanishing and my new life as a brain-injured or dead person beginning. "I am going to be one of the people that my dad would talk about over dinner as being in a coma after being beat up. I can't believe this is happening to me," was all I could think.

> *"I am very brave generally," he went on in a low voice, "only today I happen to have a headache."*
>
> LEWIS CARROLL

It seemed like the kicking went on forever, and I just kept trying to get up, only to be knocked down, again and again. The whole thing probably lasted only forty-five seconds. Finally, I flipped over on my butt and looked one of them right in the eye. They started shouting and I shouted back, in my loudest voice, "If you would stop kicking me for a second, I'll give you all the money I have." I wasn't going down quietly. But I didn't have anything. I had a lot of adrenaline pumping and was as angry as I was terrified. The kicking slowed. I reached in my pocket for my wallet, but all I had was a pack of spearmint Dentyne Ice and a $5 bill. That was it. Change from the cheeseburger and some gum. I remember handing one of the guys the money and the gum, and thinking OK, now they shoot me. But they ran away.

> *A good scare is worth more to a man than good advice.*
> **NADINE GORDIMER**

As I got up, I looked for my cell phone, but it was gone. I was in shock. I headed for the emergency room at Beth Israel Hospital, a half a block away. I remember thinking that my head must have been gouged open, beyond repair, because there was blood streaming into my eyes and down my nose. There was blood all over my jeans and my favorite sweatshirt. But I was OK.

Once I was inside the ER, they took good care of me. A brain scan found no brain damage, just external bruises and bleeding, a gouge in the back of my head and some scrapes on my forehead. My friends and family rallied around me. The mugging made me realize, really realize, how much they loved me, and how much I loved them, too.

> *Every morning I wake up saying, I'm still alive; a miracle.*
> *And so I keep on pushing.*
> **JACQUES COUSTEAU** (CAPTAIN OF *CALYPSO*)

I was actually in a great mood the next day. Anytime I started to slip into the victim mind-set even for a second, I said, "Don't go there, Chris." The experience made me so grateful for things I had formerly taken for granted. I felt like I had been given a second chance. I also learned to watch my back when I'm blabbing on my cell phone. I had my cerebellar street smarts back again.

> *We must become aware in order to choose the good—but no*
> *awareness will help us if we have lost the capacity to be moved by*

*the distress of another human being, by the friendly gaze of another
person, by the greenness of the grass.*

ERICH FROMM

FACING YOUR FEAR
FEAR CONDITIONING AND AVOIDANCE LEARNING

*I was very, very shy as a younger girl, just petrified of people. Tennis
helped give me an identity and made me feel like somebody.*

CHRIS EVERT

Fear is stored deep in your cerebellum and amygdala (Latin for almond, the
shape of this part of the brain). Any traumatic memory is automatically
stored in your implicit, unconscious memory in the cerebellum. There is a
protein called *glutamate* that sears synapses together in any unique or traumatic experience. This is how fear conditioning is hardwired. Glutamate
bonds are hard to dissolve. I believe sweat literally helps to break glutamate
down.

Let's not get panicky.

BRANCH RICKEY
(MAJOR LEAGUE BASEBALL EXECUTIVE)

When you see a coiled-up garden hose and think it's a snake, very deep
fear memories held in your genes are being passed up to your cerebrum
from the collective unconscious of your cerebellum. Specific trauma, like
getting mugged, is held in your conscious mind but also in your nonthinking cerebellum as part of your personal unconscious. For weeks afterward,
when I passed the park I had a visceral, physiological response of sweaty
palms and elevated heart rate. That response came from my down brain.
This fear was bottom-up processing. I needed to tackle it from the top down
to change it. That is what being human is about. We can get on top of our animal instincts and shape ourselves.

*I expect to pass through the world but once. Any good therefore that
I can do, or any kindness that I can show to any fellow creature, let*

me do it now. Let me not defer or neglect it, for I shall not pass this
way again.

STEPHEN GRELLET (QUAKER MISSIONARY)

I knew the most important thing for me to do to get over the deeply rooted fear conditioning was to go back to the scene of the crime to let my animal brain begin to think it was safe again. Right after the attack, if I got within a two-block radius of the scene, which I had to do in order to get home, my adrenaline and cortisol would go crazy. I would start shaking and have heart palpitations. Avoidance learning on a lesser scale is the key aspect of exercise aversion.

I approached the gates of the park with my friend Nikki Haran. My body went into spasms. She and I stood on the big slab of stone around the fountain where I had been beaten up. We stood there for a few minutes holding hands and my heart calmed down. I had conquered the fear—and it made me feel OK. Not great, but at least I could cope. It bonded Nikki and me, and our friendship took on a deeper meaning and significance.

We should be careful to get out of an experience only the wisdom that
is in it—and stop there; lest we be like the cat that sits down on a hot
stove-lid. She will never sit down on a hot stove-lid again—and that is
well; but also she will never sit down on a cold one anymore either.

MARK TWAIN

Every day for weeks, I went out of my way to go back to that slab of stone to stand on it, alone, look around, and proceed home. It was like a pilgrimage, a very therapeutic one. To this day, every time I walk through the park I walk directly over that very same stone, and it makes me feel really strong. Going back to the place that scares me most and facing it head-on makes me feel as if I am the ruler of my destiny. And creates a self-fulfilling prophecy.

The bravest thing you can do when you are not brave is to profess
courage and act accordingly.

CORRA HARRIS

LEVEL ONE: THE BEHAVIORAL APPROACH
REPROGRAMMING YOUR "HABIT BRAIN"

Action seems to follow feeling, but really action and feeling go to-
gether; and by regulating the action, which is under the more direct
control of the will, we can indirectly regulate the feeling, which is not.

WILLIAM JAMES

The memory system of your lower brain is a nonintellectual center that learns through repetition, practice, and emotional responses. In addition to being the seat of all athletic performance, I believe the cerebellum is also the seat of your implicit unconscious memories and habits.

Habit forming is the act of consciously identifying motives and routinizing them to a point at which they are sent to the depths of down brain. Bad habits often slip past our gate control, and I encourage you to be a detective in terms of decoding the series of cues that lead to undesired behavior, dissecting them, and then rebuilding. If you can break a part of the cycle, the neural net becomes disengaged and will begin to atrophy. You must disengage and break apart the bad habits.

Whatever you can do, or dream you can do, begin it. Boldness has
genius, power, and magic in it.

W. H. MURRAY (SCOTTISH HIMALAYAN EXPLORER)

FOUR STAGES TO CHANGING BEHAVIOR
IDENTIFY, DESCRIBE, PREDICT, CONTROL

Between stimulus and response there is a space. In that space is our
power to choose our response. In our response lies our growth and
our freedom.

VIKTOR E. FRANKL

Neuroscience has reinforced the behaviorist perspective by proving in recent years that the roots of all conditioned behavior are in the synaptic connections between neurons.

A pattern of behavior (like a thought or emotion) is literally a neural network. To make old patterns of behavior extinct, you must break apart the neural nets associated with them. Likewise, to acquire new behavior you shape those neurons methodically through repetition and positive reinforcement.

Over time the conditioned response becomes imprinted and encoded in the neural nets of your unconscious mind. Remember that continuous positive reinforcements, repeated frequently, result in the fastest learning. Be consistent by setting up a daily routine that reinforces exercise as a consistently agreeable experience. The key for training your down brain is repetition, repetition, repetition—and practice, practice, practice. This is how this brain learns.

> The longer I live, the more I realize the impact of attitude on life. Attitude to me is more important than facts. It is more important than the past, than failures, than successes, than what other people think or say or do. It is more important than appearance, giftedness or skill. It will make or break a company . . . a church . . . a home. The remarkable thing is we have a choice every day regarding the attitude we will embrace for that day. We cannot change the inevitable. The only thing we can do is play on the one string we have, and that is our attitude. I am convinced that life is 10 percent what happens to me and 90 percent how we react to it. And so it is with you . . . we are in charge of our attitudes.
>
> CHARLES SWINDOLL

The Key to Changing Habits

> A habit cannot be tossed out of the window; it must be coaxed down the stairs one step at a time.
>
> MARK TWAIN

1. IDENTIFY: What is the target behavior? What is the actual behavior?

2. DESCRIBE: How does this behavior manifest itself?

3. PREDICT: What is the expected pattern surrounding this behavior?

4. CONTROL: What internal and external modifications could change outcome?

There are four stages to changing your habits surrounding athletic behavior. The first is to identify it. Learn to be aware of the behavior you are hoping to achieve in a given day and the actual behavior that is occurring. Pinpoint it. And give it a name. Second, describe the behavior in more detail to yourself. What does it feel like? Are you being driven by declarative conscious thoughts of your cerebrum or unconscious implicit forces of the cerebellum? Can you isolate what is causing it? Third, predict various scenarios of playing out the behavior. Narrow it down to two choices. Play out the contiguity scenario and the steps that lead you down a beaten path of behavior. Last, figure out ways to control the behavior by breaking the cycle and achieving the desired outcome. Be methodical and look for the forks in the track where you tend to derail your own train.

The implicit habit systems of our animal brain are conditioned every day by the bells, whistles, and gongs on our cars, household electronic gadgetry, and computers. The sound effects your computer makes as you transfer documents, upload, and download, are all positive and negative reinforcers. A gong sound that lets you realize something has gone wrong with the important file you were trying to download triggers a feeling of bad stress, adrenaline, and cortisol. The tone of a bell dinging after 100 percent of a document is sent or received, coupled with the words "Files done," allows you to release a sigh of relief and experience the rush of success.

Perk up your ears and listen for the ways that your behavior is conditioned every day. Sounds that alert you of success give you a direct hit of dopamine and a winning-the-jackpot Las Vegas kind of feeling. The next time you are uploading an important file, pay attention to the difference between 99 percent complete and 100 percent complete. The victorious feeling you get is dopamine in action. Systematically releasing dopamine when you exercise by setting and achieving goals will create positive associations and lead to conditioning that will change habits.

THE FOUR METHODS OF BEHAVIORAL CONDITIONING

All human actions have one or more of these seven causes: Chance, nature, compulsion, habit, reason, passion and desire.

ARISTOTLE

Below are detailed explanations of the four methods of conditioning that you can apply to reshape your athletic behavior. You should look at these four and pick and figure out ways to incorporate them into your life. Stay adaptable, as your circumstances and motivation can change over time and from day to day. You can refer back to this section as a user's guide.

- CLASSICAL CONDITIONING: *Conditioned response: seek pleasure/ avoid pain*

- OPERANT "REWARD" CONDITIONING: *The Skinner Box reward model*

- CONTIGUITY THEORY: *Doing things in a sequence*

- TOKEN ECONOMY: *Earning tokens in exchange for behavior*

Classical Conditioning

The most basic form of animal behavior training is called classical conditioning. You want to condition yourself to associate as much of the exercise process with pleasure as possible. You need to put the perspective in place to create the reality.

Classical conditioning is your gut response to a stimulus. If the smell of chlorine makes you shiver with dread about jumping into a cold pool, that is a classically conditioned response. When you enter the changing room at the pool and smell the chlorine (stimulus), you might have flashes of summer camp and dread changing into your swimsuit, because you remember feeling vulnerable or self-conscious. Those memories are linked to the smell of chlorine and maybe even make you feel sick to your stomach (response). This is a conditioned response.

> *You desire to know the art of living, my friend? It is contained in one phrase: Make use of suffering.*
>
> HENRI-FRÉDÉRIC AMIEL

If you had never been to a pool as a kid you might just associate chlorine with the smell of cleaning supplies or something totally neutral. On the flip side, if you were the star of the swim team or loved swimming when you were younger, entering the pool deck might flood you with very positive memories. Classical conditioned responses are stored in our nonthinking lower brain and are part of the implicit memory system. You can learn to use executive function to shape the gut instinct behavior.

As an athlete, you want to create conditioned responses to exercise that reinforce the positive. That is why it is so important that you coddle your animal instincts by making the experience of working out feel safe, comfortable, and under your control at a very deep subconscious level. Remember, it is your animal brain that is picking up the conditioned vibes surrounding exercise and whispering commands into your thinking brain, while also affecting your physical response.

> *The habit of persistence is the habit of victory.*
> HERBERT KAUFMAN

If it is snowing outside and freezing cold, my animal brain wants to stay at home by the heater where it is very cozy. But I know I am prepared for the cold. I have warm clothes, a hat, gloves, and a playlist of balmy summer music and desert tunes on my iPod. I will make the animal experience of working out comfortable, and will be able to coax my down brain out of my slippers and out the door. I will also prepare some hot tea and take a bath when I get home. That is the deal I make as I fire up the iPod and get ready to head out the door. These are all animal conditioned responses.

A person anticipating a workout will have a myriad of classically conditioned responses to the exercise process that guide his behavior. These feelings usually manifest themselves as a gut instinct of exercise aversion. The implicit memory of the cerebellum deals in visceral cravings and aversions it seeks or avoids. As the big boss, your job is to attach a sense of pleasure to as many aspects of the exercise process as you can and undo the aversion by using the four behavioral methods.

Operant (Reward) Conditioning

> *Everyone has a success mechanism and a failure mechanism. The failure mechanism goes off by itself. The success mechanism only goes off with a goal. Every time we write down and talk about a goal we push the button to start the success mechanism.*
> CHARLES JONES

You constantly want to create rewards and positive reinforcement as you go thorough your athletic process. They could be actual rewards, like a bottle of Gatorade or a hot shower or just a feeling of accomplishment that will release a hit of dopamine. This is called *operant conditioning*. Invented by B. F. Skinner, the term *operant* is based on the verb to *operate*, as in "to

push on a lever" to receive a food pellet, as rats learned to do in the famous
Skinner box. I call this reward conditioning.

Skinner realized that animal behavior is voluntary, goal oriented, and
directly influenced by its consequences. There are many ways to look at exercise as a reward, aside from physical things. The reward can be based on
neurobiology (dopamine, serotonin, lower cortisol), self-esteem, weight
loss, or lower cholesterol. Decide what you find rewarding about your workout and think of the athletic process as a Skinner box that automatically rewards behavior. You can do the same with everything surrounding the
athletic process by constantly setting up a system of rewards.

*Success consists of going from failure to failure without losing enthu-
siasm.*

                                                   WINSTON CHURCHILL

As you look at the gym and exercise from a behaviorist perspective,
think of ways of creating a Skinner gym by constantly setting and achieving
goals. The goal (finishing a set of arm curls) is the lever, and the reward pellet you get is the hit of dopamine you receive after accomplishing the goal.
Successful reward conditioning in exercise depends on creating hundreds
of mini goals, dangling the carrot, as you go through a workout and consciously sounding bells and whistles inside your head when you accomplish
them.

Contiguity (Sequence) Conditioning

*First comes thought; then organization of that thought, into ideas
and plans; then transformation of those plans into reality. The beginning, as you will observe, is in your imagination.*

                                                   NAPOLEON HILL

Contiguity means connected in a sequence; the order that you go about
preparing to work out is going to carve grooves into your synapses that will
create a chain reaction. In athletics, contiguity conditioning is the process of
ritual and routine that you play out every day, creating a self-fulfilling
prophecy by training your nervous system to follow through to completion.

If you don't know where you're going, you might not get there.

                                                   YOGI BERRA

E. G. Guthrie coined the term *contiguity*, believing that your sequence of movements becomes actual patterns associated with a target behavior. Guthrie studied cats in a box who would systematically escape through the exact same pattern of movements once they figured out that the pattern worked. They repeated the movements automatically the same way every time by rote. You can do the same as you go through the process of getting ready to exercise. These neurons become imprinted into neural nets through repetition.

Action to be effective must be directed to clearly conceived ends.

JAWAHARLAL NEHRU

Structure your personal routine and carve it into your muscle memory because repetition creates a chain reaction of neurons firing in a predicted sequence. I have a tendency to have the same contiguity pattern every day for a few weeks, and then on a whim I'll change it one day. But then I'll go back to it again later. My routines are always in a rotation. I mix them up but they are systematic and cerebellar. You want to have a variety of routines that you can tap into on different days to avoid getting bored or stuck in a rut. Contiguity routines are key to avoiding procrastination because by tipping the first domino, which is easy, you can trigger a chain reaction that leads to follow-through and goal achievement, which is tougher.

Only put off until tomorrow what you are willing to die having left undone.

PABLO PICASSO

The sequence of events helps me click over into my ideal athletic self. All these things come together to reinforce a target mind-set and behavior. This is the constant "down-up" dialogue. Each of them is a trigger that will be encoded over the next few weeks. A transformation will take place; you will have an athletic conversion every day you begin and finish breaking a sweat.

Token Economy: Earning Chips Through Success

I believe that "Thou shalt earn the bread by the sweat of thy face" was a benediction and not a penalty. Work is the zest of life; there is joy in its pursuit.

BRANCH RICKEY

You will want to create a token economy as a form of positive reinforcement. Whenever you achieve long-term and short-term target behavior, keep track of your achievements. Rewards can be diverse. Be creative. A token of achievement doesn't have to be physical. A reward may even be internal, just the feeling of accomplishment. Create a personalized token economy in which you identify your implicit tokens, like hits of dopamine or being able to say, "I did it," as well as explicit rewards, such as a massage, a huge, ice-cold glass of water, a cheeseburger. . . .

Use token markers to symbolize success. Try things like a gold star, a check on a checklist, an elastic added to a rubber-band ball, a record of your achievements in your notebook. Like many things having to do with behaviorism and habitual behavior, there is a thin line between becoming compulsive and rigid or using these rewards in a casual, fun-loving way. Be on the lookout for obsessive behavior. Remember to lighten up and keep it playful.

The idea of earning a token as a reward for behavior is a highly effective way of reinforcing and tracking behavior across the board. Again, it can be specific, like having a piece of cake for dessert and committing to run an extra mile the next day, or rewarding yourself with a smoothie after a workout.

My mom wanted to lose ten pounds after the holidays so we built a pyramid out of ten boxes of butter she'd used to make cookies. Every time she lost a pound over the next six months, she threw a box out. That pyramid was a huge reminder staring her in the face every day and it made the goal more tangible. Another tactic I've used is to put coins in a Ziploc plastic bag with the task at hand written on it. The weight of the bag grows to symbolize my investment. Rubber bands added to a rubber-band ball, checkmarks off your to-do list are other token economy measures that provide feedback and reinforcement.

The Minute Minder
Egg Timer, Stopwatch, or Hourglass

Well begun is half done. A whole is that which has beginning, middle and end.

ARISTOTLE

My trademark conditioning tools are rubber bands and Lux Brand Minute-Minder timers. You want to get in the habit of putting a rubber band on your wrist every morning. As you commit to a goal, watch the rubber-band ball grow. Each day you succeed, add that morning's rubber band to the existing ball and you will be motivated by the reward of being able to complete a task and stretch a new band onto the ball. This is basic conditioning. Two other methods of conditioning I'll discuss here are egg timers and ankle weights.

On the ledge of my stove, I keep the Lux Minute-Minder timer my Yankee grandmother had in her kitchen. She used it for cooking and to time my mom when she was on the phone as a kid. I use that timer every day to time my writing, cleaning, and sit-ups. I know it sounds regimented and rigid, but it's actually liberating, because it gives everything a structure with a beginning, middle, and end. I like the ticking sound. It puts me in a trance, like white noise. The ding always gives me a hit of dopamine, too. And frees me to get on to something new.

I use a traditional hourglass for my yoga/stretching period, which is quiet and reminds me of *The Wizard of Oz*. My editor at St. Martin's Press, Diane Reverand, says that she maintains a laserlike focus on what she is reading amid stacks of papers piling up on her desk by imagining each word in front of her as a grain of sand in an hourglass. I think of this metaphor when I'm stretching. The hourglass reminds me to stay in the moment. The single grain of sand in the wasp waist of the glass represents the present tense.

If you don't have a timer, I suggest buying one and using it for things that you love to do that are guilty pleasures like playing a video game or chatting online, that keep you from doing things you should be doing. Use a timer to set limits. You can also use a timer or stopwatch to compartmentalize the time doing the things you dread like cleaning, and make the time frame of misery finite.

> *Begin with the end in mind.*
> STEPHEN COVEY

Timers are also a way to force yourself to take breaks. I use a timer when I write, so that I make sure to get up every hour and move around and do some jumping jacks and push-ups. Otherwise I could sit in front of the computer completely absorbed for five hours straight and never take a break. The timer forces me to come up for air. I've conditioned myself that way. I sometimes give out Lux Minute-Minder timers (model CP 2428) at workshops. These timers and rubber bands are my trademarks and both get a great response. Try it and see if it works for you.

Ankle Weights
Gravity and Relativity

When I pick up the ball and it feels nice and light and small I know I'm going to have a good day. But if I picked it up and it's big and heavy, I know I'm liable to get into a little trouble.

BOB FELLER

If you don't have a pair of ankle weights I recommend buying some and using them as a way to feel grounded, build stronger legs, and condition yourself. There is nothing like the theory of relativity when you take off the ankle weights and feel as free as a bird and like you're filled with helium and lifting up off the ground.

I wear ankle weights when I need to feel grounded. I wear them at work sometimes to make myself feel centered. No one can see them under my bootlegs or baggy sweatpants. I also wear my ankle weights every Friday night when I do my deep housecleaning before I go out dancing at the Pyramid Club, which I try to do every Friday. Taking off the Velcro when the cleaning is done is always a signal to me that the weekend has officially begun and that I am as free as a bird. Yes, I am a creature of habit.

LEVEL TWO: THE COGNITIVE APPROACH
BUILDING YOUR ATHLETIC ALTER EGO

Be careful what you pretend to be because you become what you pretend to be.

KURT VONNEGUT

In order to tackle changing mind-set, we are going to identify ideal athletic character traits and use these as a template to impose onto your own existing web of neurons. You will be creating an alter ego. In discussing mind-set, we are addressing the up brain. You have many ideas of mind-set in place. The goal here is to clean the slate—make your mind-set a tabula rasa—and begin to imprint a new mind-set by looking at role models and mentors.

What follows shows you how I have molded my mind-set after people that I admire and gives you clues about doing it for yourself.

You have to create a system of belief that causes you to associate exercise with agreeable experiences across the board. We will also look at fear conditioning and avoidance learning as potential obstacles. The process of exercise is viewed by many as a suffer-test: physically challenging, mentally exhausting, and disagreeable overall. In this section we'll look at ways to change your mind-set with a variety of mental tricks you can use to rewire your thinking.

Character Traits of the Spartans and Olympians
Identify a Trait, Give it a Name: "Tag it"

To me, we must learn to spell the word respect. We must respect the rights and properties of our fellow man. And then learn to play the game of life, as well as the game of athletics, according to the rules of society. If you can take that and put it into practice in the community in which you live, then, to me you have won the greatest championship.

JESSE OWENS

Ideal character traits for athletes are universal. In a detailed survey of Olympians conducted at the 2000 Olympic Games, researchers got inside the athletic mind by having Olympians describe the core values that they credited with getting them to the games. The most important common denominator was that each athlete believed he or she had the ability to influence his or her success. The athletes did not suffer from learned helplessnes or take a backseat approach; they were proactive rulers of their destiny.

Do some brainstorming in your journal and think of words that sum up who you do and don't want to be. Below the list below are the five Olympic traits that I have written on a note card and posted on the fridge as a daily reminder of my code of conduct.

- *Dedication and persistence*
- *Passion and love of the game*
- *Competitiveness*
- *Focus*
- *Strong work ethic*

All of these characteristics are within an athlete's locus of control, which is what makes them empowering. You can choose to apply these traits to whatever you pursue, whether you're an aspiring Olympian, businessperson, or athlete trying to stay motivated on the Stairmaster or Life-Cycle. The mind-set is transferable.

Make a decision to bring idealized characteristics to your athletic process. Even if it is imaginary at first, those characteristics will become a reality. Decide who you want to be and begin to forge that character. Make your list of ideal character traits a canon. How does this character think? How does he move? What does he eat, drink? This is what Lee Strasberg taught his method actors to do. They would live, breathe, and sleep the character to the point they could turn that person on or off by using a few mental or physical triggers. Think the way a method actor would think when creating a character for screen or stage. In making these traits part of your behavior, you will be reshaping the synaptic connections of your brain.

When asked to single out the most important factors that led to long-term achievement, the top-ranked response from Olympians was dedication and persistence. These two words should serve as your mantra. When you are unmotivated or want to quit, remind yourself of these words, and they will trigger your neurons. Other characteristics like optimism, passion, high motivation, and resilience are going to be critical building blocks for achieving athletic success. I would add adaptability, camaraderie, and mental toughness. Start distilling the traits of people you admire and jot them down.

Remember, naming things and giving a character trait a tag is the first step to making it a reality. We all have the ability to improve our attitude and mind-set surrounding sport. The repetition and routinization of a belief system played out day in, day out causes neuroplastic changes in our brains. With time, these grooves are carved and become the natural path your mind follows, but you must keep traveling it to keep it beaten, like a trail through the woods.

Life Is a PlayStation, Too
"Character Bibles"

*Success or failure depends more upon attitude than upon capacity.
Successful men act as though they have accomplished or are enjoying something. Soon it becomes a reality. Act, look, feel successful,*

conduct yourself accordingly, and you will be amazed at the posi-
tive results.

WILLIAM JAMES

When creating a character for a video game, programmers refer to the amalgamation of traits as a *character bible.* I like the term as a way to describe the ideal traits that an athlete incorporates into an alter ego on the playing field. I read an interview with Serena Williams in which she described her alter ego, Sheila, as being a tough-as-nails competitor she refers to in third person. My friend Adam calls himself Slice. Just as Serena Williams talks to Sheila, Adam talks to Slice, who is molded after Lance Armstrong. My dad called himself EZ in a similar fashion. Anytime he was scared he calmed himself by pretending that everything came easy to him, which created a self-fulfilling prophecy.

I encourage you to create a character bible that describes your athletic alter ego. Make a list of traits to describe your ideal athletic self and incorporate these characteristics into your own life. Maybe even give this person a name. But never lose sight of yourself. Part of the tightrope walk of *The Athlete's Way* is being able to modify who you are while staying true to your core being at all times. It can be a juggling act at times.

Give yourself a name if you want to. Take note of specific characteristics you see in the athletic role models whom you admire. I was just captivated again in 2006 watching Roger Federer blaze to another Grand Slam victory at the U.S. Open; his ability to keep his eye on the ball like a heat-seeking missile is phenomenal. I learn about the power of concentration by tracking the Swiss precision of his eyes on HDTV. Look for the nuances of the behavior of the athletes you admire. How do these play out in that athlete's game? Write them down in your journal/notebook. Often the key to their game is in the subtleties, the tilt of the head, the shift of the eyes, body language, or grunts. I often find that watching an athlete before and between points, or when they're on the sidelines, to be as informative as how he plays on the field.

Act as if what you do makes a difference. It does.

WILLIAM JAMES

When committing to reshape your mind-set, remember that you can be or already are a mentor for somebody. Reach out to other people who might be looking for a role model; lead by example. Pride yourself on how you think and behave, knowing that how you conduct your life can inspire people. Realize that you could be serving as a role model to people you don't even know.

Character Work
Captain Fantastic and the Brown Dirt Cowboy

The thing about performance, even if it's only an illusion, is that it is a celebration of the fact that we do contain within ourselves infinite possibilities.

DANIEL DAY-LEWIS

Being an athlete is a lot like being an actor. It is a performance. You have a role to play, and you bring an alter ego to the stage or the playing field. I learn a lot about the mental method by listening to actors. They have analyzed the stages of performance mind-set more than athletes or coaches, and so I have adopted their insights to sport. You become what you pretend to be. I have a Superman magnet on my fridge; he's flying out over the Manhattan skyline. I look at it every morning and say, "Play like a champion today, Chris." And I put my arm in the air like he does, and make a fist; then I envision that I can leap tall buildings in a single bound while I'm waiting for the water to boil.

Imagination, Industry, and Intelligence—The three "I's"—are all indispensable to the actress, but of these three the greatest is, without doubt, imagination.

ELLEN TERRY

Use a superhero for your alter ego. The minute you put on your workout gear you'll have the mind-set of Captain Fantastic or She-Ra, Princess of Power. Use your imagination. Think of it as a performance at first. As an athlete you want to create an alter ego based on your ideal athletic self. And don't allow a seed of self-doubt to enter the picture. If you do, the house of cards will crumble.

Ask yourself: How does this person move, how does he think? What are the props you need to get into character? What are the external and internal triggers and reinforcers that help you become this character? Remember very much of it is cerebellar, not cerebral. It takes time and practice to make the shift into your alter ego happen automatically. You should feel a shift in mind-set when you put on your workout clothes. You need to believe that you are intrepid and invincible, even if it's a facade.

> *Acting is not about dressing up. Acting is about stripping bare. The whole essence of learning lines is to forget them so you can make them sound like you thought of them that instant.*
>
> GLENDA JACKSON

As an athlete you have external reinforcers like your uniform, glasses, jewelry, and pictures on the fridge that can trigger a mind-set, but you also have body language. Shifting the tilt of my ankles on race morning to walk more like a cat ready to pounce shifts my mind-set. Use these tools to help you click over. Put the cart before the horse.

I heard Richard Gere speaking about gymnastics as a metaphor for acting. He was a gymnast as a kid. Gere said that there were many parallels between being an actor and being a gymnast in terms of rehearsal, visualization, the performance, showmanship, knowing the scene or routine like the back of your hand but then making it seem spontaneous, beginning a performance, and then finishing the scene or the routine.

> *You have to perform at a consistently higher level than others. That's the mark of a true professional.*
>
> JOE PATERNO

The Calypso Rule
Aim High—but Fly the Middle Way

> *Life is always a tightrope or a feather bed. Give me the tightrope.*
>
> EDITH WHARTON

When deciding how to sculpt your alter ego, remember that we are the sum of our actions. To Aristotle our habits made us who we were. He was referring to habits of thinking and habits of doing, habits of mind-set, and habits of behavior. Aristotle used the term *moral virtue* to describe mind-set and believed that how you think is reflected in your actions, and vice versa. Thought and action work together to shape the person you become.

Aristotle alluded to the feedback loop of behavior and neurobiology in his *Nicomachean Ethics*, in 330 B.C., long before neuroscientists were able to prove it in a laboratory with brain-imaging scans. Synaptic plasticity is also a feedback loop; your behavior shapes mind-set and mind-set shapes be-havior. Synaptic plasticity is the outcome of repetitive thoughts and actions, of habits. This process is the foundation of all learning and memory.

In deciding to shape your ideal athletic mind-set, you have to consider what behavior to make illicit. Who do you want to be? How will you get there? Aristotle's answer lies in his explanation of the mean. By determin-ing which vice (extreme) we tend toward and then moving toward the other extreme, we reach the middle or the mean.

Ever tried. Ever failed. No matter. Try again. Fail again. Fail better.
                                                    SAMUEL BECKETT

In my coaching vernacular I refer to finding the mean as *The Calypso Rule*. When I was a kid we had a small, two-person sailboat, a Sunfish, that we sailed around Buzzard's Bay on Cape Cod. My mom christened it *Ca-lypso* after Jacques Cousteau's famous vessel, which is where I got the name for this rule. The *Calypso* Rule is ultimately about sailing full speed ahead and maintaining an even keel by finding your mean. The universal rule for sailing a small vessel in a straight line is to pull hardest against the yaw of the wind or currents. You learn to let your sails in or out and to shift your center of gravity, to lean back or crouch down in a ball if necessary. You adapt to the conditions intellectually and intuitively and improve with prac-tice. You find the mean of your vessel using your cerebellum and your cere-brum, as all athletes do.

In life, if you have a tendency to do something in excess—like eat chocolate cake, don't stop eating chocolate cake altogether. Instead of eating two pieces, have one. If you drink only a couple of glasses of water a day, don't aim for drinking eight right off the bat. Aim for four. The goal is to find a place that is challenging but doable. This is the idea of balanced achievement in setting goals and finding your mean.

Only you know your personal, and often private, vices and how you can move toward the other extreme to find the mean. Identify the yaw of your life vessel and take appropriate actions. Knowing your mean allows you to sail through tempests and tidal waves. Find your mean so that you can venture far from shore and explore new territories. Finding your mean is about gaining self-knowledge so you can live life to its fullest.

The following excerpts from Aristotle's *Nicomachean Ethics* serve as a model for charting your course:

FOUR KEY POINTS FROM ARISTOTLE FOR SHAPING YOUR MIND
THE ATHLETE'S WAY

1. Whatever we learn to do, we learn by actually doing it: men
    come to be builders, for instance, by building, and harpists by
    playing the harp. In the same way, by doing just acts we come to
    be just; by doing self-controlled acts, we come to be self-controlled;
    and by doing brave acts, we become brave.

2. In all conduct, the mean is the most praiseworthy state. But as a
    practical matter, we must sometimes aim a bit toward excess and
    sometimes toward deficiency, because this will be the easiest way
    of hitting the mean, that is, what is right.

3. How we act in our relations with other people makes us just or
    unjust. How we face dangerous situations, either accustoming
    ourselves to fear or confidence, makes us brave or cowardly. In a
    word, then, activities produce similar dispositions. Therefore we
    must give a certain character to our activities. In short, the habits
    we form make no small difference, but rather they make all the
    difference.

4. We must watch the errors that have the greatest attraction for us
    personally. For the natural inclination of one man differs from that
    of another, and we each come to recognize our own by observing
    the pleasure and pain produced in us (by the different extremes.)
    We must then draw ourselves away in the opposite direction, for
    by pulling away from error we shall reach the middle, as men do
    when they straighten warped timber.

Listen to the Song of Life
Music and Brain Wiring

*Music is a moral law. It gives soul to the universe, wings to the mind,
flight to the imagination, and charm and gaiety to life and to everything. Music and rhythm find their way into the secret places of the
soul.*

PLATO

Music is the number one motivating tool for most athletes and the most powerful source of inspiration you have at your disposal. Using music as a motivating force is the best tool that you have to get and stay motivated. The combination of music, motion, and sweat cannot be beat. I always listen to music when I work out, and notice that most people I cross paths with do the same. If you like working out with music, choose anthems that create the mind-set or mood that fits your target behavior. I find in general that any song that evokes a strong emotional response is good to work out to. The music is visceral and difficult to talk about. If you love to listen to music when you exercise, you know its power. It motivates people and pushes them into the mystic, or to a higher ground.

Stay hungry.
MADONNA

Most athletes I know listen to music when they train; it enhances the experience and makes them perform better. Exactly what music does in the brain that makes it so powerful remains a mystery. We all know from first-hand experience that music has a profound impact on our state of mind. You can use it to shape your mood and reshape your mind-set. In 2004, neuro-scientists Anne Blood and Robert Zatorre of McGill University documented by using brain imaging what we have known all along: music evokes pleasure. When they scanned the brains of musicians who had chills of euphoria when listening to music, they found that music activated some of the same reward systems that are stimulated by food, sex, and addictive drugs. Dancing, which has been a part of human life since the earliest times, also is one of the most pleasurable ways to get exercise, bond with people, and enjoy music.

In a grand piano, 243 tight strings exert a pull of 40,000 pounds on an iron frame. It is proof that out of great tension may come great harmony.

THEODORE STEINWAY

One of the most interesting studies on music came from the University of Tsukuba in Japan. Neuroscientists Denetsu Sutoo and Kayo Akiyama found that "music for string orchestra by Mozart shifted the physiology of rats clearly towards relaxation or recreation. Systolic blood pressure decreased, and various tests indicated that this was due to an increase in serum calcium levels and brain dopamine levels."

Scientists have found that listening to music improves dopamine production and affects the electrical firing rate of synapses. People playing musical instruments are much like athletes in that the process is cerebellum-driven. We all know that music causes positive changes in people's brains that result in an improved mood and a sense of well-being. Exactly how it works is something that neuroscientists are still trying to figure out. They have identified that randomness releases more dopamine, which is why people like shuffle mode and the radio. Not knowing what song you are going to hear produces larger amounts of dopamine due to the lottery effect of unpredictability and reward. If you ever get tired of the songs or playlists on your iPod, mix it up. Switch to the radio, or any random source, to keep it refreshing. Know that you will be increasing your dopamine based on unpredictability.

> *Without music, life would be an error.*
> **FRIEDRICH NIETZSCHE**

Music, movement, and sweat make an unbeatable combination. Use music to add meaning and significance to your exercise experience. Find songs that enhance the experience. Use music as a catalyst to deliver you to that place—to get you through the pinhole. For me it's often a small fragment of a song—a drumbeat, a pause, or a grunt—that I play over and over again when I'm running that helps me slip through.

Any song is great to work out to if it's emotional. It doesn't have to be 180 beats per minute. Make playlists that capture the mind-set and mood you want to be in and pound them into your head. Remember to mix it up and use shuffle mode sometimes to keep the unpredictability pumping dopamine. Dial anthems on demand. Music can be used to create a shift in mind-set and a state of peak performance.

Game Face: "Physiognomy"
The Facial Feedback Loop

Your wrinkles either show that you're nasty, cranky, and senile, or that you're always smiling.

CARLOS SANTANA

Physiognomy is the study of facial expressions and body language as they are linked to a person's character. As an athlete you can use your facial expressions to send a signal to your nervous system. You can also use facial expressions to psyche out your opponent by keeping him guessing, but remember you are doing the same inside your own nervous system. Facial expression is part of a feedback loop. The *pons* (Latin for bridge) between cerebrum and cerebellum connects to muscles through the cerebellum to put an expression on your face as a reflex to the circumstances. This has evolved for millions of years as a natural way of communicating.

You can enter the facial feedback loop from the front end, called *top-down processing,* by consciously deciding to put a smile on your face. In doing so you put the cart before the horse and trick the visceral receptors in your lower brain that associate smiling with being happy. Or, you can enter it from the bottom up. Something visceral, from the cerebellum, will fill you with unconscious joy and a smile will spread across your face. Either way the loop creates a chain reaction and snowball effect. Your body will send out signals to all systems in your body that you are happy.

Neuroscientists have found that when you interpret another's facial expressions the emotions are read by your emotional brain. These signals bypass the conscious up mind and go straight to the intuitive brain.

I learned early on as an athlete that if I grimaced or scowled when I was perspiring, the perception of burden and struggle would fill my bones and grow exponentially. That made me feel tired and weak. So I learned to have a constant inner smile smeared across my face, because it made me go faster. I watched my mentor Natascha Badmann win six Hawaiian Ironman with a broad grin across her face. She made it look easy because the smile on her face make her think it was easy, too.

> Pretend that every person you meet has a sign around his or her neck that says, "Make me feel important." Not only will you succeed in sales, you will succeed in life.
>
> MARY KAY ASH

I purposely walk around with a smile on my face. Ninety-nine percent of people smile back. It's a reflex. Try it. Smile and the world smiles with you. A smile being created by nerves from my down brain tells your up brain that life is A-OK.

Pretend Big Brother Is Watching
Imagine CNN Broadcasting Your Most Private Moments

All my life people told me I wasn't going to make it.

TED TURNER

As part of character work it is helpful to use actual movie characters to mold yourself, and then pretend that you're starring in your own movie. Imagine Big Brother and the whole world are watching you. Anytime you feel like dogging it or not doing the right thing, imagine you are being observed. This was something I would picture as a fourth grader when I had my first conversion experience, which was a religious one. My fourth grade teacher, Christina Neff, was a Mennonite and converted our classroom into *Narnia*, *Little House on the Prairie*, and *A Wrinkle in Time*. She planted the spiritual seeds of knowing right from wrong and the knowledge that even when no one can see, someone is watching. She played the Cat Stevens record "Morning Has Broken" on a 45 every morning after we pledged allegiance. And her lessons stuck. Call it karma, call it hell—I will always strive to do the right thing from the lessons I learned in that classroom in 1975.

Sometimes I make believe I am in a reality show like *The Truman Show*, where Jim Carrey's whole life is actually set up on a soundstage and broadcast to millions of people. I'll pretend that there are invisible cameramen following me everywhere and sending my actions out onto a Webcast. When I'm alone on a long run in the woods and feel sometimes I'm just not that into it, I always think first of Muhammad Ali saying, "I hated every minute of training, but I said, 'Don't quit. Suffer now and live the rest of your life as a champion.' I run alone on the road, long before I dance under the lights."

Try this method of imaging that Big Brother is watching you. Create high expectations for yourself and define your character traits. On days that doing it for yourself isn't enough, do it for someone else.

The Secretariat Effect
Think Like Secretariat, Run Like Secretariat

Seven to eleven is a huge chunk of life, full of dulling and forgetting. It is fabled that we slowly lose the gift of speech with animals, that birds no longer visit our windowsills to converse. As our eyes grow accustomed to sight they armor themselves against wonder.

LEONARD COHEN

Ironman champion Chris Legh from Australia has spoken repeatedly about thinking like a horse when he races. If there are animals you relate to as an athlete, emulate the characteristics that you see in them. Copy the body language and eye movements of your favorite animals. Looking hungry like a wolf will tap your down brain. I like to think of my conscious mind as the trainer and the jockey on Secretariat, and then I treat my body with respect as I would a Thoroughbred. I treat it well, exercise it, feed it right, work it out hard, and pamper it afterward.

To me Secretariat, the greatest Thoroughbred racehorse that ever lived, illustrated the ideal character traits of *The Athlete's Way* as much as any human being. I still remember his race at Belmont when he won the Triple Crown by more than thirty-one lengths. That was the most exciting athletic event I've ever seen. I often pretend I am Secretariat, or my childhood horse, Commander, when I run. There is a certain stride and bobbing head thing I do that is like a galloping horse. This got ingrained into my cerebellum as a young person running wild through the fields on solo rides I'd take with Commander.

> Put things in their place,
> my mother shouts. I am looking
> out the window, my plastic soldier
> at my feet. The sky is blue
> and empty. In it floats
> the roof across the street.
> What place, I ask her.
> **DAVID IGNATOW** ("THE SKY IS BLUE")

When I was a kid I had a poster of Snoopy on a surfboard atop a big wave screaming "Cowwwaaabunngaaaa!" which is something I still say to myself every time I let go of the brakes and tuck into a cannonball to zoom down a steep hill on my bike at fifty miles per hour.

V-Formation of Geese
A Teamwork Analogy

Aerodynamically, the bumble bee shouldn't be able to fly but the bumble bee doesn't know it so it goes on flying anyway.

MARY KAY ASH

Geese have always been a role model for me as an athlete. They embody teamwork, loyalty, and a great sense of aerodynamics. When geese migrate south in the fall, they make a V formation—each bird takes turns leading, breaking the wind so that the geese behind can draft like in a bicycle race and conserve their energy. Each goose also takes turns pulling. The other geese honk and squawk from behind as a sign of encouragement to rally those in the front. Each goose pulls his own weight over the long haul by taking a turn at the front. Individualism and collectivism in perfect harmony.

When a goose gets sick or is wounded by gunshot and has to fall out of formation, two other geese accompany it to the ground. They stay with the goose until it is able to fly again or dies. Then they try to catch up to the lead pack, each taking turns pulling. To me geese and the V formation symbolize teamwork.

Suck It Up
Ever Heard a Sherpa Whine?

When I'd get tired and want to stop, I'd wonder what my next opponent was doing. I'd wonder if he was still working out. I tried to visualize him. When I could see him still working, I'd start pushing myself. When I could see him quit, I'd push myself harder.

DAN GABLE

The Sherpas who work as guides for mountaineers in the Himalayan slopes of Nepal are like Spartans in many ways. Sherpas often lug seventy-pound packs up and down the world's highest peaks and have excellent mountaineering skills. Often wearing only thin clothing in freezing cold temperatures, they show incredible mental toughness and physical stamina. Any time I start to whine or feel sorry for myself I get the image of a Sherpa in my head and say, "Think like a Sherpa, Chris. Think like a Sherpa." It is one of my favorite and effective mottos for sucking it up and not feeling sorry for myself, regardless of the physical discomfort. Sherpas are raised to embrace the challenge of hardship. I aspire to do the same in life and sport.

Let thy discontents be thy secrets.

BENJAMIN FRANKLIN

A study done in 1982 compared the responses to pain of Western trekkers to that of their Sherpa guides and gear bearers. The Sherpas endure physical discomfort silently, whereas the Westerners, whose culture allowed vocal expressions of physical discomfort, were more inclined to complain. The Sherpas were often barefoot and lugging huge backpacks with the Westerners' supplies, a much heavier load. Next time you feel like you're carrying the weight of the world on your back, think of the Sherpas and it may help to lighten your load.

If you don't like something, change it. If you don't change it, change your Attitude. Don't complain.

MAYA ANGELOU

CHAPTER ELEVEN

THE SLEEP REMEDY

He was part of my dream, of course—but then I was part of his dream too.

LEWIS CARROLL

THE DREAM WEAVER
SLEEP, DREAM, AND SPORT

S leep is one of the most sublime states of existence, and it's also a key to better health and improved athletic performance. So dive under the covers, cuddle up, and indulge in sleep whenever you can. It is superfluid and sublime every time.

Exercise and sleep make a perfect circle. Exercising helps people sleep better, and sleeping helps athletes perform better. Obviously, daily athletic practice is important, but dream work is equally important. In the daytime, the athlete is a neural sketch artist who makes a mental template of the patterns of his or her sport. At night, he or she becomes a dreamer, a memory artist with a hammer and blowtorch who carves the deep grooves of muscle memory. The process of reshaping memory is how we improve and become masters of sport, art, music, or surgery.

All human beings are designed to spend one-third of their lifetime sleeping. Ideally you should sleep about eight hours a night, which adds up to 122 days a year of solid sleep. Your body will function best on a two-to-one ratio of wake-to-sleep. This should be your sleep formula moving forward: for every two hours awake, you need one hour of sleep. Ideally, by the time you are sixty years old you will have spent about twenty years of your life asleep, and about five solid years in REM (rapid eye movement) sleep, dreaming.

In this chapter we will explore the importance of sleep. Although we will touch on the physical implications of not getting enough sleep, the focus here is on the positive benefits. The goal is to explain how sleep works and to convince you just how important it is. Humans are designed to be dreamers and athletes. The more exercise, the better we dream, and the more we dream, the better we get at living lives filled with activity and joy.

SLEEPLESS IN AMERICA
WE ARE A SLEEP-DEPRIVED NATION

The critical ingredient is getting off your butt and doing something. It's as simple as that. A lot of people have ideas, but there are few who decide to do something about them now. Not tomorrow. Not next week. But today. The true entrepreneur is a doer, not a dreamer.

ROBERT BROWNING

As a modern culture we sleep less and less every year, and the long-term effects of this deprivation are just beginning to reveal themselves. According to the 2005 study by the National Sleep Foundation, in 1998 35 percent of Americans got eight or more hours of sleep a night, while in 2005 that number was down to 26 percent. As people struggle to pay the bills, juggle family, career, and even exercise, sleep becomes the first disposable commodity to go. This is a dangerous tradeoff. It doesn't make sense to starve yourself of sixty minutes of sleep in order to get up and run. My advice is: If you must choose, sleep, don't run. Find a way to squeeze in twenty to thirty minutes of exercise later in the day. If you are operating on a sleep deficit, hit the snooze button instead of working out. Sleep is ultimately more important.

Humans sleep for 17–18 hours a day at birth, 10–12 hours at age 4 and 7–8.5 hours by age 20.

PRINCIPLES OF NEURAL SCIENCE

The Sleep Foundation's survey found that 75 percent of American adults experience some form of sleep problem at least a few nights per week. If you are reading this in an unrested state from a poor night's sleep, you are not alone. Make getting sleep a top priority. Find the root of what is keeping you up at night. Remember, regular exercise will help you sleep better. I will give you more ways to fall asleep later in this chapter but now let's focus on your best antidote for getting a good night's sleep. Adenosine, the sleep molecule that is stored up during exercise, works like a flip switch and knocks you out at bedtime.

So, we'll go no more a-roving so late into the night, though the heart be still as loving,
And the moon be still as bright though the night was made for loving, the day returns to soon, Yet we'll go no more a-roving by the light of the moon.

GEORGE GORDON (LORD) BYRON

ADENOSINE: THE SLEEP MOLECULE
NATURE'S NATURAL SLEEPING PILL

Onward through life he goes. Each morning sees some task begun, each evening sees its close!
Something attempted, something done, has earned a night's repose.

HENRY WADSWORTH LONGFELLOW

More than a third of all Americans suffer from some type of sleep disturbance. If you have trouble sleeping or just want to improve your odds of getting a good night's rest, exercise is the all natural sleeping tablet. Adenosine levels build up throughout the day as you move around. When the level gets high enough in your brain, it flips a switch that knocks you out. One reason you wake up in the morning is that adenosine levels drop when you don't move. When these levels get low enough, a switch goes off that wakes you up. Adenosine is the on-off switch for sleep states and wake states.

Adenosine is a byproduct of ATP, the fuel that your muscles use for energy. Adenosine builds up throughout the day and is the catalyst for a complex domino effect, the first trigger in a cascade that releases melatonin, which puts you to sleep. Released by the pituitary in connection with the pineal gland, melatonin has been linked to sleep and circadian rhythms for years. Adenosine is a new discovery as the switch that turns melatonin on and off. You could picture adenosine as the switch and melatonin as the lightbulb that makes the rooms inside your brain actually light or dark.

The more exercise you do during the day, the more adenosine you will create and the better you will sleep. Since researchers know that sleep is key to learning and memory, aim to move every day and create more adenosine.

More exercise means more adenosine, better sleep, better dreams, better mind, better body. Sleep is as important as practice to the athlete.

CIRCADIAN RHYTHMS: "ABOUT A DAY"
FROM SUNRISE TO SUNSET

Trying to sneak a fastball past Hank Aaron is like trying to sneak the sunrise past a rooster.

JO ADCOCK

Homo sapiens are one of worst-equipped nocturnal animals. We don't have particularly good night vision, hearing, or sense of smell. We rely on our eyes. At the beginning of time, man as a species was probably at home in his cave sleeping once the sun went down and was up with the dawn. The cycles of light and dark have guided our biology and evolution for millions of years. With the invention of the lightbulb, the possibility of a twenty-four-hour, round-the-clock world of light became possible.

The first twenty-four-hour power plant was opened by Thomas Edison on Pearl Street in Manhattan in 1882, less than 130 years ago. Our biology has not had time to adapt to this rapid shift in circadian cycles.

The study of our twenty-four-hour circadian cycles is at the core of most scientific sleep research. Make a point every day to get some light. I take a few minutes in the winter mornings to sit on the windowsill and let the light blast against the backs of my eyes every day—for my mental health. This is something I learned from my grandmother.

My sun sets to rise again.
ROBERT BROWNING

Seasonal affective disorder is real. As a Scandinavian, I see the winter and summer mood swings in my relatives. I call Norway the "land of the midnight sun and noontime moon syndrome." In summertime, when the sun never sets, moods become manically elevated. In the winter, people in Nordic countries tend to become violently depressed, or drink too much. I think there may be a link to these extremes and the statistically higher levels of bipolar disorder and mania among Scandinavians, and why suicide levels in Scandinavia skyrocket in the wintertime. My family history has shown me that there is no denying circadian cycles affect every cell in your body and how that affects your life.

Chronobiology
The Internal Timekeeper

Wait for those unguarded moments. Relax the mood and, like the child dropping off to sleep, the subject often reveals his truest self.

BARBARA WALTERS

Your body has more than one hundred circadian rhythms that lull you to sleep like a baby every night and either arouse or jolt you out of bed. Each unique twenty-four-hour cycle influences an aspect of your body's function, including body temperature, hormone levels, heart rate, blood pressure, even pain threshold. Every area of your body is affected by circadian rhythms. It may seem you sleep when you're tired and wake when you're alarm clock goes off, but your sleep patterns follow a circadian rhythm encoded in every cell of your body.

Humans are most likely to sleep soundly when their temperature is lowest, in the early hours of the morning. You're also most likely to awaken when your temperature starts to rise, around 6 to 8 A.M. These changes are all caused by hormonal shifts based on your circadian rhythms. Almost all hormones are regulated to some degree by circadian rhythms.

Cortisol levels are highest between 6 and 8 A.M. and gradually decline throughout the day, but tend to go up again at around 4 P.M. If you change your daily sleeping schedule, the peak of cortisol's cycle changes accordingly. Production of neurochemicals peaks during the first two hours of sleep. If you're sleep deprived, production of growth hormone drops, another reason for athletes to get plenty of sleep.

Human growth hormone is released in the deepest stage of sleep (stage 4), which comes around about every ninety minutes throughout the night. You want to aim for at least five ninety-minute sleep cycles a night to release this stored-up hormone in each stage 4 round of sleep. You have five, ninety-minute periods of sleep each night with five stages inside each period. If you miss one by sleeping less than seven hours, your system will get weaker, slower, sicker, and dumber.

Athletes seem to perform best in the late afternoon, when strength, body temperature, and flexibility peak. Athletes who compete late in the day may perform better because pain tolerance is highest in the afternoon. Changes in daily habits, like a short night's sleep, can disrupt your circadian rhythms. To live *The Athlete's Way* you want to stay in sync by keeping a consistent daily schedule.

The bottom line is that sleeping well keeps all species alive longer. Among humans, there is a much higher death rate for people who sleep fewer than seven hours. Those who slept between seven and nine hours have overall the lowest mortality rate. Normal biological function relies on sleep. The immune system is particularly vulnerable to sleep deprivation. Sleep is also crucial to rebuilding the muscles you break down when you lift weights.

Did you know that human beings are the only animals that can sleep on their backs? Use that fact to your advantage next time you find yourself leaning back in a chair to take a nap. Or flying business class on some traded-in miles.

Athletes, Pianists, Surgeons, Artists
All Rely on Practice, Then Sleep to Master Skills

I don't know if I practiced more than anybody, but I sure practiced enough. I still wonder if somebody—somewhere—was practicing more than me.

LARRY BIRD

Practice, practice, practice should really be practice-sleep, practice-sleep, practice-sleep. Sleep is an integral part of absorbing practice by your body and brain. Neuroscientific evidence is mounting that sleep, even a nap, appears to enhance information processing and learning. New experiments show that a midday snooze reverses information overload and that a 20 percent overnight improvement in learning a motor skill is largely traceable to a late stage of sleep that some early risers might be missing. Overall, studies suggest that the brain uses a night's sleep to consolidate the memories, actions, and skills learned during the day.

When I was a young tennis player, my dad was my coach. He used to tell me to practice my tennis game in my head just before I went to sleep. He taught me to commit my day's work to muscle memory by replaying it just before bed. I encourage you to spend the first few minutes before bed reviewing your day's work and filling your head with the words, ideas, and images that you want to shape your sleep state. The thoughts you have just before bed can seep deep into your head and replay themselves in your dreams. Dream-time brainwashing can be a clean and actually fun thing, if you are the master and commander of the desired result. Review your note cards and workbook before bedtime.

Robert Stickgold has dedicated his life to researching sleep as it relates to memory and learning. He explains, "Suppose you are trying to learn a passage in a Chopin etude, and you just can't get it. You walk away and the next day (after a good night's sleep), the first try, you've got it perfectly. We see this with musicians and with gymnasts. There's something about learning motor activity patterns, complex movements: they seem to get better by themselves."

If you want to get better at sports you have to get plenty of sleep. Sleep consolidates memories so that your brain can be streamlined and run like a well-tuned engine. You become what you do and what you dream about. I say live it, dream it, become it.

STOP THE RIDE! I WANT TO GET OFF
ROLLERCOASTERS, TRAMPOLINES, AND BODY SURF

Though we seem to be sleeping, There is an inner wakefulness that directs the dreams And that will eventually startle us back to the truth of who we are.

RUMI

Remember when you were a kid after spending the day at the beach, or at an amusement park on a rollercoaster, or on a trampoline. When you first closed your eyes to fall asleep that night, you felt your body relive the physical sensation of these activities. With a jerk you would bolt up in bed to catch yourself from falling.

Your body reliving these experiences would trigger a feeling that you were falling out of bed, the sense of gravity and momentum were like the bottom falling out. The novel experience was already embedded in your cells; your cerebellum captured it but hadn't figured it out yet.

The beauty of the cerebellum is that once you get a procedural/muscle memory, like riding a bike or serving a tennis ball, it is locked in. It is hardwired through sleep. The muscle memory may get very rusty, but it has been laid down forever. The beach waves you felt as a kid that made you seasick when you got in bed don't happen as an adult, because your cerebellum has processed that unfamiliar sensation and will remember it forever.

Get Five Full Rounds of Each Sleep Stage

*Morphine, the analgesic (pain reliever) drug from the opium poppy,
is named after the Greek god of dreams, Morpheus. Endorphin is
self-produced (endo) from 'Mor-phine." Morpheus was the son of the
Greek god of sleep named Somnus.*

WIKIPEDIA

Remember to beef up your cerebellum during the day, expose it to light, and then give it time to recuperate by getting five full cycles of sleep. Every ninety minutes you have a cycle of sleep that ends with the all-important REM (rapid eye movement) every night by getting seven to eight hours of solid sleep. The fifth round of sleep is the most important, and the period of heaviest dreaming and learning. If you wake up before seven hours of sleep, you cannot complete the fifth round.

REM sleep is the most mysterious and most important period in our daily twenty-four-hour cycle. Adults spend about 25 percent of their nightly sleep state in REM sleep. The cycles of REM come around every ninety minutes and last for about twenty to twenty-five minutes. Within the rapid eye movement cycle, your eyes move in bursts occupying about one-third of REM sleep.

Four of the five stages are non-REM, and the final one is REM itself. The cycle repeats itself five times a night. If you go to bed at 11 P.M. you would enter a twenty-minute REM cycle every seventy minutes, roughly at 12:10, 1:40, 3:10, 4:40, and 6:10. The last cycle of REM, from 6:10 to 6:30 A.M., would correspond to the fifth stage of sleep in eight hours and would hold all the dreams you would remember as you begin to wake up.

If you were able to take note of your shifts in body position every night, you would see the gateways of your own REM cycles. You shift position on either side of REM. Night terrors, for example, are indicative of stage 2 sleep in the second cycle and will usually occur about ninety to one hundred minutes after falling asleep. The key is to nestle in and get that last, complete, fifth round from six and a half to eight hours after your head hits the pillow.

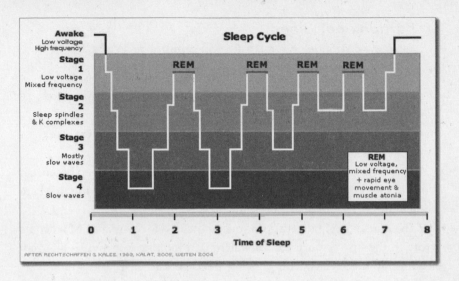

AFTER RECHTSCHAFFEN & KALES. 1968, KALAT, 2005, WEITEN 2004

We Learn When We Dream
Dreamscapes Shape Long-term Memories

We are such stuff as dreams are made on, and our little life, is rounded with a sleep.

WILLIAM SHAKESPEARE

People who play the video game Tetris before bed dream of Tetris in their sleep and are better at it the next morning when they wake up. Poets who read or write iambic pentameter before they go to bed dream in iambic pentameter and write poems in their sleep. Take advantage of the time before bed to prep your dreams by deciding how you want to launch yourself into dreams. Conjure the things you would like to think about or work on in your sleep, and it will become a dreamscape reality.

You might want to try keeping a dream journal. The scientist Claude Bernard pioneered this technique. He wrote extensive medical notes in a red book he kept by his bed and claimed to come up with most of his medical insights during his dreams. Not surprisingly, it turns out that the cerebrum and hippocampus play a role in cerebral long-term memory when you sleep. The cerebellum also plays a key role in procedural memory when you sleep. I wrote the majority of this book inside the athletic process or in a journal I kept by my nightstand, much like Claude Bernard.

Paradoxical Sleep
During REM Sleep Your Up Brain Appears to Wake Up

Now all the cloudy shapes that float and lie. Within this magic globe we call the brain fold quite away, condense, withdraw, refrain, and show it tenantless—an empty sky.

THOMAS WENTWORTH HIGGINSON

Rapid eye movement sleep is referred to as paradoxical sleep because it is one of the deepest stages of dream sleep. Yet brain waves during REM are firing at the same rate as in a person who is wide awake.

The Roman poet Lucretius was one of the first to observe REM when he wrote in the first century B.C. of watching a hunting dog twitch as it lay sleeping by the fire. Watching its eye dart, he said that "the animal was chasing some kind of phantom prey in its mind." Modern scientists didn't realize the significance of REM sleep until 1951, when the modern era of sleep research began.

Since a researcher in another room reading an EEG in a sleep lab would think that the subject had woken up when the REM phase began, researchers need to measure other feedback to ensure the subject has, in fact, not awakened. Luckily there are other measurable changes in the body that occur during REM. A person usually shifts body position—rolls over, adjusts the pillow—just before going into REM and upon exiting it.

To test REM, sleep researchers place electrodes around the eyes to detect the rapid eye movements, but they also put a detector over muscles in the chin and neck in order to measure the loss of tonus in these muscles during REM. For reasons that are not understood, the muscles of the throat and tongue relax profoundly during REM sleep. As the eyes move back and forth, tonus in the throat is lost. One reason may be so that people don't scream out their dreams or talk in their sleep.

Another interesting inherent condition of REM sleep is called atonia, which is the paralysis of voluntary muscle movement. Your body is paralyzed for REM sleep so that your cerebellum can go offline. Whenever you enter or exit REM sleep, it is marked by a significant readjustment of body position, because your body is paralyzed during REM.

During REM, the cerebellum is signing off on its duties so that it can focus on sending information elsewhere in your brain to be processed. Since the cerebellum controls proprioception, it doesn't have to keep tabs on your body's position in space if you are paralyzed. The cerebellum is also in charge of tongue, throat, eye, and body movements. Another interesting thing about REM is that the VOR reflex (vestibulo-ocular reflex) shuts off, too, so that your eyes *are* able to dart around. You can reverse VOR in the daytime by fixing on an object in front of you (like a red "power on" switch when you're running on the treadmill). Poke your tongue out a little bit and move your head back and forth and you can pull the same thing off, in reverse.

All animals sleep. Fish, which need to keep swimming in order to breathe, shut down half their brain at a time. They sleep with half their brain, while the other half keeps them moving, and then flip it. Neuroscientists think that the different stages of human sleep may be doing a similar thing in terms of giving parts of the human brain a period offline to regroup and consolidate during the five stages of the human sleep cycle.

REM is most likely about bottom-up processing. Researchers at MIT have shown that our primitive brain (the cerebellum) actually teaches our thinking brain (the cerebrum). At night, it is a tutoring session, a chance for the cerebellum to go over the lessons of the day with the cerebrum in the form of dreams and to catalogue and store them for our intellect.

Beyond Counting Sheep:
Real Methods for Beating Insomnia

Wrench'd and sweaty—calm and cool then my body becomes,
I sleep—I sleep long.

WALT WHITMAN

Hrayr P. Attarian, M.D., reviews ways to diagnose and treat insomnia, a symptom of several sleep disorders. "Insomnia is a prevalent and serious condition that is often missed or dismissed. Most of the time, it is treated with ineffectual means, frustrating both patient and physician," says Attarian, an assistant professor of neurology at Washington University School of Medicine in St. Louis and a member of the school's Sleep Disorders Center. In "Helping Patients Who Say They Cannot Sleep—Practical Ways to Evaluate and Treat Insomnia," published in the *Postgraduate Medicine* journal, Attarian lists the following rules for a good night's sleep:

- *Restrict the time you spend in bed so you're tired when you try to fall asleep.*

- *Don't nap.*

- *Leave your bedroom if you've been awake for more than fifteen minutes.*

- *Don't overachieve right before bedtime—no housework or balancing the checkbook.*

- *Increase the amount of exercise you get each day.*

- *Remove clocks from your bedroom.*

- *Use distracting activities when you're trying to get to sleep.*

- *Cut down on coffee, and avoid nicotine and alcohol.*

- *Go to bed and get up at the same time each day, even on weekends and even if you haven't slept.*

- *Use prescribed medications, but don't dose yourself with over-the-counter sleep aids.*

Another common form of insomnia is triggered by sleep apnea. Charles Czeisler points out, "We're seeing an epidemic of sleep apnea. It's related to being overweight. Older, obese men are at higher risk." During REM sleep, the muscles in the upper throat relax. As the muscles around the neck relax in overweight people, the passage can be partially or completely closed, which results in loud snoring, labored breathing, and in some cases the cessation of breath (apnea) for up to ten seconds. The loss of valuable REM sleep due to sleep apnea will deprive you of the most crucial part of sleep. If you have sleep apnea because you are overweight, you can add that as another reason to work out, eat right, and lose weight. Losing as little as ten to twenty percent of your current body fat can cut the incidence of sleep apnea in half.

Neurobiologists at UCLA have found that humans lose tissue in key parts of their brains as a result of sleep apnea. The sudden intermittent hypoxia of oxygen levels spiking and plummeting in the brain as it enters REM sleep has been shown to be very injurious to the cerebellum in animals, according to Ron Harper of UCLA.

Sleep Come Free Me
Sleep's Dark and Silent Gate

The darkness drops again; but now I know that twenty centuries of stony sleep Were vexed to nightmare by a rocking cradle, And what rough beast, its hour come round at last, Slouches towards Bethlehem to be born?

W. B. YEATS

Sleep is not the absence of consciousness. The cerebellum generates sleep, according to my father. Sleep is a positive mechanism, a job that is performed by the cerebellum. Forget the old idea that sleep is simply a state of reduced activity that occurs by default when brain activity subsides. Rather, sleep is an actively induced, highly organized brain state that is dictated from the down brain.

Sleep researchers have found that the brain cannot think and process at the same time. The cerebellum absorbs everything during the day, using its remarkable processing powers to teach the up brain declarative things via the hippocampus, and then replaying this information to the cerebrum during REM sleep. This is why the brain reads awake during REM sleep. During this reenactment, we dream as the brain rewires the synaptic connections using ZIF-268 and other proteins—as the brain relives and stores long-term memory during REM dreams.

Allan Hobson, a professor of psychiatry at Harvard Medical School points out, "Studies show that hallucinatory mental content is lowest during active waking and highest during REM sleep. The incidence of thinking is highest during quiet waking and lowest during REM sleep. The implication of these findings is that the sleeping brain can either generate its own perceptions or it can think about them. It cannot do both at the same time." The sleeping and waking dream state is like a trance; it is hallucinatory and thoughtless. The primitive brain is actually generating the perceptions. The knowing is in the nonthinking cerebellum.

Crossing the Mid-Brain
The Royal Road to Dreams

That we come to this earth to live is untrue: We come but to sleep . . . to dream.

AZTEC PROVERB

The mid-brain is the gatekeeper between our conscious and our unconscious mind. In his 1900 book *The Interpretation of Dreams,* Freud theorized that dreams are the royal road to understanding the unconscious mind. That view has come under fire during the past thirty years as scientists have probed the neural bases of dreaming. New findings from brain-imaging studies are beginning to show that there may be some truth behind Freud's hypothesis.

In dream and sport we slip through the mid-brain's net. We "go behind the veil" as Lance Armstrong might say. Without the ability to open the channels at mid-brain, we are locked out of dream states. We cannot sleep, we cannot dream. When we exercise, the strings in the cerebellum send jamming frequencies up into the cerebrum, which is why we are able to create a waking dream state through sport. The same happens anytime we lose ourselves in something cerebellar—music, art, religion or love, and, of course, when we sleep.

> *Every child is an artist. The problem is how to remain an artist once he grows up. . . . The artist is a receptacle for the emotions that come from all over the place: from the sky, from the earth, from a scrap of paper, from a passing shape, from a spider's web. . . . The purpose of art is washing the dust of daily life off our souls. . . . We all know that art is not truth. Art is a lie that makes us realize the truth.*
>
> **PABLO PICASSO**

CHAPTER TWELVE

SUPERFLUIDITY: CHASE YOUR BLISS

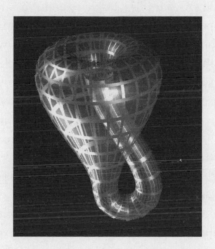

Looking back on my own experiences, they all converge towards a kind of insight to which I cannot help ascribing some metaphysical significance. The keynote of it is invariably a reconciliation. It is as if the opposites of the world whose contradictoriness and conflict make all our difficulties and troubles, were melted into unity. Not only do they, as contrasted species, belong to one and the same genus, but one of the species, the nobler and better one, is itself the genus, and so soaks up and absorbs its opposite into itself.

WILLIAM JAMES (*THE VARIETIES OF RELIGIOUS EXPERIENCE*)

THE DAILY ATHLETIC QUEST
CHASE YOUR BLISS!

With all your science can you tell how it is, and whence it is that light comes into the soul?

HENRY DAVID THOREAU

Joseph Campbell always said to "follow your bliss." As an athlete I say, chase your bliss. The idea of following has always seemed too passive to me. You need to hunt down your bliss, tackle it, and pin it to the ground. The athletic process is more than just getting from point A to point B, achieving goals, bolstering confidence or self-esteem. There is always a very strong spiritual aspect to the process. The deliverance you feel when you connect to your own biology is too powerful to be denied. This mystical aspect is the most fascinating aspect of breaking a sweat every day. You never know where it will take you, but when you get there you know. Exercise is a vehicle for transporting your being to someplace else.

The prime motivating force for me to exercise every day, beyond the nuts and bolts of achievement and feeling good, is to experience some type of enlightenment. Each day's athletic journey is working toward achieving some type of rapture, a feeling of connectedness to other people, myself, and the world around me. It's biological, and it is easy to get there. All roads lead to this place; you just need to get on the road. When you get there—feeling like a creature enraptured—you'll know.

Precisely the least, the softest, lightest, a lizard's rustling, a breath, a flash, a moment—a little makes the way of the best happiness.

FRIEDRICH NIETZSCHE

Remember, life in the human body was designed to be an ecstatic process. You have all the molecules at your disposal to create this state. You just need to put the key in the ignition and turn it.

Since going to this very real special place has been my prime motivating force and destination in life since I was seventeen, I can click into a trancelike state in about seven to eight minutes once I start sweating and stay there for hours, or even days. This is why I became an ultra-runner. I wanted to see how long I could exist in this Nirvana-like place. It's what makes me able to work out for so long. If you make it a destination, you'll find your way there, too, I guarantee.

SUPERFLUIDITY
NO FRICTION. NO VISCOSITY

Everything vanishes around me, and works are born as if out of the void. Ripe graphic fruits fall off. My hand has become the obedient instrument of a remote will.

PAUL KLEE (SWISS ARTIST)

Where neurobiology, science, mysticism, religion, and sport overlap is the most interesting territory to me as an athlete. I call it soul biology. When these coalesce, it creates superfluidity. Superfluidity sounds like it feels. Peak experience, epiphany, rapture, and ecstasy are other terms that work. Superfluidity really begins where language ends.

If language does not work for you, perhaps an image can help you to visualize the transcendent superfluidity of athletic bliss. That's where the Klein bottle comes in. A friend of mine, a mathematician, drew a picture of the Klein bottle on the placemat at dinner one night, and then sort of made one out of a dinner napkin. I said, "Eureka! Yes, that looks how superfluidity feels."

The Klein bottle is a vessel existing in four dimensions with no inside and no outside. It is a tangible, visual, mathematical concept that illustrates how peak experiences, epiphanies, ecstasy, and superfluidity feel. It is actually just two Möbius strips stuck together. When you dive into the Klein bottle, you tap into the present tense—and beyond.

I say to the moment: "Stay now! You are so Beautiful!"
JOHANN WOLFGANG VON GOETHE

Superfluidity and the Klein bottle both express what piercing through feels like, like the looking glass in *Alice's Adventures in Wonderland*. These things all describe the pinhole to another plane that I see as being directly linked to the cerebellum and unconscious minds.

EXCELSIOR! TAKE IT HIGHER
PEAK EXPERIENCES

When I hit that note—if I hit it correctly—I'm just as important as Jimi Hendrix, Eric Clapton, or anybody. Because when I hit that note, I hit the umbilical cord of anybody who is listening.

CARLOS SANTANA

Abraham Maslow defined a peak experience as a profound moment of love, understanding, happiness, or rapture. Or when a person feels more whole, alive, self-sufficient, and yet a part of the world, more aware of truth, justice, harmony, and goodness. I call this a state of superfluidity, which is a level above and beyond the regular fluid experience of flow. Superfluid performance is when you deeply recognize the radiance of life and feel a sense of oneness through sports.

It was an ocean of adventure and full of obstacles and sea monsters probably. All that disappeared when I set foot on the cable. But it was not a surprise. It was not a new condition. . . . The wire is a safe place for me to be. The street is not. Life is not. It's a rigorous and simple path. It's straight. . . . I was finally finding myself living, because I had now opened the door to living on the edge, living the only place where it's worth living, which is fully, and grabbing my life and carrying my life across.

PHILIPPE PETIT
(ON CROSSING BETWEEN THE WORLD TRADE CENTER TOWERS IN 1974)

The peak experience that Maslow referred to, or what James Joyce describes as an *epiphany,* is the highest level of athletic bliss, and is sublime. You can have multiple peak experiences in a single workout, or have at least one every time.

One point of this program is to make it accessible to everyone and to demystify the idea of self-actualization and the pursuit of peak experiences, which seem unattainably lofty to most. I can almost guarantee that if you break a sweat, whether in a fancy health club or wearing beat-up sweats in a public park, you will create superfluidity if you push against your own limits on a regular basis. Take it up a notch every day. Turn up the volume in your life, and you are more likely to experience higher highs. Constantly challenging yourself will bring you close to superfluidity. You don't have to kill yourself. Just nudge up against the comfort cusp and you'll open up the door.

Mine was it in the fields both day and night, and by the waters, all the summer long.
And in the frosty season, when the sun was set, and, visible for many a mile,
The cottage-windows through the twilight blazed, I heeded not the summons: happy time
it was indeed for all of us; for me it was a time of rapture.

WILLIAM WORDSWORTH

It is not necessary to have arrived at a state of enlightenment or self-actualization as an athlete to experience an epiphany. You just have to put your time in. The more you sweat the more primed you are to make it happen. The skill really is just mastering your ability to make it more likely to occur by noticing when it happens.

That is why I break flow into two tiers. Regular fluid performance is easy to dial up if you choose balanced challenge. But superfluidity is much more episodic and comes in waves. If you aspire to create fluidity, that is the launching pad to the next level. If you keep pushing against the door it will open up and you'll cross over to moments of superfluidity. William Blake touches on this when he says, "If the doors of perception were cleaned, man would see everything as it is, infinite." Explore superfluidity. Put your antennae up—look for it in other people's performances and then define what it means to you.

Every religion emphasizes human improvement, love, respect for others, sharing other people's suffering. On these lines every religion has more or less the same viewpoint and the same goal.

THE DALAI LAMA

A SENSE OF MYSTERY
THE MEANING OF LIFE

People say that what we're all seeking is a meaning for life. I don't think that's what we're really seeking. I think that what we're seeking

*is an experience of being alive, so that our life experiences on the
purely physical plane will have resonances within our own innermost being and reality, so that we actually feel the rapture of being
alive. That's what it's all finally about, and that's what these clues
help us to find within ourselves.*

JOSEPH CAMPBELL

Ultimately the biggest question for most people is "What am I doing here?
What is my purpose for being alive?" The most rewarding aspect of *The Athlete's Way* is that it leads to a better understanding of self, and a feeling of
being connected to something within yourself that is also part of a much
bigger picture. Superfluid experiences happen when you realize that you
and the other are one.

Joseph Campbell talks about athletics as a modern-day opportunity to
explore peak experiences and claims that the peak experiences in his own
personal life were mostly through sports. In *The Power of Myth,* Campbell
says, "When I was running at Columbia I ran a couple of races that were just
beautiful. I just knew I was going to win. And it was my peak experience.
Nobody could beat me that day. That's being in full form and really knowing it. I don't think I have ever done anything in my life as competently as I
ran those two races—it was the experience of really being at my full and doing a perfect job." His description reminds me of just how Roger Bannister
described his four-minute mile or how I felt when I won the Triple Iron Man
the first time.

Campbell continues, "The place to find is within yourself. I learned
about this in athletics. The athlete who is in top form has a quiet place
within himself and it's around this somehow that his action occurs. If he's
all out there in the action field, he will not be performing properly. My wife
is a dancer, and she tells me that this is true in dance as well. There's a center of quietness within, which has to be known to be held. If you lose that
center, you are in tension and begin to fall apart."

The real power of sweat and sport is that by using your body you
are connecting to your biology. You connect to your body, and by connecting to your body, you connect to your source, and then you connect to the
Source. If you don't use your body to open these doors, you never tap
the cerebellum. I don't think you can know God intellectually through
your declarative thinking in your cerebrum. That is why yoga, art, music,
and sport create the real epiphanies, the real moments of superfluidity.
Just thinking will not generally induce rapture. You cannot experience

the rapture of being alive sitting on the couch watching TiVo and eating Cheetos.

When you face a fork in the road, step on the exhilarator!

PAT RILEY

Sometimes I huff and I puff and try to knock the door down to pierce through to a state of superfluidity, to get into the Klein bottle, and it doesn't happen. I feel shut out, firmly planted in the humdrum workaday world. Usually I get my first wave of superfluidity around twenty-two to twenty-four minutes into a workout. That's when my brain is ripe to click over. But sometimes I don't feel superfluid for the first time until thirty-six minutes. When that door does open I do what I always do, which is say, *"Yes,"* with a mix of triumph and surrender.

Cherish your vision; cherish your ideals; cherish the music that stirs your heart, the beauty that forms in your mind, the loveliness that drapes your purest thoughts, if you remain true to them your world will at last be built.

JAMES ALLEN

The feeling of superfluidity is like biological tumblers lining up in your brain, which is why they occur in flashes, like all the keys slipping into the right doors with perfect synchronicity. If you have plumped up your microtubules, this state is more likely to occur. This is what Carl Jung referred to as "The Dream": "a little hidden door in the innermost and most secret recesses of the soul, opening into that cosmic night which was psyche long before there was any ego-consciousness, and which will remain psyche no matter how far our ego conscious may extend."

The universe is change; our life is what our thoughts make it.

MARCUS AURELIUS ANTONINUS

YOU ARE A TOUR DE FORCE
BELIEVE IT

I get the greatest feeling when I'm singing. It's other-worldly. Your feet are anchored into the Earth and into this energy force that comes up through your feet and goes up the top of your head and maybe you're holding hands with the angels or the stars, I have no idea. When I sing I don't feel like it's me. I feel I am fabulous, like I'm ten feet tall. I am the greatest. I am the strongest. I am Samson. I'm whoever I want to be.

CYNDI LAUPER

I love this Cyndi Lauper quote because it captures the feeling of superfluidity as universal and transferable. Also, the sense that in moments of superfluid performance the ego dissolves, or is transformed. Ecstasy comes from the Greek "to stand outside oneself." In moments of superfluidity your ego blends with some outside energy source and you are one with the other. The power of that union makes you feel like a tour de force. You become one. I can feel the tumblers in my brain shift tectonically as I slip through the pinhole into a state of superfluid performance.

Recently, using fMRI imaging technology, brain researchers have been able to watch the brain switch off "self," or what could be considered the ego. Researchers Rafael Malach and Ilan Goldberg at the Weizmann Institute of Science in Israel found that during sensory tasks that create a state of fluid performance—one in which subjects "lose themselves" in what they are doing—the prefrontal cortex becomes very quiet on the fMRI. During sport or sex, or when creating art, making music, or meditating, fMRI suggests that blood flow to the prefrontal cortex is reduced. Consciousness is shifted from the front of the brain, and the seat of your "self" is moved. My educated guess is that it is shifted into the cerebellum. No one knows for sure.

The researchers above propose, "The picture that emerges from the present results is that, during intense perceptual engagement . . . the term 'losing yourself' receives a clear neuronal correlation echoing in Eastern philosophies such as Zen teachings, which emphasize the need to enter into a 'mindless,' selfless mental reality." This much is clear—shutting down the amount of neural activity in the prefrontal cortex by being fully engaged in a sensory task appears to facilitate losing yourself in whatever you're doing, and will increase the chances of having a superfluid episode.

The noun of self becomes a verb. This flashpoint of creation in the present moment is where work and play merge.

STEPHEN NACHMANOVITCH

*Any genuine philosophy leads to action and from action back again
to wonder, to enduring fact of mystery.*

HENRY MILLER

THE ECSTATIC PROCESS
ECSTASY IN SECULAR AND RELIGIOUS EXPERIENCES

*Thus, the task is not so much to see what no one has seen before, but
to think what no one has thought about what everybody sees.*

ST. GEORGI

In the early 1960s a professor named Marghanita Laski wrote a book called
Ecstasy in Secular and Religious Experiences that was one of my favorite books
in college. As a scientist and mystic obsessed with pleasure, pain, and rapture, Laski touched on many things that fit with *The Athlete's Way: Sweat and
the Biology of Bliss.*

Below are the findings that Laski identified in samplings of a 1961 survey on feelings of secular and religious ecstasy. Use this checklist to help define the state of superfluidity. These descriptions can serve as a road map to
describe where you want to go.

PEOPLE DESCRIBING PERCEPTIONS OF ECSTASY
WORDS FOR HOW SUPERFLUIDITY FEELS

1. DIFFERENCE: *The hard lines around one's individuality are gone;
   undefined existence; the soul loses all distinction in things.*

2. TIME: *Complete absence of a sense of specific time.*

3. PLACE: *You're not anywhere; detached from every earthly thing
   and place.*

4. LIMITATION: *Transcends your normal limitation; the flesh begins to
   feel the change, the soul transcends the limit of its natural way of
   existence.*

5. WORLDLINESS: *Removed from consideration of earthly things.*

6. DESIRE: *All human desires and purposes shriveled; seeking naught,
   desiring naught.*

7. *SORROW: Complete separation from trouble; "the vicissitudes of life had become indifferent to me; all my past wretchedness and pain is forgotten."*

8. *SELF: A loss of the sense of being yourself; "I lost myself; temporary loss of my own identity."*

9. *WORDS: "I don't know how to put it into words; the more I seek words the more I feel the impossibility of describing this thing; the tongue does not speak; hard to distinguish between thought and feeling. Impossible to articulate."*

10. *SENSES: overwhelming all senses and superseding thought; sensation . . . melted . . . into one.*

11. *UNITY, EVERYTHING: A sense of the oneness of things; you understand that everything in reality is connected to one thing; saw nothing and everything; all the separate notes have melted into one swelling harmony. "I saw, and knew the being of all things in that moment."*

12. *RELEASE: Complete sense of liberation; new doors, and beginning to open—glory seemed to open.*

13. *SATISFACTION: Complete satisfaction.*

14. *JOY: Extreme happiness; exultation; immense joyousness.*

15. *SALVATION, PERFECTION: Something being perfected, feeling nothing but the pureness, innocence, and righteousness.*

16. *GLORY: Sudden glory; passed from gloom to glory; unspeakable, divine glory.*

17. *CONTACT: A sense of being in touch with the Creator; communion with something else; joined to God; the universe is a living presence.*

18. *KNOWLEDGE BY IDENTIFICATION: In touch with the Creator; the knowledge of the reality of things; the inner and outer meaning of the earth and sky and all that is in them. "I fit exactly. I saw that the Divine universe is a living presence in everything."*

Please visit www.theathletesway.com if you are interested in sharing your description of superfluidity. I am compiling my own research to carry on the work of Laski, and your input would be greatly appreciated. I want to isolate the components that make it a universal and timeless experience in all human beings. The Web site will lead to a simple questionnaire.

THE GOD SQUAD
ZEN AND THE ART OF BRAIN SCULPTING

The Buddha, the Godhead, reside quite as comfortably in the circuits of a digital computer or the gears of a cycle transmission as he does at the top of a mountain or in the petals of a flower.

ROBERT M. PIRSIG (ZEN AND THE ART OF MOTORCYCLE MAINTENANCE)

In the *Nicomachean Ethics*, Aristotle speaks of happiness as being directly linked to physical well-being, science, and ultimately to God. Taking care of your body with proper nourishment, exercise, and rest is the key to both physical and mental health. In closing, we have come full circle from the introduction, the Möbius strip of interconnectedness of mind and body summed up by *mens sana in corpore sano*. In Aristotle's view, the health of the body is a means to learn to perform moral actions, which in turn leads to moral health.

You can lose yourself in *The Athlete's Way* and the biology of bliss anywhere, in things profound or the seemingly inane. Seek the bliss out; use your imagination. Superfluidity can and should happen anywhere, from peeling potatoes to taking a bath. In order to have a profound experience, you need to have a profound sense of mystery, but the mystery can be found in everyday things.

Explore higher heights. Push the envelope in your life. Break a sweat as many days a week as you can. Recognize the rapture of being alive; try reciting "The Athlete's Recognition" the next time you find yourself inside the athletic process as an affirmation of the benefits of living *The Athlete's Way*. The adventure of the athlete is really just the adventure of being alive.

THE ATHLETE'S RECOGNITION

BY CHRISTOPHER BERGLAND

Recognize that god is alive in every cell.
Recognize that god is in us all.

Recognize this source of power—every hour, here.
Recognize with strength and love there is no fear.

Recognize the light in every eye and soul.
Recognize the sun lives in us all.

Recognize your thoughts and actions every day.
Recognize the passion—always give your all.

Recognize One Blood, One Sun, One Hope, One Love.
Recognize the collective conscience of humankind.

Recognize that god is living everywhere.
Recognize that god is you and I.

Recognize a trance like this.
As you break a sweat—
Drip, Drip, Drip.

EPILOGUE

SOLO CROSSINGS
TELESCOPES AND ISLANDS

I close with a quote from Charles Lindbergh describing his solo crossing of the Atlantic in 1927. This quote has been on a corkboard by my computer for years. It captures the sense of wonder I have often felt near the end
of a big race like the Kiehl's Badwater Ultramarathon, Hawaii World Championships, or a Triple Iron Man triathlon. Lindbergh's words reiterate that it
is the process itself that is most fulfilling, not the victory, or actually reaching the destination.

The Athlete's Way is not just about trophies, standing on mountaintops,
winning medals, or crossing a finish line. It is about what happens along the
way. The connections to friends, family, and community that you build as
you go matter most.

Yes, it is a solo journey and there is beauty and reward in the personal
achievement, and the rapture that Lindbergh describes below. The pure bliss
in those times, when your own cells connect you to your biology and bring
you to a place of pure peace, are sublime and very seductive. But superfluidity is short-lived and episodic. It is a vacuous state ultimately. Being "in the
world but not of it" is not an ideal state of existence. The city on the hill can
be a lonely place.

We need friends and we need community more than anything else.
Find the balance between your individual life experience and that of the collective. Reach out, give back, and share it with other human beings, but also
treasure your success inside the individual process. That is the ultimate
tightrope walk, and mastering that paradox is *The Athlete's Way*.

Within the hour I'll land, and strangely enough I'm in no hurry to have it pass. I haven't the slightest desire to sleep. There's not an ache in my body. The night is cool and safe. I want to sit quietly in this cockpit and let the realization of my completed flight sink in. . . . It's like struggling up a mountain after a rare flower, and then, when you have it within arm's reach, realizing that the satisfaction and happiness lie more in the finding than in the having. Plucking the flower and having it wither are inseparable. . . . I almost wish Paris were a few more hours away. It seems a shame to land with the night so clear and so much fuel in my tanks.

CHARLES LINDBERGH

ACKNOWLEDGMENTS
THANK YOU, THANK YOU, THANK YOU

If the only prayer you said in your whole life was, "thank you," that would suffice.

MEISTER ECKHART (GERMAN PHILOSOPHER)

Sheila Curry Oakes and **Alyse Diamond:** For seeing this book across the finish line. John Karle, Alice Baker, and to everyone else at **St. Martin's Press** for being such a dream team.

Andrew Goetz: How about Thursday? NYH maternity ward. Bouvier Des Flandres. Sneaking down below Chambers Street on 9/12. Biking over the Brooklyn Bridge at sunrise into oncoming traffic. The Bench. **Angela Ellsworth:** Tania. Hampshire. Badwater. Drawing on Breath. **Andréa Tasha:** AXT. Tattoo you. Springtime on a February morning. Tasha Hill. Qantas. Spiritus. Un tuta café. **Anthony Catala:** Evidence of Brilliance. Putting the kettle to the mettle. "Drink this and you'll grow wings on your heels." **Anthony Marsowicz:** That's GREEAAAT! Jumping turnstiles. Kill Bill. Nice moustache! **Ben Barnz:** Spring of '89. Shep's Like a Prayer DJ only Promo. Nonstop cowbell, choir, and bazooka bass beats in the basement of MARS. Churchapella conversion experiences on the dance floor. Joan Armatrading. Sinéad. "I Do Not Want What I Haven't Got." The Little Prince. **Bob Buchanan:** Green note cards. A stool in the corner and superfluidity.

Bob and Nancy Hurlbut and all my teachers at The Park School: Mr. Conway. Nancy Faulkner . . . Thank you for educating with "live-life" exuberance. You imprinted the ideals of your visionary "hidden curriculum" of "boundary-less" teaching into my head at an impressionable age. Hopefully this book carries that torch. **Bo Arlander:** Frick and Frack. Sisu Squared. "Same time next year." Swimming stride for stride in waters all over the world. **Bobby Lavelle:** ILYSM! The hovel in Los Feliz. P-CHA. Bunny's Greatest Hits. Saca de Resaca. Culebra and Vieques. Hairspeak. "Every hour-hair here" **Cammie Cannella:** For leading by example and teaching me what being a good manager was all about. Ordering me flowers in times good and bad.

Charles Francis: For stabbing your index finger into my sternum and saying sternly, "You better not de-gay your book, Christopher. Don't be a coward. 'Trust yourself, Every heart vibrates to that iron string.'" **Cheryl Walker:** For coaching me and pulling me over the threshold. **Chris Kostman:** For race directing Badwater superbly. AdventureCORPS. **Christina Neff:** For opening my eyes to a sense of wonder in the fourth grade and pouring a concrete foundation of belief at a young age. "In the name of God, go to the right or go to the left." **Darius Kohan at NYU Medical:** For giving me a bionic ear after I blew a gasket early on. I thank you every time I hear stereophonic sound. **David Matesanz:** Inspector Gadget. Benny's, Mama Buddha, Sapore, Chumley's, or the Village Den? All things Swedish, or preppy. Your "half-a-laugh." Next-door neighbors.

Daniel Pelavin: For capturing the "Art Deco, Greek, Rockefeller Center, W.P.A., 1930s, Clark Kent, Charles Atlas (without being intimidating) feeling" I struggled to articulate so elegantly in your illustrations. **David Ketterling:** One of these days I'll make it out to L.A. Moulin Rouge at the Ziegfield. The Cactus Tree Motel. **Chip Duckett:** For keeping 1984 and the Pyramid Club going for all these years. Anytime I feel like dancing I know where to go. **David at Rebel Rebel Records** on Bleecker St. for keeping me well supplied with vinyl and live concert CDs in a digital age. **David Ryan:** Wax boxes. The Klepper kayak. White Street. Never Knew Love Like This Before. **Dean Karnazes:** For your camaraderie and sticking it out for twenty-four hours on the treadmill. Staying grounded and leading a running revolution. **Susan Dell:** For your generous spirit and hard work to made this world a better place.

Diane Reverand: You are the quintessential editor. Thank you for seating yourself in my spine and editing from that place. This one's for you. I am the luckiest author in the world to have had the opportunity to create this seminal book for me, with you. **Dominic Barty-King:** Jonbour! James. Never being boring. Love Won't Wait. Right back where we started from . . . Stock-Aitken-Waterman. All the pop music we're not embarrassed to love. Goodbye Yellow Brick Road. Thursday lunches in the West Village. Weekends in Asbury. Memorial days in P-town. Dancing on Charles Street. Squealing like Michael Jackson with torrets moonwalking down Greenwich Avenue.

Donald Capoccia: Doubles, Triples, The Treadathalon. This book would never have happened without you. Thank you for reading my manuscript early on and giving me such poignant feedback. Sacher (puffed cheeks) Torte. Fondue. Fantasy Island. Compass Point. We must never be parted. "Cheese" Burgers. NoHo Star. Five Points. Mo'hair. La-Z-Boy. Stuy Town. "Step on the pedal and never look back month." **Deirdre and Bella Tasha:** For providing me with food, shelter, and a cottage in Provincetown so that I could completely immerse myself in this book. Thank you for going to the grocery store and putting up with me as I became an invalid of sorts. Offering me companionship when I came out of my hole . . . and for throwing my laundry in the wash when I forgot. **Ed Dulac:** For confirming that the pinhole and superfluidity are universal. Running stairs at 7 World Trade and everything else. **Ed Tedeschi:** For believing in me early on and getting me set up with my first bike and eager to race. **Eric Nies:** Crunch. RopeSport. The Grind. Thanks for always being supportive, for talking the talk and walking the walk. **Penny Burnett:** Cheeze Balls. Aged Gouda and Chimaya. When are we moving to Tahiti?!?

Elizabeth Bergland: Please don't move back to Australia! New York will be so lonely without you. You have been a pillar of support for me for over twenty-four years. From Beacon Hill to Tuxedo Park, to East End Ave. and some less highbrow situations—We are family. Pippin. Godspell. **Adam Geyer:** Provincetown. Boston marathon. Mixed tapes for Kona. Neurosurgery and dermatology. **Garrett McKechnie:** Handing me Gatorade in Death Valley, cheering me on at 5 A.M. during Treadathalon.

Lee Silverman and everyone at JackRabbit Sports: Thank you for the opportunity to help shape an athletic hub and a great place to work. **Marilyn Silverman:** Wordcenter! You're the best. **Melanie Brown:** For writing and sharing your "Great" book with all its wonderful advice and insights. **Monica Scholz:** Light really does come out of your mouth whenever you speak. Shine on! Stayin' Alive. Nightfever. Rock on gold dust woman! Meet me at Whitney Portals or Furnace Creek anytime. **Giles Anderson:** You are a fantastic literary agent. Thank you for helping me craft a sellable proposal, being patient about not rushing it to market until we had it right, and hooking me up with a perfect match: Diane Reverand and St. Martin's Press.

Gracia Walker: For being my rock of Gibraltar through the Kiehl's year . . . Badwater, Treadathalon, and introducing me to your mom. **Laura Franklin:** For slamming your hands on the wooden floor again and again and screaming "Get up!" at the top of your lungs after I hit the wall. . . . Your voice broke through the fog and got me back on my feet. Thank you. **Freddy:** For "Iron Man Barbie"

Mary Jo Litchard (my mom): For leading such an admirable life and always being so much fun to be with. You have the bravest, most generous heart I know. You celebrate life every day—and that is contagious. "Live Thy Life Nobly," "Promise Little Do Much," "Want Not, Need Not." You are still changing the shutters on your Saltbox house—and painting the barn at the age of seventy. I guess we have Gabby and Grampa to thank for putting that Yankee fire in our veins. I can't wait to grow old together!

Jami Morse and **Klaus von Heidegger:** For welcoming me into the World of Kiehl's at such a pivotal point and appreciating the power of physicality. **Jason Frye at Equinox:** For access to the best gyms in America. **Joe Fanelli:** For making such spectacular paintings and helping me find the "there, there." **Jonathan Cane:** Without you I never would have gotten started or achieved any of my dreams. **Julia Hansen:** Kaija and Allette! Erik. Union Square deck. Your gourmet meals. Always having my back, bringing a smile to my face and fun times. **Kenny Gatta:** B.S.U.R. The only ways is up, for us. **Mirabel:** Welcome to the world! I love you and can't wait to know you more as you grow.

Louise Demirjian: Summers in Quogue as a kid. The Surf Club. "American Pie" performances in the backyard by the trampoline. Being such a dedicated and talented artist. Putting up butcher block paper during The Treadathalon so Dean and I didn't roast like rotisserie chickens in the window. **Mark Klion:** The best orthopedist in New York. Thank you for helping to heal my sprained spinal situation weeks before the Treadathalon. **Abbie Schiller:** For making stuff really get cooking at Kiehl's. Badwater. Ona Rae! **Mark Stumer:** The best lawyer in New York. Thank you for handling all the contracts, trademarks, S-corps and everything else litigious. **Aunt Mart Lamar:** I see myself in you and learn so much every time we speak. I adore you. **Aunt June Keener Wink:** For the trips to the Red Lighthouse under the Washington Bridge as a kid. And the Blue Plates.

MLVCR: For laying the brainchips of excellence and fearlessness in my head when I was seventeen and for being rocket fuel during every workout ever since. **Nikki Haran:** UR my sunlight and my rain. Don't fall in love with a dreamer. Are you serious? You don't bring me flowers. The Hours . . . Let's Go! I've got two tickets to Paradise. I'm heading for the border. Are you in or out? **Nora Burns:** Fred. Bruno. Pedro. Come back to New York. We need you and the Nellie Oleson's here not in Maui. Thank you for the daily calls, e-mails and your constant support. I think of you every time the sun sets over the West Side highway or in P-town as I'm jogging along . . . or eat salsa. **Paula Lee:** On my Honor. Let's do the Time

Warp. Off the Wall. Homeroom of '78 was a long time ago. Park, Choate, Santander, L. A. Joy es Lava. Verano '82. Mecano. Looks like we're both still standing. Thank you for being there for me every time I really cracked and needed a friend who has understood me since the age of twelve. **Patti O'Brien:** For being a rock star triathlon goddess I could idolize, emulate—and for letting me into your life, and sharing everything you knew.

Richard Bergland: For passing on your dynamic—albeit very intense—Viking genes. For showing me that hanging on to the edge of a cliff and pulling oneself up by one's fingernails, with one hand tied behind the back, is guaranteed to "add sweet perfume to the task." You made it look easy, always. Thanks for letting me bounce ideas about mind science around with you, too . . . and for responding to my daily queries about the brain within minutes while I was writing this book. I miss you. Rest in peace. **Renée Bergland:** Annelise. Kim. You have the biggest brain and largest memory bank of anyone I've ever encountered. . . . Remind me never to play Trivial Pursuit with you. You're my older sister and so calm, steady, and wise in your approach to life. . . . You make me feel safe and sound even when I'm a big mess. You always catch my fall when the wheels fly off the bus. **Sandy Bergland:** For being such a maverick and the coolest little sister a guy could have. I am so proud of you for piloting FedEx MD-11s around the globe. "Who's the boss around here, Amelia? You or you?" ☺ Thanks for taking charge whenever I unraveled. You help me achieve higher highs. **Geoff at Macrostate:** For building an awesome Web site. **Lisa Romerin, Steve Snider, and David Baldeosingh Rotstein:** For creating a perfect book cover.

Rob Morea: I forgive you for eating all my salt and vinegar potato chips at the Double Ironman. **Sheila O'Keefe:** Love Potion #9—Lime, Basil, Mandarin, and D'Hadrien . . . I think of you every day. Why?!? I drop to my knees and throw my hands to the sky and ask myself that question every day.

Stephen B. Savage: From a muse to daily Le Creuset upside down and clean in the kitchen sink. Living with you is great. **Sue Remes:** Nice boots! I'll look for you on the Sunny Side of the street. **Tim Holderbaum and Ali Zake:** For cheering me on every inch of the way. **Tom Pucci:** Summer jobs on Cape Cod and the rope bracelet I never take off. **Vicki Holmes:** From Chelsea Piers to JackRabbit Sports, I owe you. Kailua-Kona, Lake Placid, Florionopolis. I kiss the ground you walk on. The Sports Center at Chelsea Piers is an *Athlete's Way* Paradise, thanks to you. **Youssif Eid:** For the Third Eye and the Microwave. Rain and the silk-screened picture with the chain.

Aima Walsh: A month of blue Sundays. Forever in blue jeans. Spring Vac '79. The Park School. 52 Hedge/2496 Beacon . . . Circle Cinema, Defender, Galaxian. Jacomo. Just an illusion. **The Wises:** For letting me stay in Winchester for summers when home life was too strained. And offering help whenever I needed it. Eat to the Beat. Fame. The White Farm in Blandford.

Mr. Yankus (my dean in high school): For trying to convince me that I would amount to nothing. Whether it was reverse psychology or not, you forced me to make something of my life just to prove you wrong. I needed to succeed at first just to spite you. I didn't *ever* want you to be able to say, "I told you so." My resentment toward you was the seed that sparked my athletic conversion. At the end of the day, I am grateful to you for being so hard on me even though it really sucked at the time. Thank you.

Christina Rago: For granting permission to include your father's work. Here, in its entirety, as promised:

THE KNOWLEDGE OF LIGHT

BY HENRY RAGO

I

The willow shining
From the quick rain,
Leaf, cloud, early star
Are shaken, light in this water:
The tremolo of their brightness: light
Sung back in light.

II

The deep shines with the deep.
A deeper sky utters the sky.
These words waver
Between sky and sky.

III

A tree laced of many rivers
Flows into a wide slow darkness
And below the darkness, flowers again
To many rivers, that are a tree.

IV
Wrung from silence
Sung in lightning
From stone sprung
The quickening signs
Lines quivered
Numbers flew

Darkness beheld
Darkness and told
Each in each
The depths not darkness.

V
To know
Meaning to celebrate:
Meaning
To become "in some way"
Another; to come
To a becoming:
To have come well.

VI
Earth wakens to the word it wakens.

These dancers turn half-dreaming
Each to the other, glide
Each from a pool of light on either side
Below the dark wings
And flutter slowly, come slowly
Or drift farther again,
Turn to the single note, lifted,
And leap, their whirling lines
Astonished into one lucidity:
Multiples of the arc.

Shapes of the heart!

VII
The year waits at the depth of summer.
The air, the island, and the water
Are drawn to evening. The long month
Is lost in the long evening.

If words could hold this world
They would bend themselves to one
Transparency; if this
Depth of the year, arch of the hour
Came perfect to
The curving of one word
The sound would widen, quietly as from crystal,
Sphere into sphere: candor
Answering a child's candor
Beyond the child's question.

INDEX